PERIODS OF SUSCEPTIBILITY TO TERATOGENESIS

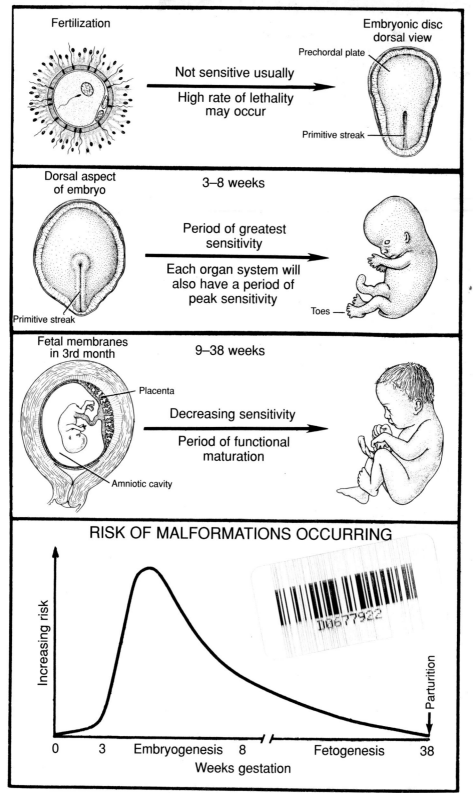

EMBRYONIC DEVELOPMENT IN DAYS

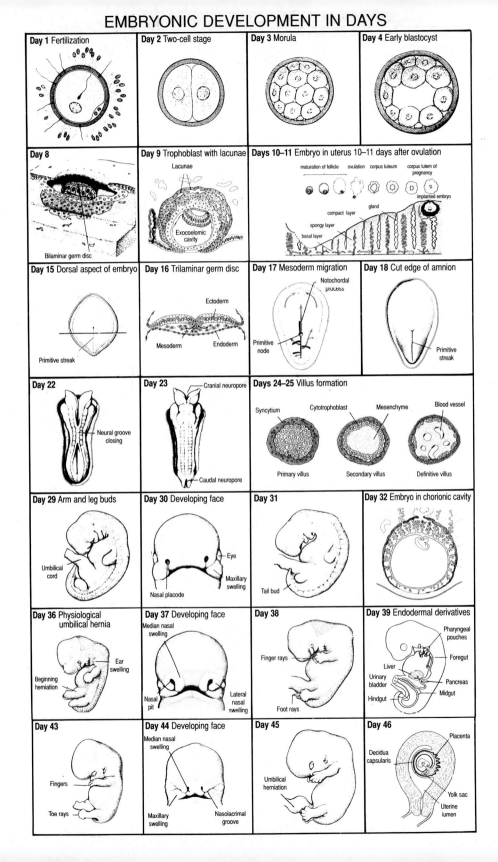

EMBRYONIC DEVELOPMENT IN DAYS

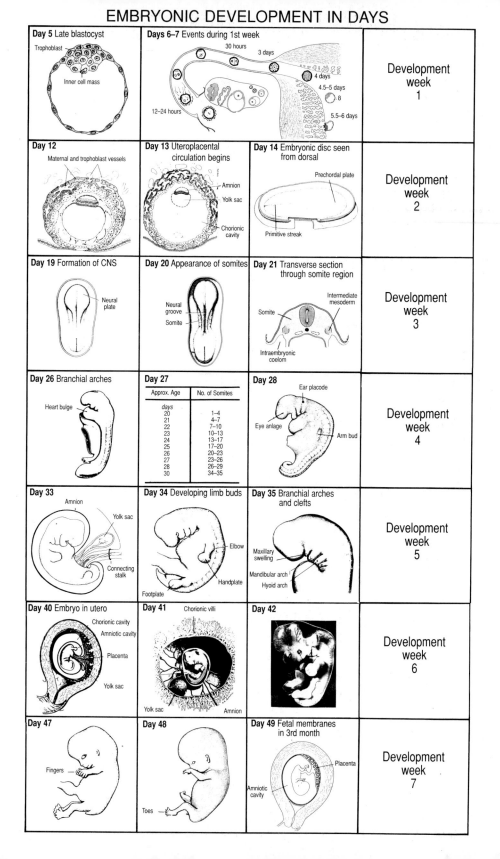

Day 5 Late blastocyst	**Days 6–7** Events during 1st week		Development week 1
Day 12	**Day 13** Uteroplacental circulation begins	**Day 14** Embryonic disc seen from dorsal	Development week 2
Day 19 Formation of CNS	**Day 20** Appearance of somites	**Day 21** Transverse section through somite region	Development week 3
Day 26 Branchial arches	**Day 27**	**Day 28**	Development week 4
Day 33	**Day 34** Developing limb buds	**Day 35** Branchial arches and clefts	Development week 5
Day 40 Embryo in utero	**Day 41**	**Day 42**	Development week 6
Day 47	**Day 48**	**Day 49** Fetal membranes in 3rd month	Development week 7

Day 5 Late blastocyst: Trophoblast, Inner cell mass

Days 6–7 Events during 1st week: 30 hours, 3 days, 12–24 hours, 4 days, 4.5–5 days, 8, 5.5–6 days

Day 12: Maternal and trophoblast vessels

Day 13 Uteroplacental circulation begins: Amnion, Yolk sac, Chorionic cavity

Day 14 Embryonic disc seen from dorsal: Prechordal plate, Primitive streak

Day 19 Formation of CNS: Neural plate

Day 20 Appearance of somites: Neural groove, Somite

Day 21 Transverse section through somite region: Intermediate mesoderm, Somite, Intraembryonic coelom

Day 26 Branchial arches: Heart bulge

Day 27:

Approx. Age	No. of Somites
days	
20	1–4
21	4–7
22	7–10
23	10–13
24	13–17
25	17–20
26	20–23
27	23–26
28	26–29
30	34–35

Day 28: Ear placode, Eye anlage, Arm bud

Day 33: Amnion, Yolk sac, Connecting stalk

Day 34 Developing limb buds: Elbow, Handplate, Footplate

Day 35 Branchial arches and clefts: Maxillary swelling, Mandibular arch, Hyoid arch

Day 40 Embryo in utero: Chorionic cavity, Amniotic cavity, Placenta, Yolk sac

Day 41: Chorionic villi, Yolk sac, Amnion

Day 42:

Day 47: Fingers

Day 48: Toes

Day 49 Fetal membranes in 3rd month: Placenta, Amniotic cavity

SUSCEPTIBILITY TO TERATOGENS FOR SELECTED ORGAN SYSTEMS

(Peaks represent periods of sensitivity. Each organ system may have a single or multiple periods of sensitivity.)

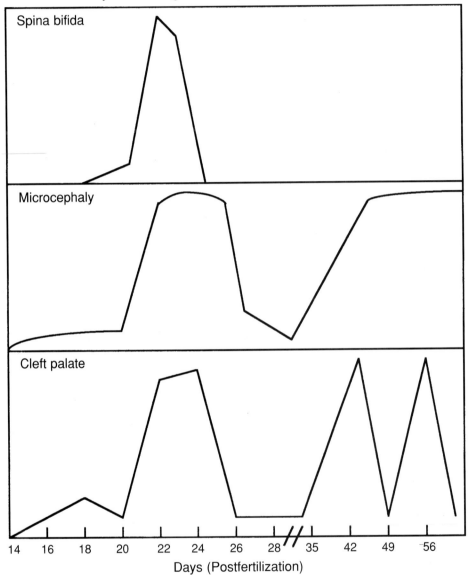

Days (Postfertilization)

LANGMAN'S
MEDICAL
EMBRYOLOGY

Seventh Edition

LANGMAN'S MEDICAL EMBRYOLOGY

Seventh Edition

T. W. SADLER, Ph.D.

Professor, Cell Biology and Anatomy
Director, UNC Birth Defects Center
The University of North Carolina at Chapel Hill
Chapel Hill, North Carolina

Original Illustrations by Jill Leland
Computer Illustrations by Susan L. Sadler-Redmond
Cover Illustration by Kathleen K. Sulik

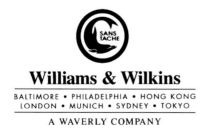

Williams & Wilkins

BALTIMORE • PHILADELPHIA • HONG KONG
LONDON • MUNICH • SYDNEY • TOKYO

A WAVERLY COMPANY

Editor: Patricia Coryell
Managing Editor: Crystal Taylor
Copy Editor: Bill Cady
Designer: Norman W. Och
Illustration Planner: Wayne Hubbel
Cover Designer: Tom Scheuerman
Production Coordinator: Raymond E. Reter

Copyright © 1995
Williams & Wilkins
428 E. Preston Street
Baltimore, Maryland 21202, USA

All rights reserved. This book is protected by copyright. No part of this book may be reproduced in any form or by any means, including photocopying, or utilized by any information storage and retrieval system without written permission from the copyright owner.

Printed in the United States of America

First edition, 1963
   Reprinted 1964, 1965, 1966, 1967
Second edition, 1969
   Reprinted 1970, 1971, 1972, 1973
Third edition, 1975
   Reprinted 1975, 1976, 1977, 1979, 1980

Fourth edition, 1981
   Reprinted 1982, 1983, 1984
Fifth edition, 1985
   Reprinted 1986, 1987, 1988
Sixth edition, 1990
   Reprinted 1991, 1992, 1993, 1994

English language co-editions
   Asian, 1966, 1969, 1975
   Indian, 1966, 1969, 1976
   Korean student, 1966, 1981

Translations
   Dutch, 1966, 1970, 1975, 1981
   French, 1965, 1971, 1976, 1984
   German, 1970, 1975, 1984
   Indonesian, 1981
   Italian, 1967, 1970, 1978

   Japanese, 1967, 1971, 1976, 1982
   Persian, 1971
   Portuguese, 1966, 1970, 1977
   Spanish, 1963, 1969, 1976, 1981

Library of Congress Cataloging-in-Publication Data

Sadler, T. W. (Thomas W.)
   Langman's medical embryology. — 7th ed. / T. W. Sadler; original illustrations by Jill Leland; cover micrograph by Kathleen K. Sulik.
      p.—cm.
   Includes bibliographical references and index.
   ISBN 0-683-07489-X
   1. Embryology, Human. 2. Abnormalities, Human—Genetic aspects. I. Langman, Jan. II. Title. III. Title: Medical embryology.
      [DNLM: 1. Abnormalities. 2. Embryology. QS 604 S126m 1995]
   QM601.L35 1995
   612.6′4—dc20
   DNLM/DLC
   for Library of Congress
                          94-29937
                          CIP

97 98 99
3 4 5 6 7 8 9 10

Dedicated to each and every child

I would like to express my gratitude to Dr. Kathleen Sulik for her love, support, and inspiration. She is a superb embryologist who has added greatly to my knowledge of the subject and its clinical significance. Her scanning electron micrographs appear throughout the book and are also presented, together with many drawings from this text, as a collection in Embryo Images, *a computer tutorial available through The Slice of Life at the University of Utah in Salt Lake City.*

Preface to the Seventh Edition

This edition of *Langman's Medical Embryology* continues to focus on the essentials of clinically relevant aspects of embryology. The goal is to provide students with an understanding of the principles of embryogenesis that can be used in the diagnosis, care, and prevention of birth defects. Birth defects are the leading cause of infant mortality and a major contributor to disabilities. Their prevention is, in part, dependent on educated health care professionals who understand the genetic and environmental origins of congenital malformations. Therefore, the amount of clinical material in this edition has been expanded, and a section on problems to solve that have a clinical and embryological basis has been included. In addition, three-dimensional renderings and scanning electron micrographs have been incorporated to simplify difficult concepts. Molecular aspects of developmental biology have been left to texts in cell and developmental biology so that topics of clinical relevance can be emphasized in the short time allotted courses in embryology.

T. W. S.
Chapel Hill, North Carolina
January 1995

Preface to the First Edition

Recent advances in embryology, radioautography, and electron microscopy have been so overwhelming that the medical student often has difficulty in grasping the basic facts of development from the highly complicated picture presented to him. The aim of this book, therefore, is to give the future doctor a concise, well-illustrated presentation of the essential facts of human development, clarifying the gross anatomical features without omitting the recent advances or changing concepts in the basic sciences. Furthermore, since embryology has become of great practical value because of the enormous progress made in surgery and teratology, each chapter on the development of the organ systems has been complemented by a description of those malformations important to the student in his further training. As a further reflection of the increased clinical importance of embryology, an entire chapter has been devoted to the etiology of congenital defects.

Of the many colleagues who have been of help in the writing of this book, I particularly wish to thank Dr. C. P. Leblond for his continuous interest and encouragement; Dr. F. Clarke Fraser, for his help in discussing the various aspects of the congenital malformations; and my friends, Dr. Harry Maisel, Dr. Robert van Mierop, and Dr. Yves Clermont, who have spared no effort in assisting with the design of the drawings and the checking of the text.

I wish to express my sincere thanks to Miss Jill Leland, who prepared all the illustrations in this book, and to Mrs. E. Dawson, who has been of such excellent support to me in setting up the manuscript.

Contents

PART I

General Embryology

chapter 1

Gametogenesis: Conversion of Germ Cells Into Male and Female Gametes

The development of a human begins with fertilization, a process by which the **spermatozoon** from the male and the **oocyte** from the female unite to give rise to a new organism, the **zygote.** In preparation for fertilization, both male and female germ cells undergo meiosis and cytodifferentiation. The purpose of these processes is twofold:

① To reduce the number of chromosomes from the **diploid** number of 46, observed in somatic cells, to the **haploid** number of 23, observed in the gametes. (**Ploidy** refers to the number of copies of each chromosome.) This is accomplished by **meiotic** or **maturation** divisions and is necessary, since fusion of a male and a female germ cell would otherwise result in an individual with twice the number of chromosomes of the parent cells.

② To alter the shape of the germ cells in preparation for fertilization. The male germ cell, initially large and round, loses practically all of its cytoplasm and develops a head, neck, and tail. The female germ cell, on the other hand, gradually becomes larger as the result of an increase in the amount of cytoplasm. At maturity, the oocyte has a diameter of about 120 μm.

The human somatic cell contains 23 pairs or a **diploid** number of chromosomes. There are 22 pairs of matching chromosomes, the **autosomes,** and 1 pair of **sex chromosomes.** If the sex pair is **XX,** then the individual is genetically female; if the pair is **XY,** the individual is genetically male. One chromosome of each pair is originally derived from the mother, and the other, from the father. The members of a chromosome pair are generally not in close proximity to each other either in the resting cell or during mitotic divisions. The only time that they come in intimate contact with each other is during meiotic or maturation divisions of the germ cells.

To make the events occurring during meiotic divisions easier to understand, the most important features of these divisions are compared with those of a **mitotic** division. Similarly, although reduction in the number of chromosomes and cytoplasmic changes are both integral parts of germ cell maturation, each process is described separately.

Chromosomes During Mitotic Division

Before a cell enters mitosis, each chromosome replicates its DNA, which becomes doubled. During the DNA replication phase, chromosomes are extremely long, diffusely spread through the nucleus, and cannot be recognized with the light microscope. With the onset of mitosis, chromosomes begin to coil, contract, and condense, and these events mark the beginning of prophase. Each chromosome consists of two parallel subunits (**chromatids**) that are joined at a narrowed region common to both called the **centromere.** Throughout prophase, chromosomes continue to condense and become shorter and thicker (Fig. 1.1*A*), but only at prometaphase will the chromatids become distinguishable (Fig. 1.1*B*). During metaphase, chromosomes line up in the equatorial plane, and their doubled structure is clearly visible (Fig. 1.1*C*). Each is attached by **microtubules** (**mitotic spindle**) extending from the centromere to the centriole. Soon, the centromere of each chromosome divides, marking the beginning of anaphase, followed by migration of chromatids to opposite poles of the spindle. Finally,

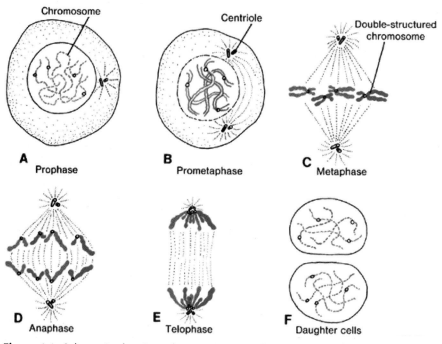

Figure 1.1. Schematic drawing of various stages of mitosis. In prophase, chromosomes are visible as slender threads. Doubled chromatids become clearly visible as individual units during prometaphase. At no time during division do members of a chromosome pair unite. *Blue,* paternal chromosomes; *red,* maternal chromosomes.

during telophase, chromosomes uncoil and lengthen, the nuclear envelope reforms, and division of the cytoplasm occurs (Fig. 1.1, *D* and *E*). Each daughter cell receives one-half of all the doubled chromosome material and thus maintains the same number of chromosomes as the mother cell.

Chromosomes During Meiotic Divisions

FIRST MEIOTIC DIVISION

As in a mitotic division, the female as well as the male primitive germ cells (primary oocyte and primary spermatocyte) replicate their DNA just before the 1st meiotic division begins. Hence, at the beginning of the maturation divisions, germ cells contain double the normal amount of DNA, and each of the 46 chromosomes is a double structure (Fig. 1.2).

The *first characteristic feature* of this meiotic division is **pairing (synapsis) of homologous chromosomes,** which are referred to as **bivalents** (Fig. 1.2*A*). The pairing is exact and point for point except for the X-Y combination. Centromere regions of homologous chromosomes do not pair. Since each individual chromosome is double-structured and contains two chromatids, each homologous pair consists of four chromatids (Fig. 1.2*B*). **In a mitotic division, homologous chromosomes never pair.**

The *second characteristic feature* of the 1st meiotic division is called **crossover** and consists of the **interchange of chromatid segments** between two paired homologous chromosomes (bivalents) (Fig. 1.2*C*). When, subsequently, each (double-structured) member of the homologous pair splits longitudinally, one or more transverse breaks occur in the chromatids, and an interchange of chromatid segments between two homologous chromosomes occurs (Fig. 1.2*C*). During separation of the homologous chromosomes, points of interchange temporarily remain united, and the chromosomal structure then has an X appearance known as a **chiasma** (Fig. 1.2*C*). During the chiasma stage, blocks of genes are exchanged between homologous chromosomes. In the meantime, separation continues, and the two members of each pair become oriented on the spindle (Fig. 1.2*D*). In subsequent stages the members migrate to the opposite poles of the cell (Fig. 1.2*E*).

After the 1st meiotic division has been completed, each daughter cell contains one member of each chromosome pair and thus has 23 double-structured chromosomes (Fig. 1.2*F*). Since each chromosome is still double-structured except at the centromere, the amount of DNA in each daughter cell equals that of a normal somatic cell.

SECOND MEIOTIC DIVISION

Shortly after the 1st meiotic division, the cell begins its 2nd maturation division. In contrast to the 1st meiotic division, **no DNA synthesis occurs in advance of this division.** The 23 double-structured chromosomes divide at the centromere, and each of the newly formed daughter cells receives 23 **chromatids** (Fig. 1.2*G*). The amount of DNA in the newly formed cells is now half that of the normal somatic cell. Hence, the purpose of the two meiotic or maturation

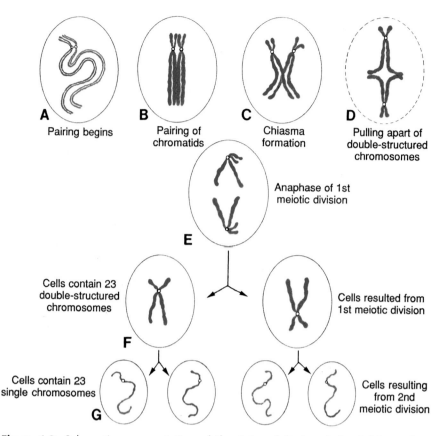

Figure 1.2. Schematic representation of the 1st and 2nd meiotic divisions. **A.** Homologous chromosomes approach each other. **B.** Homologous chromosomes pair, and each member of the pair consists of two chromatids. **C.** Intimately paired homologous chromosomes interchange chromatid fragments (crossover). Note the chiasma. **D.** Double-structured chromosomes pull apart. **E.** Anaphase of the 1st meiotic division. **F** and **G.** During the 2nd meiotic division, the double-structured chromosomes split at the centromere. At completion of division, chromosomes in each of the four daughter cells are different from each other.

divisions is twofold: *(a)* to provide for genetic variability through the processes of crossover, which creates new chromosomes, and random distribution of homologous chromosomes to the daughter cells; and *(b)* to provide each germ cell with both a haploid number of chromosomes and half the amount of DNA of a normal somatic cell (2nd meiotic division).

As a result of the meiotic divisions, one primary oocyte eventually gives rise to four daughter cells, each with 22 + 1 X chromosomes (Fig. 1.3*A*). Only one of these develops into a mature gamete, the oocyte; the other three, the **polar bodies,** receive hardly any cytoplasm and degenerate during subsequent development.

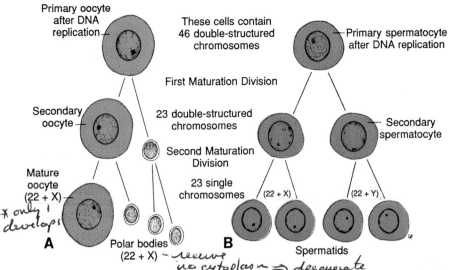

Figure 1.3. Schematic drawing showing events occurring during the 1st and 2nd maturation divisions. **A.** The primitive female germ cell (primary oocyte) produces only one mature gamete, the mature oocyte. **B.** The primitive male germ cell (primary spermatocyte) produces four spermatids, all of which develop into spermatozoa.

The primary spermatocyte gives rise to four daughter cells; two with 22 + 1 X chromosomes and two with 22 + 1 Y chromosomes (Fig. 1.3B). All four develop into mature gametes.

CLINICAL CORRELATES

Abnormalities in chromosome number may originate during meiotic divisions. Normally, two members of a homologous chromosome pair separate during the 1st meiotic division, so that each daughter cell receives one component of each pair (Fig. 1.4A). Sometimes, however, separation does not occur **(nondisjunction),** and both members of a pair then move into one cell (Fig. 1.4B). As a result of nondisjunction of the chromosomes, one cell receives 24 chromosomes, and the other receives 22 instead of the normal 23 chromosomes. When, at fertilization, a gamete having 23 chromosomes fuses with a gamete having 24 or 22 chromosomes, the result will be an individual with either 47 chromosomes (trisomy) or 45 chromosomes (monosomy). Nondisjunction occurs during either the 1st or the 2nd meiotic division of the germ cells and may involve any of the chromosomes.

The incidence of chromosomal abnormalities increases after a woman reaches age 35. Cases of monosomy and trisomy occur more

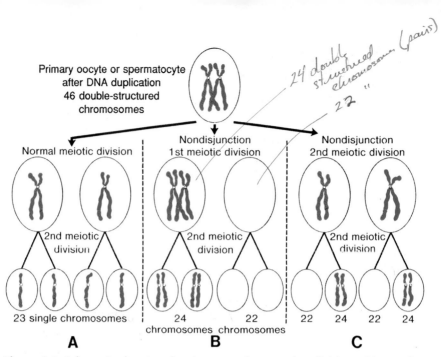

Primary oocyte or spermatocyte after DNA duplication 46 double-structured chromosomes

24 double structured chromosomes (pairs)
22 "

Normal meiotic division

Nondisjunction 1st meiotic division

Nondisjunction 2nd meiotic division

2nd meiotic division

2nd meiotic division

2nd meiotic division

23 single chromosomes

24 chromosomes · 22 chromosomes

22 · 24 · 22 · 24

A

B

C

Figure 1.4. Schematic drawing showing normal maturation divisions **(A)**, nondisjunction in the 1st meiotic division **(B)**, and nondisjunction in the 2nd meiotic division **(C)**.

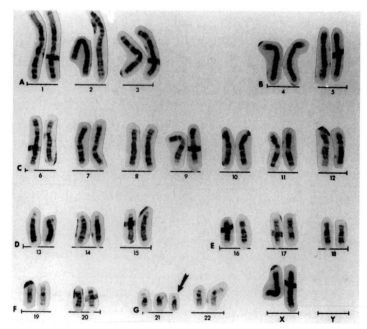

Figure 1.5. Karyotype of an individual with trisomy 21 *(arrow),* Down syndrome.

frequently and may involve the sex chromosomes or autosomes (see Chapter 8). Down syndrome is an example of trisomy in which there is an extra chromosome 21 (Fig. 1.5). In 80% of cases, the defect is caused by nondisjunction during meiosis in the mother, with the remainder of cases due to nondisjunction of paternal chromosomes. Trisomy 21 is not the only chromosome involved, however, in production of trisomy-induced abnormalities. Trisomies 8, 9, 13, and 18 also cause syndromes of abnormal development (see Chapter 8).

Occasionally, nondisjunction of chromosome 21 occurs during mitosis **(mitotic nondisjunction)** in an embryonic cell during the earliest cell divisions. In such cases, **mosaicism** results, with some cells having an abnormal chromosome number and others being normal. Affected individuals may exhibit few or many of the characteristics of Down syndrome, depending on the number of cells involved and their distribution.

Sometimes, chromosome breaks occur, and pieces of one chromosome become attached to another. Such **translocations** may be **balanced,** in which case breakage and reunion occur between two chromosomes, but no critical genetic material is lost and individuals are normal; or they may be **unbalanced,** in which case part of one chromosome is lost and an altered phenotype is produced. For example, unbalanced translocations between the long arms of chromosomes 14 and 21 during meiosis I or II produce gametes with an extra copy of chromosome 21, which, when fertilized, provide another etiology for Down syndrome (Fig. 1.6). Translocations are particularly common between chromosomes 13, 14, 15, 21, and 22 because they cluster during meiosis.

In some cases, chromosome breaks occur, and the pieces do not attach to other chromosomes. These pieces may result in partial trisomies or monosomies such as in the cri-du-chat (5p) syndrome where a portion of chromosome 5 is missing.

Gene mutations also occur with increasing maternal and paternal age and may result in aberrant phenotypes. Achondroplasia, where individuals have shortened stature and limbs, is an autosomal dominant disorder resulting from a mutation. Older paternal age is a contributing factor to the risk for this disorder.

Many major chromosomal abnormalities result in spontaneous abortion. In fact, 50–60% of all conceptions terminate in spontaneous abortion, and approximately 50% of these have major chromosomal defects. The most common chromosomal abnormalities of abortuses are trisomy 16, triploidy (usually due to fertilization of an egg by two sperm), and 45,X.

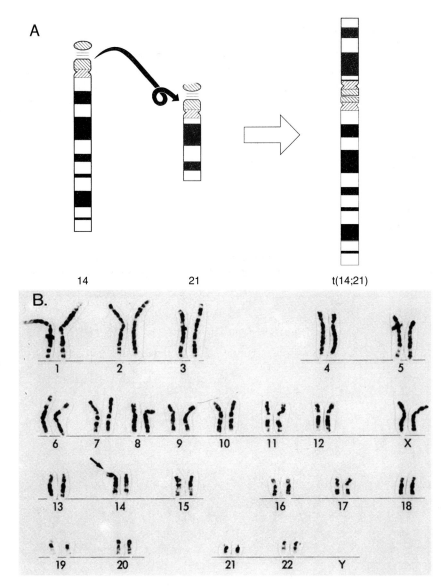

Figure 1.6. A. Illustration of the translocation of the long arms of chromosomes 14 and 21 at the centromere. Loss of the short arms is not clinically significant, and these individuals are clinically normal, although they are at higher risk for producing offspring with unbalanced translocations. **B.** Karyotype of an individual with translocation of chromosome 21 onto 14, resulting in Down syndrome.

Morphological Changes During Maturation

PRIMORDIAL GERM CELLS

Mature male and female germ cells are direct descendants of primordial germ cells, which in human embryos appear in the wall of the yolk sac at the end of the 3rd week of development (Fig. 1.7). These cells migrate by ameboid movement from the yolk sac toward the developing gonads (primitive sex glands), where they arrive at the end of the 4th or the beginning of the 5th week (see Chapter 15).

OOGENESIS

Prenatal Maturation

Once primordial germ cells have arrived in the gonad of a genetic female, they differentiate into **oogonia** (Fig. 1.8, *A* and *B*). These cells undergo a number of mitotic divisions and, by the end of the 3rd month, become arranged in clusters, surrounded by a layer of flat epithelial cells (Fig. 1.9*A*). Whereas all of the oogonia in one cluster are probably derived from a single primordial germ cell,

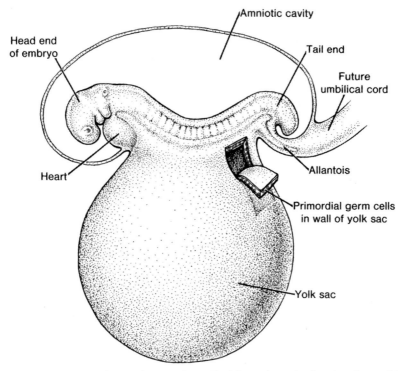

Figure 1.7. Drawing of an embryo at the end of the 3rd week, showing the position of primordial germ cells in the wall of the yolk sac, close to the attachment of the future umbilical cord.

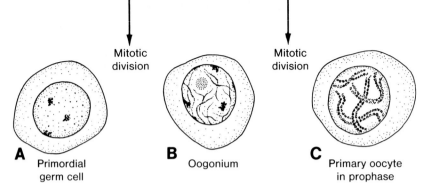

Figure 1.8. Differentiation of primordial germ cells into oogonia begins shortly after their arrival in the ovary. By the 3rd month of development, some oogonia give rise to primary oocytes that enter prophase of the 1st meiotic division. This prophase may last 40 or more years and will finish only when the cell begins its final maturation. During this period, it carries 46 double-structured chromosomes.

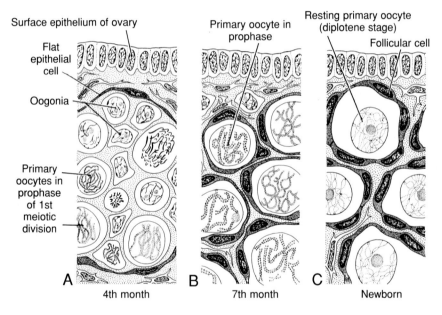

Figure 1.9. Schematic representation of a segment of the ovary at different stages of development. **A.** At 4 months. Oogonia are grouped in clusters in the cortical part of the ovary. Some show mitosis; others have already differentiated into primary oocytes and have entered prophase of the 1st meiotic division. **B.** At 7 months. Almost all oogonia are transformed into primary oocytes in prophase of the 1st meiotic division. **C.** At birth. Oogonia are absent. Each primary oocyte is surrounded by a single layer of follicular cells, thus forming the primordial follicle. Oocytes have entered the diplotene stage, in which they remain until just before ovulation. Only then do they enter metaphase of the 1st meiotic division.

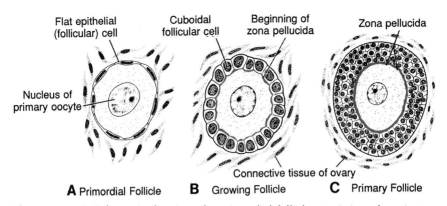

Figure 1.10. A. Schematic drawing of a primordial follicle consisting of a primary oocyte surrounded by a layer of flattened epithelial cells. **B.** As maturation of the follicle proceeds, the follicular cells become cuboidal. They now begin to secrete the zona pellucida, which is visible in irregular patches on the surface of the oocyte. **C.** With further maturation, the follicular cells form a stratified layer of granulosa cells around the oocyte, thus transforming the primordial follicle into a primary follicle, and the zona pellucida is well defined.

the flat epithelial cells, known as **follicular cells,** originate from surface epithelium covering the ovary.

The majority of oogonia continue to divide by mitosis, but some of them differentiate into much larger **primary oocytes.** Immediately after their formation, they replicate their DNA and enter prophase of the 1st meiotic division (Figs. 1.8*C* and 1.9*A*). During the next few months, oogonia increase rapidly in number, and by the 5th month of development, the total number of germ cells in the ovary reaches its maximum, estimated at 7 million. At this time, cell death begins, and many oogonia as well as primary oocytes become atretic. By the 7th month, the majority of oogonia have degenerated except for a few near the surface. All surviving primary oocytes, however, have entered the 1st meiotic division, and most of them are now individually surrounded by a layer of flat epithelial cells (Fig. 1.9*B*). A primary oocyte, together with its surrounding flat epithelial cells, is known as a **primordial follicle** (Fig. 1.10*A*).

Postnatal Maturation

Near the time of birth, all primary oocytes have started prophase of the 1st meiotic division, but instead of proceeding into metaphase they enter the **diplotene stage,** a resting stage during prophase that is characterized by a lacy network of chromatin (Fig. 1.9*C*). **Primary oocytes remain in prophase and do not finish their 1st meiotic division before puberty is reached,** apparently because of **oocyte maturation inhibitor (OMI),** a substance secreted by follicular cells. The total number of primary oocytes at birth is estimated to vary from 700,000 to 2 million. During the following years of childhood, the majority of the oocytes become atretic; only approximately 400,000 are present by the beginning of puberty, and fewer than 500 will be ovulated in the reproductive lifetime of the individual.

It is important to realize that some oocytes, reaching maturity late in life, have been dormant in the diplotene stage of the 1st meiotic division for 40 years or more. Whether or not the diplotene stage is the most suitable phase to protect the oocyte against environmental influences acting on the ovary during life is presently unknown. Considering that the incidence of children with chromosomal abnormalities increases with maternal age, one may wonder whether or not the extended period in meiosis makes the primary oocyte vulnerable to damage.

With the onset of puberty, 5–15 primordial follicles begin to mature with each ovarian cycle. The primary oocyte (still in the diplotene stage) begins to increase in size, while the surrounding follicular cells change from flat to cuboidal and proliferate to produce a stratified epithelium of **granulosa cells.** The follicle is now known as a **primary follicle** (Fig. 1.10, *B* and *C*). Granulosa cells rest on a basement membrane separating them from surrounding stromal cells that form the **theca folliculi.** Additionally, granulosa cells and the oocyte secrete a layer of glycoproteins on the surface of the oocyte, thus forming the **zona pellucida** (Fig. 1.10*C*). As follicles continue to grow, cells of the theca folliculi become organized into an inner layer of secretory cells, the **theca interna,** and an outer layer of connective tissue containing fibroblast-like cells, the **theca externa.** Also, small, finger-like processes of the follicular cells extend across the zona pellucida and interdigitate with microvilli of the plasma membrane of the oocyte. These processes are thought to be important for transport of materials from follicular cells to the oocyte.

As development continues, fluid-filled spaces appear between granulosa cells, and when these spaces coalesce, the **antrum** is formed, and the follicle is termed a **secondary follicle.** Initially, the antrum is crescent shaped, but with time it greatly enlarges (Fig. 1.11, *A* and *B*). Granulosa cells surrounding the oocyte remain intact and form the **cumulus oophorus.** At maturity, the follicle, which may be 10 mm or more in diameter, is known as the **tertiary, vesicular,** or **graafian follicle.** It is surrounded by the theca interna, which is composed of cells having characteristics of steroid secretion, rich in blood vessels, and the theca externa, which gradually merges with the ovarian stroma (Fig. 1.11).

With each ovarian cycle a number of follicles begin to develop, but usually only one reaches full maturity. The others degenerate and become atretic. As soon as the follicle is mature, the primary oocyte resumes its 1st meiotic division, leading to formation of two daughter cells of unequal size, but each with 23 (double-structured) chromosomes (Fig. 1.12, *A* and *B*). One cell, the **secondary oocyte,** receives most of the cytoplasm; the other, the **1st polar body,** receives practically none. The latter is located between the zona pellucida and the cell membrane of the secondary oocyte in the perivitelline space (Fig. 1.12*B*). The 1st meiotic division resumes shortly before ovulation.

At completion of the 1st maturation division and before the nucleus of the secondary oocyte has returned to its resting stage, the cell enters the **2nd maturation division without DNA replication.** The moment the secondary

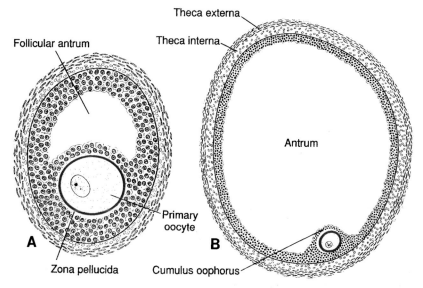

Figure 1.11. Schematic representation of a maturing follicle. **A.** The oocyte, surrounded by the zona pellucida, is eccentrically located; the antrum has developed by coalescence of intercellular spaces. Note the arrangement of cells of the theca interna and the theca externa. **B.** Mature vesicular or graafian follicle. The antrum has enlarged considerably, is filled with follicular fluid, and is surrounded by a stratified layer of granulosa cells. The oocyte is embedded in a mound of granulosa cells, known as the cumulus oophorus.

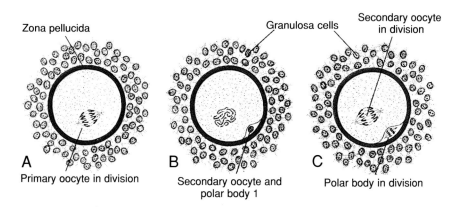

Figure 1.12. Maturation of the oocyte. **A.** Primary oocyte showing the spindle of the 1st meiotic division. **B.** Secondary oocyte and 1st polar body. Note that the nuclear membrane is absent. **C.** Secondary oocyte showing the spindle of the 2nd meiotic division. The 1st polar body is also dividing.

oocyte shows spindle formation with chromosomes aligned on the metaphase plate, ovulation occurs, and the oocyte is shed from the ovary (Fig. 1.12*C*). The 2nd maturation division is completed only if the oocyte is fertilized; otherwise, the cell degenerates approximately 24 hours after ovulation. Whether or not the 1st polar body undergoes a 2nd division is uncertain, but fertilized ova accompanied by three polar bodies have been observed.

SPERMATOGENESIS

Spermatogenesis includes all of the events by which **spermatogonia** are transformed into **spermatozoa.** In the male, differentiation of primordial germ cells begins at puberty; in the female, however, it begins in utero during the 3rd month of development. At the time of birth, germ cells in the male can be recognized in the sex cords of the testis as large, pale cells surrounded by supporting cells (Fig. 1.13*A*). The latter are derived from the surface epithelium of the gland in the same manner as follicular cells and become **sustentacular** or **Sertoli cells.**

Shortly before puberty, the sex cords acquire a lumen and become the **seminiferous tubules.** At about the same time, primordial germ cells give rise to **spermatogonia,** which consist of two types: **type A spermatogonia,** which divide by mitosis to provide a continuous reserve of **stem cells,** and **type B spermatogonia,** which give rise to primary spermatocytes. In the normal progression of events, some of the type A cells leave the stem cell population and give rise to successive generations of spermatogonia, each more differentiated than the last (Figs. 1.13, *B* and *C,* and 1.14). On completion of the last division

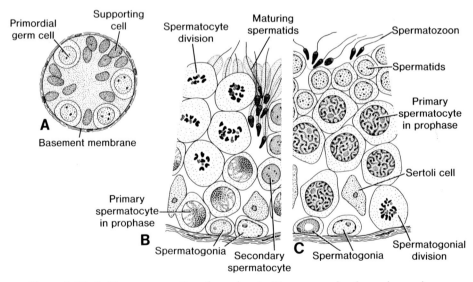

Figure 1.13. A. Transverse section through primitive sex cords of a male newborn, showing primordial germ cells and supporting cells. **B** and **C.** Two segments of the seminiferous tubule shown in transverse section. Note the different stages in spermatogenesis.

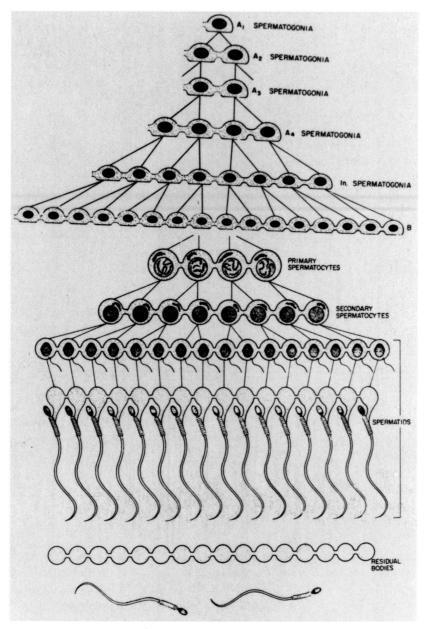

Figure 1.14. Drawing illustrating the clonal origin of male germ cells. Only the most primitive type A spermatogonia undergo complete cytokinesis to replenish the stem cell population. Once type A cells leave the stem cell population, cytoplasmic bridges join cells in each succeeding division until individual sperm are separated from residual bodies. In fact, the number of individual interconnected cells is considerably greater than depicted in this figure.

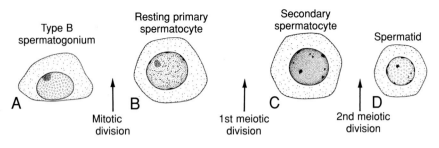

Figure 1.15. Schematic representation of spermatogenesis in humans.

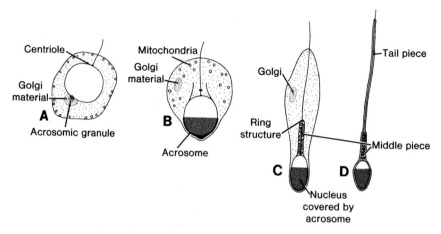

Figure 1.16. Schematic drawings showing the important stages in transformation of the human spermatid into the spermatozoon.

of type A cells, type B spermatogonia are formed; when these cells subsequently undergo mitosis, **primary spermatocytes** are created (Fig. 1.14). Primary spermatocytes then enter a prolonged prophase (22 days), followed by rapid completion of meiosis I and formation of **secondary spermatocytes.** These cells begin immediately to form **spermatids** during the 2nd meiotic division (Figs. 1.14–1.16), which contain the haploid number of 23 chromosomes. Throughout this series of events, from the time type A cells leave the stem cell population to formation of spermatids, cytokinesis is incomplete such that successive cell generations are joined by cytoplasmic bridges. Thus, the progeny of a single type A spermatogonium form a cluster of germ cells that maintain contact throughout differentiation (Fig. 1.14). Furthermore, spermatogonia and spermatids remain embedded in deep recesses of Sertoli cells throughout their development (Fig. 1.17). In this manner, Sertoli cells provide support and protection for the germ cells, participate in their nutrition, and assist in the release of mature spermatozoa.

SPERMIOGENESIS

The series of changes resulting in the transformation of spermatids into spermatozoa is known as **spermiogenesis.** These changes include *(a)* formation of the acrosome, which covers half the nuclear surface and contains enzymes to assist in penetration of the egg and its surrounding layers during fertilization (Fig. 1.16, *B* and *C*); *(b)* condensation of the nucleus; *(c)* formation of neck, middle piece, and tail (Fig. 1.16*C*); and *(d)* shedding of most of the cytoplasm (Fig. 1.16*D*). In humans, the time required for a spermatogonium to develop into a mature spermatozoon is approximately 64 days.

When fully formed, spermatozoa enter the lumen of seminiferous tubules. From there, they are pushed toward the epididymis by contractile elements in the

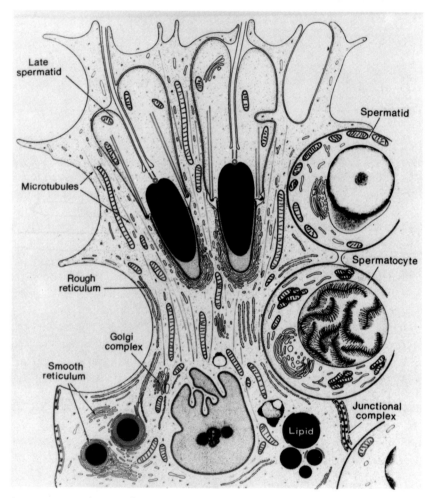

Figure 1.17. High magnification of a Sertoli cell, illustrating its relationship to germ cells. Spermatocytes and early spermatids occupy depressions in basal aspects of the cell, while late spermatids are located in deep recesses near the apex.

wall of the seminiferous tubules. Although initially only slightly motile, spermatozoa obtain full motility in the epididymis.

CLINICAL CORRELATES

In the human as well as in most mammals, one ovarian follicle occasionally contains two or three clearly distinguishable primary oocytes (Fig. 1.18A). Although these oocytes may give rise to twins or triplets, they usually degenerate before reaching maturity. In rare cases, one primary oocyte contains two or even three nuclei (Fig. 1.18B). Such binucleated or trinucleated oocytes, however, die before reaching maturity.

Contrary to atypical oocytes, abnormal spermatozoa are seen frequently, and up to 10% of all spermatozoa have observable defects. The head, as well as the tail, may be abnormal, they may be giants or dwarfs, and sometimes they are joined (Fig. 1.18C). Sperm with morphological abnormalities lack normal motility and probably do not fertilize oocytes.

SUMMARY

In preparation for fertilization, both male and female germ cells undergo a number of chromosomal and morphological changes, a process known as **gametogenesis.** The chromosomal changes occur during **meiotic divisions.** During the 1st meiotic division, **homologous chromosomes pair** and **exchange genetic material;** during the 2nd meiotic division cells fail to replicate DNA, and each cell is thus provided with a **haploid** number of chromosomes and half the amount of DNA of a normal somatic cell (Fig. 1.2). Hence, mature male and female gametes have, respectively, 22 + X or 22 + Y chromosomes.

Human germ cells, known as **primordial germ cells,** appear in the wall of the yolk sac (Fig. 1.7) at the end of the 3rd week and migrate to the

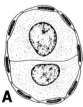

A
Primordial follicle with two oocytes

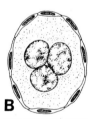

B
Trinucleated oocyte

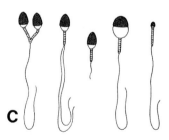

C

Figure 1.18. Drawings of abnormal germ cells in the female and male. **A.** Primordial follicle with two oocytes. **B.** Trinucleated oocyte. **C.** Various types of abnormal spermatozoa.

indifferent gonad, where they arrive in the 5th week. In the male, the maturation process from primitive germ cell to mature gamete is known as **spermatogenesis;** in the female, it is known as **oogenesis.** In the female, primordial germ cells differentiate into **oogonia.** After repeated divisions, some of these differentiate into **primary oocytes,** which, immediately after their formation, enter the 1st meiotic division. By the 7th month, all primary oocytes have entered the 1st meiotic division, and most of them are individually surrounded by a layer of flat follicular cells (Fig. 1.9). Together, they form the **primordial follicle. Primary oocytes do not finish their 1st meiotic division but remain in the diplotene stage until puberty.** At birth, their total number varies from 700,000 to 2 million.

With the onset of puberty a number of primordial follicles begin to mature with each ovarian cycle, but usually only one reaches full maturity. During this maturation process, one primary oocyte gives rise to one **secondary oocyte** plus one **polar body.** The secondary oocyte, in turn, gives rise to a mature oocyte plus another polar body. Hence, a primary oocyte develops into one mature oocyte and three polar bodies (Fig. 1.3).

In the male, primordial cells remain dormant until puberty, and only then do they differentiate into spermatogonia. These stem cells give rise to primary spermatocytes, which, through two successive meiotic divisions, produce four **spermatids** (Fig. 1.3). Spermatids subsequently go through a series of changes **(spermiogenesis)** (Fig. 1.16) including *(a)* formation of the acrosome, *(b)* condensation of the nucleus, *(c)* formation of neck, middle piece, and tail, and *(d)* shedding of most of the cytoplasm. The time required for a spermatogonium to become a mature spermatozoon is approximately 64 days.

PROBLEMS TO SOLVE

1. What is the most common cause for abnormal chromosome number? Give an example of a clinical syndrome involving abnormal numbers of chromosomes.

2. In addition to numerical abnormalities, what other types of chromosomal alterations occur?

3. What is mosaicism, and how does it occur?

SUGGESTED READINGS

Chandley AC: Meiosis in Man. *Trends Genet* 4:79, 1988.
Clermont Y: Kinetics of spermatogenesis in mammals: seminiferous epithelium cycle and spermatogonial renewal. *Physiol Rev* 52:198, 1972.
Eddy EM, Clark JM, Gong D, Fenderson BA: Origin and migration of primordial germ cells in mammals. *Gamete Res* 4:333, 1981.
Heller CG, Clermont Y: Kinetics of the germinal epithelium in man. *Recent Prog Horm Res* 20:545, 1964.
Larsen WJ, Wert SE: Roles of cell junctions in gametogenesis and early embryonic development. *Tissue Cell* 20:809, 1988.
Pelletier RA, We K, Balakier H: Development of membrane differentiations in the guinea pig spermatid during spermiogenesis. *Am J Anat* 167:119, 1983.
Russell LD: Sertoli-germ cell interactions: a review. *Gamete Res* 3:179, 1980.

Stoll C, Roth MP, Bigel P: A re-examination of paternal age effect on the occurrence of new mutants for achondroplasia. *Prog Clin Biol Res* 104:419, 1982.

Witschj E: Migration of the germ cells of the human embryos from the yolk sac to the primitive gonadal folds. *Contrib Embryol* 36:67, 1948.

chapter 2

Ovulation to Implantation
(First Week of Development)

Ovarian Cycle

At puberty, the female begins to undergo regular monthly cycles. These cycles, known as **sexual cycles,** are controlled by the hypothalamus. **Gonadotropin-releasing hormone** (GnRH) produced by the hypothalamus acts on cells of the anterior pituitary gland, which, in turn, secrete **gonadotropins.** These hormones, **follicle-stimulating hormone** (FSH) and **luteinizing hormone** (LH), stimulate and control cyclic changes in the ovary.

At the beginning of each ovarian cycle, 5–15 primordial follicles begin to grow under the influence of FSH (Fig. 2.1). Under normal conditions, only one of these follicles reaches full maturity, and only one oocyte is discharged; the others degenerate and become atretic. In the next cycle, another group of follicles begin to grow, and again only one reaches maturity. Consequently, the majority of follicles degenerate without ever reaching full maturity. When a follicle becomes atretic, the oocyte and surrounding follicular cells degenerate and are replaced by connective tissue, thus forming a **corpus atreticum.** During growth of the follicle, large numbers of follicular and thecal cells are formed. In cooperation, these cells produce estrogens that (a) cause the uterine endometrium to enter the follicular or **proliferative phase** and (b) stimulate the pituitary gland to secrete LH. A surge of this hormone is needed for final stages of follicle maturation and to induce ovulation.

Ovulation

In the days immediately preceding ovulation, the graafian follicle increases rapidly in size under the influence of FSH and LH and expands to a diameter of 15 mm. Coincident with final development of the graafian follicle, the primary oocyte, which until this time has remained in the diplotene stage, resumes and finishes its 1st meiotic division. In the meantime, the surface of the ovary begins to bulge locally, and at the apex an avascular spot, the **stigma,** appears. As a result of local weakening and degeneration of the ovarian surface, increasing intrafollicular pressure, and muscular contraction in the ovarian wall, the oocyte is extruded. Thus, the oocyte, together with surrounding granulosa cells from the region of the cumulus oophorus, breaks free and floats out of the ovary (Figs. 2.2

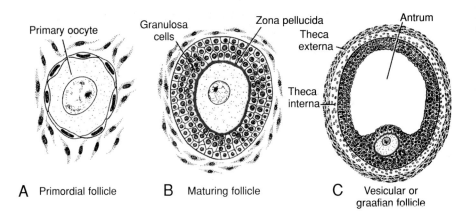

A Primordial follicle B Maturing follicle C Vesicular or graafian follicle

Figure 2.1. Drawing of changes occurring in the primordial follicle during the first half of the ovarian cycle. Under influence of FSH the primordial follicle **(A)** matures into the graafian follicle **(C).** The oocyte remains a primary oocyte in the diplotene stage until shortly before ovulation. During the last few days of the growing period, estrogens, produced by follicular and thecal cells, stimulate formation of LH in the pituitary (see Fig. 2.13).

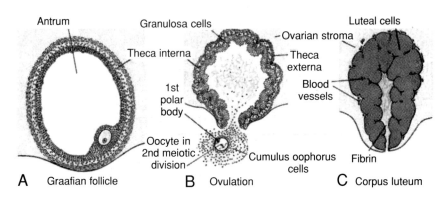

A Graafian follicle B Ovulation C Corpus luteum

Figure 2.2. A. Graafian follicle just before rupture. **B.** Ovulation. The oocyte, beginning its 2nd meiotic division, is discharged from the ovary, together with a large number of cumulus oophorus cells. Follicular cells remaining inside the collapsed follicle differentiate into luteal cells. **C.** Corpus luteum. Note the large size of the corpus luteum caused by hypertrophy and accumulation of lipid in granulosa and theca interna cells. The remaining cavity of the follicle is filled with fibrin.

and 2.3). Some of the cumulus oophorus cells then rearrange themselves around the zona pellucida to form the **corona radiata** (Figs. 2.4–2.6). At the moment that the oocyte with its cumulus oophorus cells is discharged from the ovary **(ovulation),** the 1st meiotic division is completed, and the secondary oocyte has started its 2nd meiotic division (Fig. 2.2*B*).

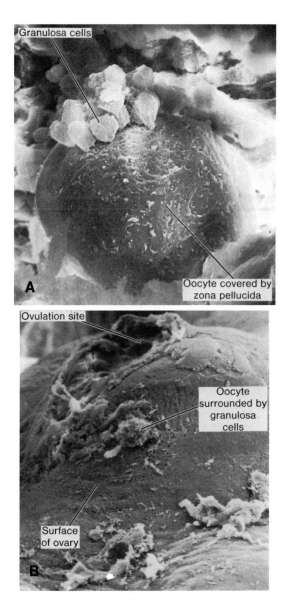

Figure 2.3. **A.** Scanning electron micrograph of ovulation in the mouse. The surface of the oocyte is covered by the zona pellucida. Note the cumulus oophorus composed of granulosa cells. **B.** Scanning electron micrograph of a rabbit oocyte 1½ hours after ovulation. The oocyte is surrounded by granulosa cells and lies on the surface of the ovary. Note the site of ovulation.

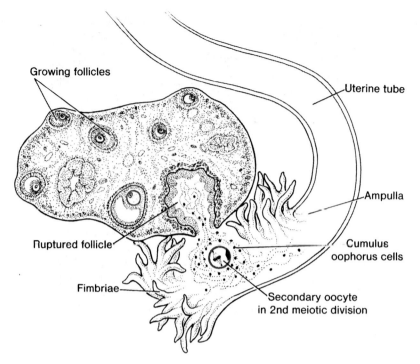

Growing follicles

Uterine tube

Ruptured follicle

Ampulla

Fimbriae

Cumulus
oophorus cells

Secondary oocyte
in 2nd meiotic division

Figure 2.4. Relationship of fimbriae and ovary. During ovulation, fimbriae are thought to sweep over the rupturing follicle, collecting the oocyte and guiding it into the uterine tube.

CLINICAL CORRELATES

In some women, ovulation is accompanied by slight pain, known as middle pain because this event normally occurs near the middle of the menstrual cycle. Ovulation is also generally accompanied by a rise in basal temperature, an event that can be monitored to aid in determining when release of the oocyte occurs. Some women fail to ovulate due to a diminished concentration of gonadotropins. In these cases, administration of an agent to stimulate gonadotropin release and, hence, ovulation can be employed. Although such drugs are effective, they often produce multiple ovulations, such that the risk of multiple pregnancies is 10 times higher in these patients.

Corpus Luteum

Following ovulation, granulosa cells remaining in the wall of the ruptured follicle, together with cells from the theca interna, are vascularized by surrounding vessels and become polyhedral. Under influence of LH, these cells develop a

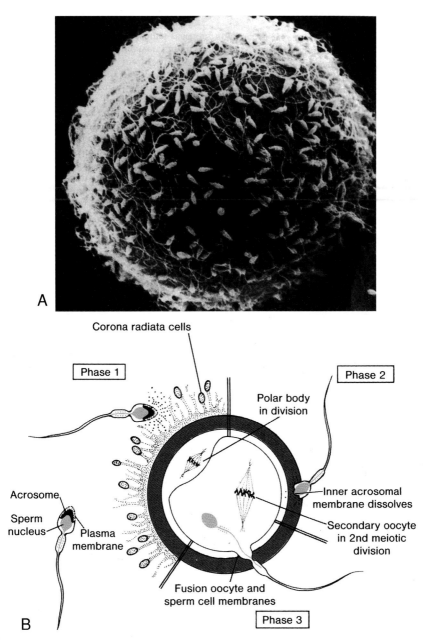

Figure 2.5. **A.** Scanning electron micrograph of sperm binding to the zona pellucida. **B.** Schematic representation of the three phases of oocyte penetration. In phase 1, spermatozoa break through the corona radiata barrier; in phase 2, one or more spermatozoa penetrate the zona pellucida; in phase 3, one spermatozoon penetrates the oocyte membrane while losing its own plasma membrane. **Inset** shows normal spermatocyte with acrosomal head cap.

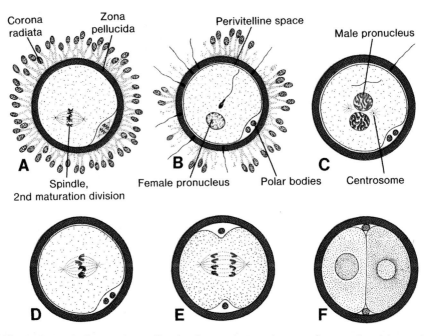

Corona radiata
Zona pellucida
Perivitelline space
Male pronucleus
Spindle, 2nd maturation division
Female pronucleus
Polar bodies
Centrosome

A   B   C

D   E   F

Figure 2.6. **A.** Oocyte immediately after ovulation, showing the spindle of the 2nd meiotic division. **B.** A spermatozoon has penetrated the oocyte, which has finished its 2nd meiotic division. Chromosomes of the oocyte are arranged in a vesicular nucleus, the female pronucleus. Heads of several sperm are stuck in the zona pellucida. **C.** Male and female pronuclei. **D** and **E.** Chromosomes become arranged on the spindle, split longitudinally, and move to opposite poles. **F.** Two-cell stage.

yellowish pigment and change into **luteal cells,** which form the **corpus luteum** and secrete **progesterone** (Fig. 2.2*C*). This hormone, together with estrogenic hormones, causes the uterine mucosa to enter the **progestational** or **secretory stage** in preparation for implantation of the embryo.

Oocyte Transport

Shortly before ovulation, fimbriae of the oviduct begin to cover the surface of the ovary, and the tube itself begins to contract rhythmically. It is believed that the oocyte surrounded by some granulosa cells (Figs. 2.3 and 2.4) is carried into the tube by sweeping movements of the fimbriae and by motion of cilia on the epithelial lining. Once in the tube, cumulus cells lose contact with the oocyte by withdrawing their cytoplasmic processes from the zona pellucida.

Once the oocyte is in the uterine tube, it is pushed toward the uterine lumen by contractions of the muscular wall. The rate of transport is somewhat affected by the endocrine status during and after ovulation, but in humans the fertilized oocyte reaches the uterine lumen in approximately 3–4 days.

Corpus Albicans

If fertilization fails to occur, the corpus luteum reaches maximum development about 9 days after ovulation. It can easily be recognized as a yellowish projection on the surface of the ovary. Subsequently, the corpus luteum decreases in size through degeneration of luteal cells and forms a mass of fibrotic scar tissue, known as the **corpus albicans.** Simultaneously, progesterone production decreases, thus precipitating menstrual bleeding.

If the oocyte is fertilized, degeneration of the corpus luteum is prevented by **chorionic gonadotropin (hCG),** a hormone secreted by the trophoblast of the developing embryo. The corpus luteum continues to grow and forms the **corpus luteum of pregnancy (graviditatis).** By the end of the 3rd month, this structure may be one-third to one-half of the total size of the ovary. Yellowish luteal cells continue to secrete progesterone until the end of the 4th month; thereafter, they regress slowly as secretion of progesterone by the trophoblastic component of the placenta becomes adequate for maintenance of pregnancy. Removal of the corpus luteum of pregnancy before the 4th month usually leads to abortion.

Fertilization

Fertilization, the process by which male and female gametes fuse, occurs in the **ampullary region of the uterine tube.** This is the widest part of the tube and is located close to the ovary (Fig. 2.4). Spermatozoa and the oocyte remain viable in the female reproductive tract for approximately 24 hours.

Spermatozoa pass rapidly from the vagina into the uterus and subsequently into the uterine tubes. This ascent is caused by contractions of the musculature of the uterus and the tube. It must be kept in mind that spermatozoa, on arrival in the female genital tract, are not capable of fertilizing the oocyte. They must undergo *(a)* **capacitation** and *(b)* the **acrosome reaction.**

Capacitation is a period of conditioning in the female reproductive tract that, in the human, lasts approximately 7 hours. During this time, a glycoprotein coat and seminal plasma proteins are removed from the plasma membrane that overlies the acrosomal region of the spermatozoa. Only capacitated sperm can pass through the corona cells and undergo the acrosome reaction.

The **acrosome reaction** occurs after binding to the zona pellucida and is induced by zona proteins. This reaction culminates in the release of enzymes needed to penetrate the zona pellucida, including acrosin and trypsin-like substances (Fig. 2.5).

The phases of fertilization include phase 1—penetration of the corona radiata, phase 2—penetration of the zona pellucida, and phase 3—fusion of the oocyte and sperm cell membranes.

PHASE 1: PENETRATION OF THE CORONA RADIATA

Of the 200–300 million spermatozoa deposited in the female genital tract, only 300–500 reach the site of fertilization. Only one of those is needed for fertilization, and it is thought that the others aid the fertilizing sperm in penetrating the barriers protecting the female gamete. Capacitated sperm pass freely through corona cells (Fig. 2.5).

PHASE 2: PENETRATION OF THE ZONA PELLUCIDA

The zona is a glycoprotein shell surrounding the egg that facilitates and maintains sperm binding and induces the acrosome reaction. Release of acrosomal enzymes allows sperm to penetrate the zona, thereby coming in contact with the plasma membrane of the oocyte (Fig. 2.5). Permeability of the zona pellucida changes when the head of the sperm comes in contact with the oocyte surface. This contact results in release of lysosomal enzymes from cortical granules lining the plasma membrane of the oocyte. In turn, these enzymes cause an alteration in properties of the zona pellucida (**zona reaction**) to prevent sperm penetration and inactivate species-specific receptor sites for spermatozoa on the zona surface. Other spermatozoa have been found embedded in the zona pellucida, but only one seems to be able to penetrate the oocyte (Fig. 2.6).

PHASE 3: FUSION OF THE OOCYTE AND SPERM CELL MEMBRANES

As soon as a spermatozoon comes in contact with the oocyte cell membrane, the two plasma membranes fuse (Fig. 2.5). Since the plasma membrane covering the acrosomal head cap has disappeared during the acrosome reaction, actual fusion is accomplished between the oocyte membrane and the membrane that covers the posterior region of the sperm head (Fig. 2.5). In the human, both the head and tail of the spermatozoon enter the cytoplasm of the oocyte, but the plasma membrane is left behind on the oocyte surface.

As soon as the spermatozoon has entered the oocyte, the egg responds in three different ways:

① **Cortical and zona reactions.** As a result of the release of cortical oocyte granules, which contain lysosomal enzymes, *(a)* the oocyte membrane becomes impenetrable to other spermatozoa, and *(b)* the zona pellucida alters its structure and composition to prevent sperm binding and penetration. In this manner polyspermy is prevented.

② **Resumption of the 2nd meiotic division.** The oocyte finishes its 2nd meiotic division immediately after entry of the spermatozoon. One of the daughter cells receives hardly any cytoplasm and is known as the **2nd polar body;** the other daughter cell is the **definitive oocyte.** Its chromosomes (22 + X) become arranged in a vesicular nucleus known as the **female pronucleus** (Figs. 2.6 and 2.7).

③ **Metabolic activation of the egg.** The activating factor is probably carried by the spermatozoon. Postfusion activation may be considered to encompass the initial cellular and molecular events associated with early embryogenesis.

The spermatozoon, meanwhile, moves forward until it lies in close proximity to the female pronucleus. Its nucleus becomes swollen and forms the **male pronucleus** (Fig. 2.6), while the tail is detached and degenerates. Morphologically, the male and female pronuclei are indistinguishable and eventually will

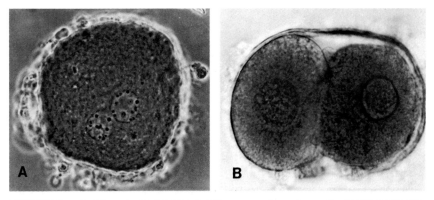

Figure 2.7. **A.** Phase contrast view of the pronuclear stage of a fertilized human oocyte. Note male and female pronuclei. **B.** Two-cell stage of human zygote.

come into close contact and lose their nuclear envelopes (Fig. 2.7*A*). During growth of male and female pronuclei (both haploid), each pronucleus must replicate its DNA. If it does not, each cell of the two-cell-stage zygote would have half the normal amount of DNA. Immediately after DNA synthesis, chromosomes become organized on the spindle in preparation for a normal mitotic division. The 23 maternal and 23 paternal (double) chromosomes split longitudinally at the centromere, and sister chromatids move to opposite poles, thus providing each cell of the zygote with the normal diploid number of chromosomes and DNA (Fig. 2.6, *D* and *E*). While sister chromatids move to opposite poles, a deep furrow appears on the surface of the cell, gradually dividing the cytoplasm into two parts (Figs. 2.6*F* and 2.7*B*).

The main results of fertilization are

1. **Restoration of the diploid number of chromosomes,** half from the father and half from the mother. Hence, the zygote contains a new combination of chromosomes different from both parents.
2. **Determination of the sex** of the new individual. An X-carrying sperm will produce a female (XX) embryo, and a Y-carrying sperm will produce a male (XY) embryo. Hence, the chromosomal sex of the embryo is determined at fertilization.
3. **Initiation of cleavage.** Without fertilization the oocyte usually degenerates 24 hours after ovulation.

CLINICAL CORRELATES

Fertilization can be prevented by a variety of contraceptive methods:

① Barrier techniques include the male condom, made of latex and often containing chemical spermicides, that fits over the penis; and the female condom, made of polyurethane, that lines the vagina. Other barriers, placed in the vagina, include diaphragms, cervical caps, and the contraceptive sponge.

② The "pill" is a combination of estrogen and the progesterone analogue, progestin, that inhibit ovulation but permit menstruation. Both hormones act at the level of FSH and LH, preventing their release from the pituitary. The pills are taken for 21 days and then stopped to allow menstruation, followed by repeating the cycle.

③ Depo-Provera is a progestin compound that can be implanted subdermally or injected intramuscularly to prevent ovulation for up to 5 years or 2–3 months, respectively.

④ IUDs are intrauterine devices that are placed in the uterine cavity. Their mechanism for preventing pregnancy is not clear but may involve effects on sperm and oocytes or inhibition of preimplantation stages of development.

⑤ The drug RU 486 will cause abortion if it is administered within 8 weeks of the previous menses. It initiates menstruation, possibly through its action as an antiprogesterone agent.

⑥ Vasectomy and tubal ligation are effective means of contraception, and both procedures are reversible, although not in every case.

Among 15–30% of couples, **infertility** is a problem. Male infertility may be due to insufficient numbers of sperm and/or their motility. Normally, the ejaculate has a volume of 3–4 mL with approximately 100 million sperm per mL. Males with 20 million sperm per mL or 50 million sperm per total ejaculate are usually fertile.

Infertility in females may be due to a number of causes, including occluded oviducts (most commonly due to pelvic inflammatory disease), hostile cervical mucus, immunity to spermatozoa, absence of ovulation, and others.

In vitro fertilization (IVF) of human ova and embryo transfer is a frequent practice conducted by laboratories throughout the world. Follicle growth is stimulated in the ovary by administration of gonadotropins. Oocytes are recovered by laparoscopy from ovarian follicles with an aspirator just prior to ovulation when the oocyte is in late stages of the 1st meiotic division. The egg is then placed in a simple culture medium, and sperm are added immediately. Fertilized eggs are monitored to the eight-cell stage and then placed in the uterus to develop to term. Fortunately, since preimplantation stage embryos are resistant to teratogenic insult, the risk of producing malformed offspring by in vitro procedures is low.

A disadvantage of the technique is the low success rate of the procedure, since only 20% of fertilized ova implant and develop to term. Therefore, in order to increase chances of a successful pregnancy, four to five ova are collected, fertilized, and placed in the uterus. This approach leads to the potential for multiple births, which have occurred.

Another technique, called **gamete intrafallopian transfer (GIFT),** introduces oocytes and sperm into the ampulla of the fallopian (uterine) tube where fertilization takes place. Development then proceeds in a normal fashion. In a similar approach, **zygote intrafallopian transfer (ZIFT),** fertilized oocytes are placed into the ampullary region. Both of these methods require patent uterine tubes.

Cleavage

Once the zygote has reached the two-cell stage, it undergoes a series of mitotic divisions, resulting in an increase in cell number. These cells, which become smaller with each cleavage division, are known as **blastomeres** (Fig. 2.8), and until the eight-cell stage, they form a loosely arranged clump (Fig. 2.9A). However, following the 3rd cleavage, blastomeres maximize their contact with each other, forming a compact ball of cells held together by tight junctions (Fig. 2.9B). This process, known as **compaction,** segregates inner cells, which communicate extensively by gap junctions, from outer cells. Approximately 3 days after fertilization, cells of the compacted embryo divide again to form a 16-cell **morula** (mulberry). Inner cells of the morula constitute the **inner cell mass,** while surrounding cells compose the **outer cell mass.** The inner cell mass will give rise to tissues of the **embryo proper,** while the outer cell mass forms the **trophoblast,** which later contributes to the **placenta.**

Blastocyst Formation

About the time the morula enters the uterine cavity, fluid begins to penetrate through the zona pellucida into the intercellular spaces of the inner cell mass. Gradually, the intercellular spaces become confluent, and finally, a single cavity, the **blastocele,** is formed (Fig. 2.10, A and B). At this time the embryo is known as a **blastocyst.** Cells of the inner cell mass, now referred to as the **embryoblast,** are located at one pole, while those of the outer cell mass, or **trophoblast,** flatten and form the epithelial wall of the blastocyst (Fig. 2.10, A and B). The zona pellucida has now disappeared, allowing implantation to begin.

In the human, trophoblastic cells over the embryoblast pole begin to penetrate between the epithelial cells of the uterine mucosa at about the 6th day (Fig. 2.10C). Penetration and subsequent erosion of epithelial cells of the mucosa result from proteolytic enzymes produced by the trophoblast. The uterine mucosa, however, promotes the proteolytic action of the blastocyst, so that implantation is the result of mutual trophoblastic and endometrial action. Hence, by the end of the 1st week of development, the human zygote has passed through the morula and blastocyst stages and has begun implantation in the uterine mucosa.

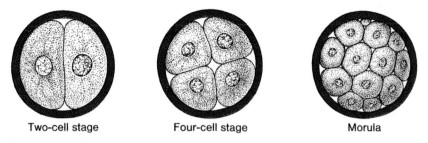

Two-cell stage   Four-cell stage   Morula

Figure 2.8. Schematic representation of the development of the zygote from the two-cell stage to the late morula stage. The two-cell stage is reached approximately 30 hours after fertilization; the four-cell stage, at approximately 40 hours; the 12- and 16-cell stage, at approximately 3 days; and the late morula stage, at approximately 4 days. During this period, blastomeres are surrounded by the zona pellucida, which disappears at the end of the 4th day.

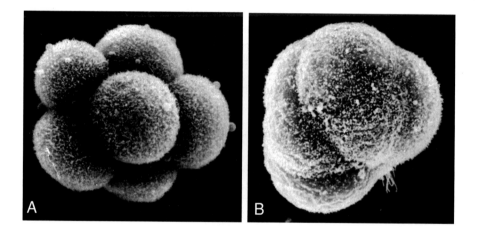

Figure 2.9. Scanning electron micrographs of uncompacted (**A**) and compacted (**B**) eight-cell mouse embryos. In the uncompacted state, outlines of each blastomere are distinct, whereas after compaction cell-cell contacts are maximized and cellular outlines are indistinct.

CLINICAL CORRELATES

The exact number of **abnormal zygotes** formed is unknown because they are usually lost early in pregnancy (within 2–3 weeks after fertilization), before the woman realizes she is pregnant, and therefore are not detected. Estimates suggest that as many as 50% of all pregnancies end in spontaneous abortion and that half of these losses

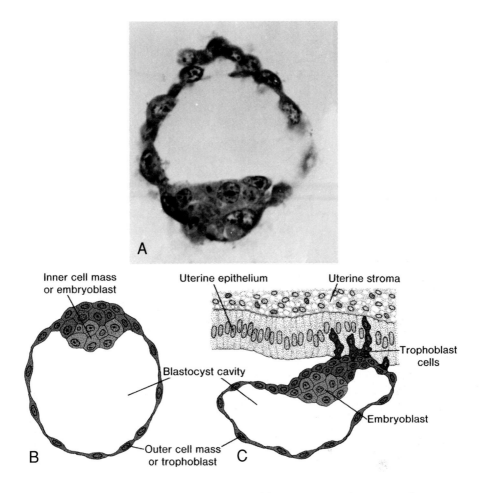

Figure 2.10. **A.** Section of a 107-cell human blastocyst. Note the inner cell mass and trophoblast cells. **B.** Schematic representation of a section through a human blastocyst recovered from the uterine cavity at approximately 4½ days. Blue cells represent the inner cell mass or embryoblast, and brown cells, the trophoblast. **C.** Schematic drawing of a section of a macaque monkey blastocyst at the 9th day of development. Trophoblast cells, located at the embryonic pole of the blastocyst, begin to penetrate the uterine mucosa. The human blastocyst begins to penetrate the uterine mucosa by the 5th or 6th day of development.

are due to chromosomal abnormalities. These abortions serve as a natural means of screening embryos for defects and in this manner reduce the incidence of congenital malformations. Without this phenomenon, approximately 12% instead of 2–3% of all infants would have birth defects.

With use of a combination of in vitro fertilization and polymerase chain reaction (PCR) techniques, molecular screening of embryos for genetic defects is being conducted. Single blastomeres from early-staged embryos can be removed, and their DNA can be amplified, for analysis. As the Human Genome Project provides more sequencing information and as specific genes are linked to various syndromes, such procedures will become more commonplace.

Uterus at Time of Implantation

The wall of the uterus consists of three layers: *(a)* **endometrium** or mucosa lining the inside wall; *(b)* **myometrium,** a thick layer of smooth muscle; and *(c)* **perimetrium,** the peritoneal covering lining the outside wall (Fig. 2.11). From puberty (11–13 years) until menopause (45–50), the endometrium undergoes

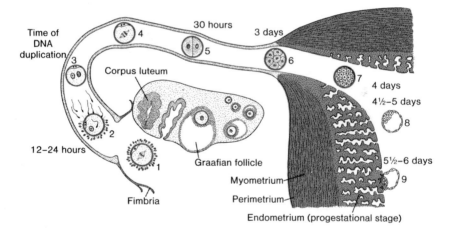

Figure 2.11. Schematic representation of events taking place during the 1st week of human development. *1,* Oocyte immediately after ovulation. *2,* Fertilization approximately 12–24 hours after ovulation. *3,* Stage of the male and female pronuclei. *4,* Spindle of the 1st mitotic division. *5,* Two-cell stage (approximately 30 hours of age). *6,* Morula containing 12–16 blastomeres (approximately 3 days of age). *7,* Advanced morula stage reaching the uterine lumen (approximately 4 days of age). *8,* Early blastocyst stage (approximately 4½ days of age). The zona pellucida has now disappeared. *9,* Early phase of implantation (blastocyst approximately 6 days of age). The ovary shows stages of transformation between a primary follicle and a graafian follicle as well as a corpus luteum. The uterine endometrium is depicted in the progestational stage.

cyclical changes that occur approximately every 28 days and are under hormonal control by the ovary. During this menstrual cycle, the uterine endometrium passes through three stages, which consist of the **follicular** or **proliferative phase,** the **secretory** or **progestational phase,** and the **menstrual phase** (Figs. 2.11–2.13). The proliferative phase begins at the end of the menstrual phase, is under the influence of estrogen, and parallels growth of the ovarian follicles. The secretory phase begins approximately 2–3 days after ovulation in response to progesterone produced by the corpus luteum. If fertilization does not occur, then shedding of the endometrium (compact and spongy layers) begins, marking the initiation of the menstrual phase. If fertilization does occur, then the endometrium assists in implantation and contributes to formation of the placenta.

At the time of implantation, the mucosa of the uterus is in the **secretory** phase (Figs. 2.11 and 2.12), during which time uterine glands and arteries become coiled and the tissue becomes succulent. As a result, three distinct layers can be recognized in the endometrium: a superficial **compact layer,** an intermediate **spongy layer,** and a thin **basal layer** (Fig. 2.12). Normally, the human blastocyst implants in the endometrium along the posterior or anterior wall of the body of the uterus, where it becomes embedded between the openings of the glands (Fig. 2.12).

If the oocyte is not fertilized, venules and sinusoidal spaces gradually become packed with blood cells, and an extensive diapedesis of blood into the tissue is

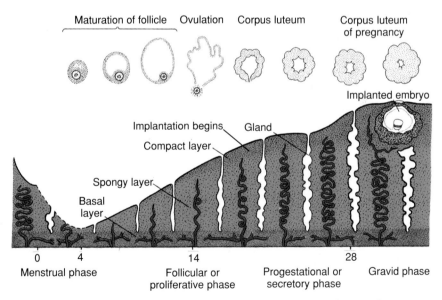

Figure 2.12. Schematic representation of the changes taking place in the uterine mucosa, correlated with those in the ovary. Note that implantation of the blastocyst has caused development of a large corpus luteum of pregnancy. Secretory activity of the endometrium increases gradually as a result of large amounts of progesterone produced by the corpus luteum of pregnancy.

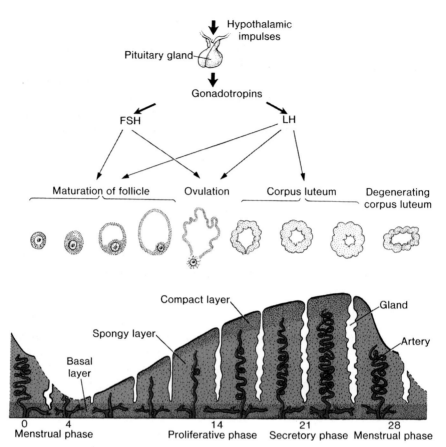

Figure 2.13. Schematic drawing of changes taking place in the uterine mucosa (endometrium) during a regular menstrual cycle in which fertilization fails to occur. Note the corresponding changes in the ovary.

seen. When the **menstrual phase** begins, blood escapes from superficial arteries, and small pieces of stroma and glands break away. During the following 3 or 4 days, the compact and spongy layers are expelled from the uterus, and the basal layer is the only part of the endometrium that is retained (Fig. 2.13). This layer is supplied by its own arteries, the **basal arteries,** and functions as the regenerative layer in the rebuilding of glands and arteries in the **proliferative phase** (Fig. 2.13).

SUMMARY

With each ovarian cycle, a number of follicles begin to grow, but usually only one reaches full maturity, and only one oocyte is discharged at **ovulation.** At ovulation, the oocyte is in its **2nd meiotic** division and is surrounded by the zona pellucida and some granulosa cells (Fig. 2.4).

Through sweeping action of tubal fimbriae, the oocyte is carried into the uterine tube.

Before spermatozoa can fertilize the oocyte, they must undergo *(a)* a **capacitation process,** during which a glycoprotein coat and seminal plasma proteins are removed from the spermatozoon head, and *(b)* the **acrosome reaction,** during which hyaluronidase and trypsin-like substances are released to penetrate oocyte barriers. During fertilization, the spermatozoon must penetrate *(a)* the **corona radiata,** *(b)* the **zona pellucida,** and *(c)* the **oocyte cell membrane** (Fig. 2.5). As soon as the spermatocyte has entered the oocyte, *(a)* the oocyte finishes its 2nd meiotic division and forms the **female pronucleus;** *(b)* the zona pellucida becomes impenetrable to other spermatozoa; and *(c)* the head of the sperm separates from the tail, swells, and forms the **male pronucleus** (Figs. 2.6 and 2.7). After both pronuclei have replicated their DNA, paternal and maternal chromosomes intermingle, split longitudinally, and go through a mitotic division, thus giving rise to the two-cell stage. The **results of fertilization** are *(a)* **restoration of the diploid number of chromosomes,** *(b)* **determination of chromosomal sex,** and *(c)* **initiation of cleavage.**

Cleavage is a series of mitotic divisions, resulting in an increase in cells, **blastomeres,** which become smaller with each division. After three divisions, blastomeres undergo **compaction** to become a tightly grouped ball of cells with inner and outer layers. Compacted blastomeres divide to form a 16-cell **morula.** As the morula enters the uterine cavity on the 3rd or 4th day after fertilization, a cavity begins to appear, and the **blastocyst** is created. The **inner cell mass,** which formed at the time of compaction, will develop into the embryo proper and is located at one pole of the blastocyst. The **outer cell mass** surrounds the inner cells and the blastocyst cavity and will form the trophoblast.

PROBLEMS TO SOLVE

1. What are the primary causes of infertility in males and females?

2. A woman has had several bouts with pelvic inflammatory disease in the past and now wants to have children. However, she has been having difficulty becoming pregnant. What might be the problem, and what would you suggest?

SUGGESTED READINGS

Archer DF, Zeleznik AJ, Rockette HE: Ovarian follicular maturation in women. II. Reversal of estrogen inhibited ovarian folliculogenesis by human gonadotropin. *Fertil Steril* 50:555, 1988.
Blandau RJ: Growth of the ovarian follicle and ovulation. *Prog Gynecol* 5:58, 1970.
Boldt J, Howe AM, Parkerson JB, Gunter LE, Kuehn E: Carbohydrate involvement in sperm-egg fusion in mice. *Biol Reprod* 40:887, 1989.
Carr DH: Chromosome studies on selected spontaneous abortions: polyploidy in man. *J Med Genet* 8:164, 1971.
Chen CM, Sathananthan AH: Early penetration of human sperm through the vestments of human egg *in vitro. Arch Androl* 16:183, 1986.
Cowchock S: Autoantibodies and fetal wastage. *Am J Reprod Immunol* 26:38, 1991.

Edwards RG: A decade of *in vitro* fertilization. *Res Reprod* 22:1, 1990.

Edwards RG, Bavister BD, Steptoe PC: Early stages of fertilization *in vitro* of human oocytes matured *in vitro. Nature (Lond)* 221:632, 1969.

Egarter C: The complex nature of egg transport through the oviduct. *Am J Obstet Gynecol* 163:687, 1990.

Enders AC, Hendrickx AG, Schlake S: Implantation in the rhesus monkey: initial penetration of the endometrium. *Am J Anat* 167:275, 1983.

Garner DL, Easton MP: Immunofluorescent localization of acrosin in mammalian spermatozoa. *J Exp Zool* 200:157, 1977.

Gilbert SF: *Developmental Biology.* Sunderland, MA, Sinauer Associates, 1991.

Grobstein D, Fowler M, Mendeloff J: External human fertilization: an evaluation of policy. *Science* 222:127, 1983.

Handyside AH, Kontogianni EH, Hardy K, Winston RML: Pregnancies from biopsied human preimplantation embryos sexed by Y-specific DNA amplification. *Nature* 344:768, 1990.

Hertig AT, Adams EC, Mulligan WJ: On the pre-implantation stages of the human ovum: a description of four normal and four abnormal specimens ranging from the second to the fifth day of development. *Contrib Embryol* 35:199, 1954.

Hertig AT, Rock J, Adams EC: A description of 34 human ova within the first 17 days of development. *Am J Anat* 98:435, 1956.

Oura C, Toshimori K: Ultrasound studies on the fertilization of mammalian gametes. *Rev Cytol* 122:105, 1990.

Pedersen RA, We K, Balakier H: Origin of the inner cell mass in mouse embryos: cell lineage analysis by microinjection. *Dev Biol* 117:581, 1986.

Propping D, Tauber PF, Zaneveld LJD: Fertilization and implantation. *In* Ludwig H, Tauber PF (eds): *Human Fertilization.* Stuttgart, Georg Thieme, 1978.

Reed M: Hypothalamic releasing factors. *In* Philipp EE, Barnes J, Newton M (eds): *Scientific Foundations of Obstetrics and Gynecology.* London, William Heinemann, 1970.

Settlage DSF, Motoshima M, Tredway DR: Sperm transport from the external cervical os to the fallopian tubes in women. *Fertil Steril* 24:655, 1973.

Talbot P: Sperm penetration through oocyte investments in mammals. *Am J Anat* 174:331, 1985.

Tarkowski AK, Wrobelwska J: Development of blastomeres of mouse eggs isolated at the 4- and 8-cell stage. *J Embryol Exp Morphol* 18:155, 1967.

Warkany J: Prevention of congenital malformation. *Teratology* 23:175, 1981.

Wasserman PM: Fertilization in mammals. *Sci Am* 259:78, 1988.

Wolf DP, Quigley MM (eds): *Human in Vitro Fertilization and Transfer.* New York, Plenum Press, 1984.

Yen SC, Jaffe RB (eds): *Reproductive Endocrinology: Physiology, Pathophysiology, and Clinical Management.* 2nd ed. Philadelphia, WB Saunders, 1986.

chapter 3

Bilaminar Germ Disc
(Second Week of Development)

In the following paragraphs, a day-by-day account is given of the major events occurring in the 2nd week of development. It must be realized, however, that embryos of the same fertilization age do not necessarily develop at the same rate. Indeed, considerable differences in rate of growth have been found even at these early stages of development.

Eighth Day of Development

At the 8th day of development, the blastocyst is partially embedded in the endometrial stroma. In the area over the embryoblast, trophoblast has differentiated into two layers: *(a)* an inner layer of mononucleated cells, the **cytotrophoblast,** and *(b)* an outer, multinucleated zone without distinct cell boundaries, the **syncytiotrophoblast** (Figs. 3.1 and 3.2). Mitotic figures are found in the cytotrophoblast but never in the syncytiotrophoblast. Thus, cells in the cytotrophoblast divide and then migrate into the syncytiotrophoblast, where they fuse and lose their individual cell membranes.

Cells of the inner cell mass or embryoblast also differentiate into two layers: *(a)* a layer of small, cuboidal cells adjacent to the blastocyst cavity, known as the **hypoblast layer;** and *(b)* a layer of high columnar cells adjacent to the amniotic cavity, the **epiblast layer** (Figs. 3.1 and 3.2). Cells of each germ layer form a flat disc and together are known as the **bilaminar germ disc.**

At the same time, a small cavity appears within the epiblast. This cavity enlarges to become the **amniotic cavity.** Those epiblast cells adjacent to the cytotrophoblast are called **amnioblasts** and, together with the rest of the epiblast, line the amniotic cavity (Figs. 3.1 and 3.3).

The endometrial stroma adjacent to the implantation site is edematous and highly vascular. The large, tortuous glands secrete abundant glycogen and mucus.

Ninth Day of Development

The blastocyst is more deeply embedded in the endometrium, and the penetration defect in the surface epithelium is closed by a fibrin coagulum (Fig. 3.3).The trophoblast shows considerable progress in development, particularly at the embryonic pole, where vacuoles appear in the syncytium. When these vacuoles fuse, they form large lacunae, and this phase of trophoblast development is therefore known as the **lacunar stage** (Fig. 3.3).

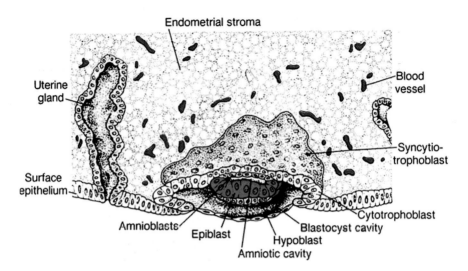

Figure 3.1. Drawing representing a 7½-day human blastocyst, partially embedded in the endometrial stroma. The trophoblast consists of an inner layer with mononuclear cells, the cytotrophoblast, and an outer layer without distinct cell boundaries, the syncytiotrophoblast. The embryoblast is formed by the epiblast and hypoblast germ layers. The amniotic cavity appears as a small cleft.

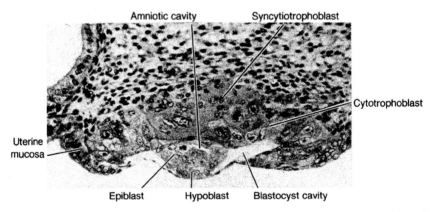

Figure 3.2. Section of a 7½-day human blastocyst (×100). Note the multinucleated appearance of the syncytiotrophoblast, large cells of the cytotrophoblast, and slit-like amniotic cavity.

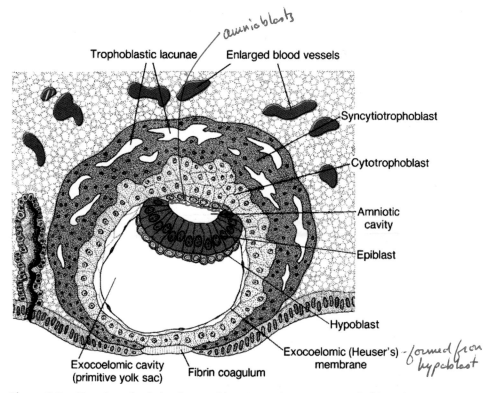

Trophoblastic lacunae   *amnioblasts*   Enlarged blood vessels

Syncytiotrophoblast

Cytotrophoblast

Amniotic cavity

Epiblast

Hypoblast

Exocoelomic (Heuser's) membrane — *formed from hypoblast*

Exocoelomic cavity (primitive yolk sac)   Fibrin coagulum

Figure 3.3. Drawing of a 9-day human blastocyst. The syncytiotrophoblast shows a large number of lacunae. Note the flat cells that form the exocoelomic membrane. The bilaminar germ disc consists of a layer of columnar epiblast cells and a layer of cuboidal hypoblast cells. The original surface defect is closed by a fibrin coagulum.

At the abembryonic pole, meanwhile, flattened cells, probably originating from the hypoblast, form a thin membrane, known as the exocoelomic (Heuser's) membrane, that lines the inner surface of the cytotrophoblast (Fig. 3.3). This membrane, together with the hypoblast, forms the lining of the **exocoelomic cavity (primitive yolk sac).**

Eleventh to Twelfth Day of Development

By the 11th to 12th day of development, the blastocyst is completely embedded in the endometrial stroma, and the surface epithelium almost entirely covers the original defect in the uterine wall (Figs. 3.4 and 3.5). The blastocyst now produces a slight protrusion into the lumen of the uterus.

The trophoblast is characterized by lacunar spaces in the syncytium that form an intercommunicating network. This is particularly evident at the embryonic pole; at the abembryonic pole, however, the trophoblast still consists mainly of cytotrophoblastic cells (Figs. 3.4 and 3.5).

Concurrently, cells of the syncytiotrophoblast penetrate deeper into the stroma and erode the endothelial lining of the maternal capillaries. These capillaries are congested and dilated and are known as **sinusoids.** The syncytial lacunae then

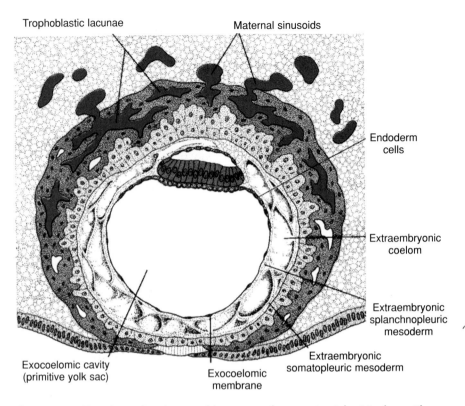

Trophoblastic lacunae

Maternal sinusoids

Endoderm cells

Extraembryonic coelom

Extraembryonic splanchnopleuric mesoderm

Extraembryonic somatopleuric mesoderm

Exocoelomic cavity (primitive yolk sac)

Exocoelomic membrane

Figure 3.4. Drawing of a human blastocyst of approximately 12 days. The trophoblastic lacunae at the embryonic pole are in open connection with maternal sinusoids in the endometrial stroma. Extraembryonic mesoderm proliferates and fills the space between the exocoelomic membrane and the inner aspect of the trophoblast.

become continuous with the sinusoids, and maternal blood enters the lacunar system (Fig. 3.4). As the trophoblast continues to erode more and more sinusoids, maternal blood begins to flow through the trophoblastic system, thus establishing the **uteroplacental circulation.**

In the meantime, a new population of cells appears between the inner surface of the cytotrophoblast and the outer surface of the exocoelomic cavity. These cells are derived from yolk sac cells and form a fine, loose connective tissue, the **extraembryonic mesoderm,** which eventually fills all of the space between the trophoblast externally and the amnion and exocoelomic membrane internally (Figs. 3.4 and 3.5). Soon, large cavities develop in the extraembryonic mesoderm, and when these become confluent, a new space known as the **extraembryonic coelom (chorionic cavity)** is formed (Fig. 3.4). This space surrounds the primitive yolk sac and amniotic cavity except where the germ disc is connected to the trophoblast by the connecting stalk (Fig. 3.6). The extraembryonic mesoderm lining the cytotrophoblast and amnion is called the **extraembryonic**

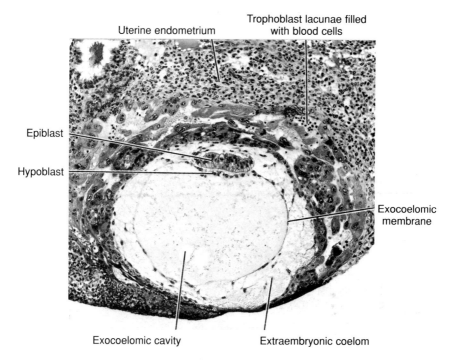

Uterine endometrium

Trophoblast lacunae filled with blood cells

Epiblast

Hypoblast

Exocoelomic membrane

Exocoelomic cavity

Extraembryonic coelom

Figure 3.5. Section of a fully implanted 12-day human blastocyst (×100). Note maternal blood cells in the lacunae, the exocoelomic membrane lining the primitive yolk sac, and the hypoblast and epiblast.

somatopleuric mesoderm; that covering the yolk sac is known as the **extraembryonic splanchnopleuric mesoderm** (Fig. 3.4).

Growth of the bilaminar germ disc is relatively slow, compared with that of the trophoblast; consequently, the disc remains very small (0.1–0.2 mm). Cells of the endometrium, meanwhile, become polyhedral and loaded with glycogen and lipids; intercellular spaces are filled with extravasate, and the tissue is edematous. These changes, known as the **decidua reaction,** at first are confined to the area immediately surrounding the implantation site but soon occur throughout the endometrium.

Thirteenth Day of Development

By the 13th day of development, the surface defect in the endometrium has usually healed. Occasionally, however, bleeding may occur at the implantation site as a result of increased blood flow into the lacunar spaces. Since this bleeding occurs near the 28th day of the menstrual cycle, it may be confused with normal menstrual bleeding and so cause inaccuracy in determining the expected delivery date.

The trophoblast is characterized by the appearance of villous structures. Cells of the cytotrophoblast proliferate locally and penetrate into the syncytiotrophoblast, thus forming cellular columns surrounded by syncytium. Cellular columns with the syncytial covering become known as **primary villi** (Figs. 3.6 and 3.7 and Chapter 4).

In the meantime, the hypoblast produces additional cells that migrate along the inside of the exocoelomic membrane (Fig. 3.4). These cells proliferate and gradually form a new cavity within the exocoelomic cavity. This new cavity is known as the **secondary** or **definitive yolk sac** (Figs. 3.6 and 3.7). This yolk sac is much smaller than the original exocoelomic cavity or primitive yolk sac. During its formation, large portions of the exocoelomic cavity are pinched off. These portions are represented by **exocoelomic cysts,** which are often found in the extraembryonic coelom or **chorionic cavity** (Figs. 3.6 and 3.7).

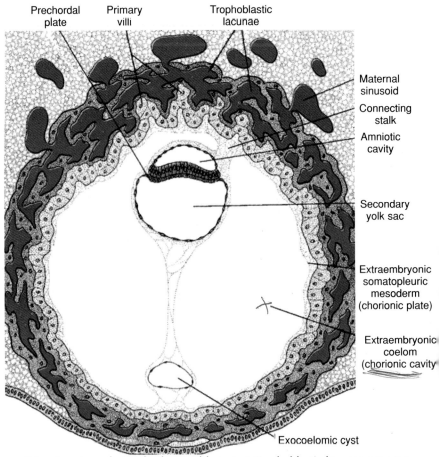

Figure 3.6. Drawing of a 13-day human blastocyst. Trophoblastic lacunae are now present at the embryonic as well as the abembryonic pole, and the uteroplacental circulation has begun. Note the primary villi and the extraembryonic coelom or **chorionic cavity.** The secondary yolk sac is entirely lined with endoderm.

Meanwhile, the extraembryonic coelom expands and forms a large cavity known as the **chorionic cavity.** The extraembryonic mesoderm lining the inside of the cytotrophoblast is then known as the **chorionic plate.** The only place where extraembryonic mesoderm traverses the chorionic cavity is in the **connecting stalk** (Fig. 3.6). With development of blood vessels, the stalk will become the **umbilical cord.**

By the end of the 2nd week, the germ disc is represented by two apposed cell discs: the epiblast, which forms the floor of the continuously expanding amniotic cavity, and the hypoblast, which forms the roof of the secondary yolk sac. In its cephalic region the hypoblastic disc shows a slight thickening known as the **prechordal plate.** This is an area of columnar cells that are firmly attached to the overlying epiblastic disc (Fig. 3.6).

CLINICAL CORRELATES

The syncytiotrophoblast is responsible for hormone production (see Chapter 7), including **human chorionic gonadotropin** (hCG). By the end of the 2nd week, sufficient quantities of this hormone are produced to be detected by radioimmunoassays, which serve as the basis for pregnancy testing.

Because 50% of the implanting embryo's genome is paternally derived, it represents a foreign body that, potentially, should be

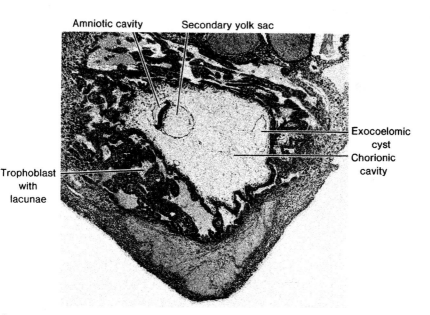

Amniotic cavity   Secondary yolk sac

Exocoelomic cyst

Chorionic cavity

Trophoblast with lacunae

Figure 3.7. Section through the implantation site of a 13-day embryo. Note the amniotic cavity, yolk sac, and exocoelomic cyst in the chorionic cavity. Most of the lacunae are filled with blood.

rejected by the maternal system. Several theories exist as to why the conceptus is not rejected, including a resistance of the syncytiotrophoblast to killer cells and absence of transplantation antigens on the syncytiotrophoblast surface. In cases of autoimmune disease in the mother, as for example systemic lupus erythematosus (SLE), rejection of the embryo occurs due to antibodies generated by the disease that secondarily attack the conceptus.

Abnormal implantation sites sometimes occur even within the uterus. Normally, the human blastocyst implants along the posterior or anterior wall of the body of the uterus. Occasionally, the blastocyst implants close to the internal opening os (opening) (Fig. 3.8) of the cervix such that at later stages of development the placenta over-bridges the opening (**placenta previa**) and causes severe, potentially life-threatening bleeding in the second part of pregnancy and during delivery.

Not infrequently, implantation sites are found outside the uterus, resulting in **extrauterine** or **ectopic pregnancy.** Ectopic pregnancies may occur at any place in the abdominal cavity, ovary, or uterine

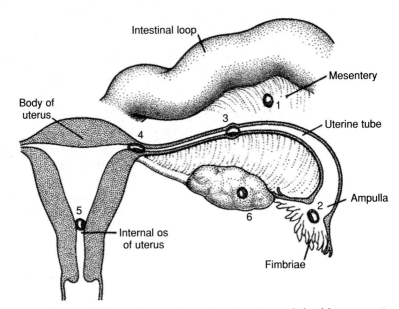

Figure 3.8. Drawing to show abnormal implantation sites of the blastocyst. *1,* Implantation site in the abdominal cavity. The ovum most frequently implants in the rectouterine cavity (Douglas' pouch) but may implant at any place covered by peritoneum. *2,* Implantation in the ampullary region of the tube. *3,* Tubal implantation, i.e., in the narrow portion of the uterine tube. *4,* Interstitial implantation, i.e., in the narrow portion of the uterine tube. *5,* Implantation in the region of the internal os, frequently resulting in placenta previa. *6,* Ovarian implantation.

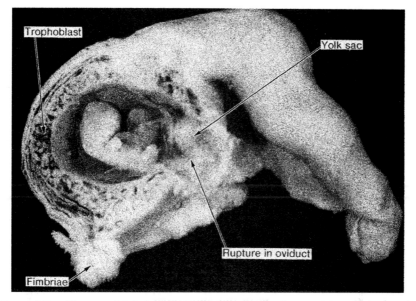

Figure 3.9. Photograph of a tubal pregnancy. Embryo is approximately 2 months old and is about to escape through a rupture in the tubal wall.

tube (Fig. 3.8). However, 95% of ectopic pregnancies occur in the uterine tube, and most of these are located in the ampulla (Fig. 3.9). In the abdominal cavity, the blastocyst most frequently attaches itself to the peritoneal lining of the **rectouterine cavity (Douglas' pouch)** (Fig. 3.10). The blastocyst may also attach itself to the peritoneal covering of the intestinal tract or to the omentum. Sometimes, the blastocyst develops in the ovary proper, causing a **primary ovarian pregnancy.** Most ectopic pregnancies result in death of the embryo around the 2nd month of gestation, resulting in severe hemorrhaging and abdominal pain in the mother.

Abnormal blastocysts occur with surprising frequency. For example, in a series of 26 implanted blastocysts varying in age from 7½–17 days, recovered from patients of normal fertility, 9 (34.6%) were abnormal. Some consisted of syncytium only, whereas others showed varying degrees of trophoblastic hypoplasia. In two, the embryoblast was absent, and in some, the germ disc showed an abnormal orientation.

It is likely that most abnormal blastocysts would not have produced any sign of pregnancy, since their trophoblast was of such inferior quality that the corpus luteum could not have persisted. These

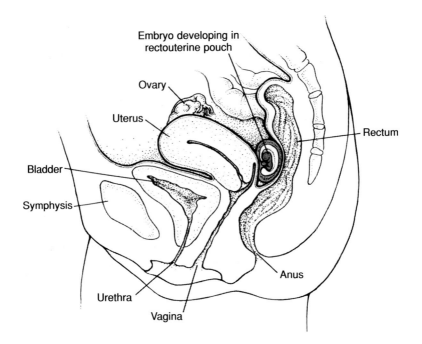

Figure 3.10. Drawing of midline section of bladder, uterus, and rectum to show an abdominal pregnancy in the rectouterine (Douglas') pouch.

embryos probably would have been aborted with the following menstrual flow, and therefore, pregnancy would not have been detected. In some cases, however, the trophoblast develops and forms placental membranes, but little or no embryonic tissue is present. Such a condition is known as a **hydatidiform mole.** Moles secrete high levels of hCG and may produce benign or malignant **(invasive mole, choriocarcinoma)** tumors.

Genetic analysis of hydatidiform moles indicates that, although male and female pronuclei may be genetically equivalent, they may be different functionally. This evidence is derived from the fact that while cells of moles are diploid, their entire genome is paternally derived. Thus, most moles arise from fertilization of an oocyte lacking a nucleus followed by duplication of the male chromosomes to restore the diploid number. These results also suggest that paternal genes regulate most of the development of the trophoblast, since in moles this tissue differentiates even in the absence of a female pronucleus.

Other examples of functional differences in maternal and paternal genes are provided by the observation that certain genetic diseases depend on whether the defective or missing gene is inherited from the father or the mother. For example, inheritance of a deletion on chromosome 11 from a father produces Prader-Willi syndrome, whereas inheritance of the same defect from the mother results in Angelman syndrome. This phenomenon, where there is differential modification and/or expression of homologous alleles or chromosome regions, depending on the parent from whom the genetic material is derived, is know as **genomic imprinting.** Imprinting involves autosomes and sex chromosomes (in all female mammals, one X chromosome is inactivated in somatic cells) and is modulated by DNA methylation. Certain diseases, such as Huntington's chorea, neurofibromatosis, familial cancer disorders (Wilms' tumors, familial retinoblastoma), and myotonic dystrophy, also involve imprinting. Fragile X syndrome, the leading cause of inherited mental retardation, may be another example of a condition based on imprinting (see Chapter 8).

Preimplantation and postimplantation reproductive failure occurs often. Even in selected fertile women under optimal conditions for pregnancy, 15% of oocytes fail to become fertilized, and 10–15% start cleavage but fail to implant. Of the 70–75% that implant, only 58% will survive until the 2nd week, and 16% of those will be abnormal. Hence, at the time when the first expected menstruation is missed, only 42% of the eggs exposed to sperm are surviving. Of this percentage, a number of cases will be aborted during subsequent weeks, and a number will be abnormal at the time of birth.

SUMMARY

At the beginning of the 2nd week, the blastocyst is partially embedded in the endometrial stroma. The **trophoblast** differentiates into *(a)* an inner, actively proliferating layer, the **cytotrophoblast,** and *(b)* an outer layer, the **syncytiotrophoblast,** which erodes maternal tissues (Fig. 3.1). By day 9, lacunae develop in the syncytiotrophoblast. Subsequently, maternal sinusoids are eroded by the syncytiotrophoblast, maternal blood enters the lacunar network, and by the end of the 2nd week, a primitive **uteroplacental circulation** begins (Fig. 3.6). The cytotrophoblast, meanwhile, forms cellular columns penetrating into and surrounded by the syncytium. These columns are **primary villi.** By the end of the 2nd week, the blastocyst is completely embedded, and the surface defect in the mucosa has healed (Fig. 3.6).

The **inner cell mass** or **embryoblast,** meanwhile, differentiates into *(a)* the **epiblast** and *(b)* the **hypoblast,** together forming the **bilaminar germ disc** (Fig. 3.1). Ectoderm cells are continuous with amnioblasts, and together they surround a new cavity, the **amniotic cavity.** Endoderm cells are continuous with the **exocoelomic membrane,** and together they surround the **primitive yolk sac** (Fig. 3.4). By the end of the 2nd week, extraembryonic mesoderm is formed, which fills the space between the trophoblast and the amnion and exocoelomic membrane, internally. When vacuoles develop in this tissue, the **extraembryonic coelom** or **chorionic cavity** is formed (Fig. 3.6). **Extraembryonic mesoderm** lining the cytotrophoblast and amnion is **extraembryonic somatopleuric mesoderm;** that surrounding the yolk sac is **extraembryonic splanchnopleuric mesoderm** (Fig. 3.6).

Implantation occurs at the end of the 1st week. Trophoblast cells then invade the epithelium and underlying endometrial stroma with the help of proteolytic enzymes. Implantation may also occur outside the uterus, such as in the rectouterine pouch, on the mesentery, in the uterine tube, or in the ovary **(ectopic pregnancies).**

PROBLEMS TO SOLVE

1. During implantation, the trophoblast is invading maternal tissues, and since it contains about 50% paternal genes, it represents a foreign body. Therefore, why is the conceptus not rejected by an immunologic response from the mother's system?

2. A woman who believes she is pregnant complains of edema and vaginal bleeding. Examination reveals high plasma hCG concentrations and the presence of placental tissue but no evidence of an embryo. How would you explain this condition?

3. A young woman who relates that she has missed two menstrual periods complains of intense abdominal pain. What might an initial diagnosis be, and how would you confirm it?

SUGGESTED READINGS

Aplin JD: Implantation, trophoblast differentiation and hemochorial placentation: mechanistic evidence *in vivo* and *in vitro. J Cell Sci* 99:681, 1991.

Cattanack BM, Beechey CV: Autosomal and X-chromosome imprinting. *Dev Suppl* 63, 1990.

Enders AC, Schlafke S, Hendrickx A: Differentiation of the embryonic disc, amnion, and yolk sac in the rhesus monkey. *Am J Anat* 177:161, 1986.

Hertig AT, Rock J: Two human ova of the previllous stage, having a developmental age of about seven and nine days respectively. *Contrib Embryol* 31:65, 1945.

Hertig AT, Rock J, Adams EC: A description of 34 human ova within the first 17 days of development. *Am J Anat* 98:435, 1956.

Holliday R: Genomic imprinting and allelic exclusion. *Dev Suppl* 125, 1990.

Luckett WP: Amniogenesis in the early human and rhesus monkey embryos. *Anat Rec* 175:375, 1975.

Luckett WP: Origin and differentiation of the yolk sac and extraembryonic mesoderm in presomite human and rhesus monkey embryos. *Am J Anat* 152:59, 1978.

Luckett WP: The origin of extraembryonic mesoderm in the early human and rhesus monkey embryos. *Anat Rec* 169:369, 1971.

Monk M, Grant M: Preferential X-chromosome inactivation, DNA methylation and imprinting. *Dev Suppl* 55, 1990.

O'Rahilly R: *Developmental Stages in Human Embryos. Part A. Embryos of the First Three Weeks (Stages One to Nine).* Washington, DC, Carnegie Institution of Washington, 1973.

Rubin GL: Ectopic pregnancy in the United States: 1970 through 1978. *JAMA* 249:1725, 1983.

Smith C, Moore HDM, Hearn JP: The ultrastructure of early implantation in the marmoset monkey *(Callitrix jacchus). Anat Embryol* 175:399, 1987.

chapter 4

Trilaminar Germ Disc
(Third Week of Development)

Gastrulation: Formation of Embryonic Mesoderm and Endoderm

The most characteristic event occurring during the 3rd week is **gastrulation,** the process that establishes all three **germ layers** in the embryo. Gastrulation begins with formation of the **primitive streak** on the surface of the epiblast (Figs. 4.1, 4.2*A*, and 4.5). Initially, the streak is vaguely defined (Fig. 4.1), but in a 15–16-day embryo it is clearly visible as a narrow groove with slightly bulging regions on either side (Fig. 4.2*A*). The cephalic end of the streak, known as the **primitive node,** consists of a slightly elevated area surrounding the small **primitive pit** (Fig. 4.2). In a transverse section through the region of the primitive groove, it is seen that the cells are flask-shaped and that a new cell layer develops between the epiblast and hypoblast (Fig. 4.2, *B* and *C*). Cells of the epiblast migrate in the direction of the primitive streak (Fig. 4.2) to form mesoderm and intraembryonic endoderm. On arrival in the region of the streak, they become flask-shaped, detach from the epiblast, and slip beneath it (Fig. 4.2*B*). This inward movement is known as **invagination.** Once the cells have invaginated, some displace the hypoblast, thereby creating the embryonic endoderm, while some come to lie between the epiblast and newly created endoderm to form mesoderm. Cells remaining in the epiblast then form ectoderm. Thus, the epiblast, through the process of gastrulation, is the source of all the germ layers in the embryo (i.e., **ectoderm, mesoderm,** and **endoderm**) (Figs. 4.2*B* and 4.4*B*).

As more and more cells move in between the epiblast and hypoblast layers, they begin to spread in lateral and cephalic directions (Fig. 4.2). Gradually, they migrate beyond the margin of the disc and establish contact with extraembryonic mesoderm covering the yolk sac and amnion. In the cephalic direction, they pass on each side of the prechordal plate to meet each other in front of this area, where they form the **cardiogenic** or **heart-forming plate** (Figs. 4.3*A* and 12.2).

Formation of the Notochord

Prenotochordal cells invaginating in the primitive pit move forward in a cephalic direction until they reach the **prechordal plate** (Fig. 4.3). These prenotochordal cells become intercalated in the hypoblast such that, for a short

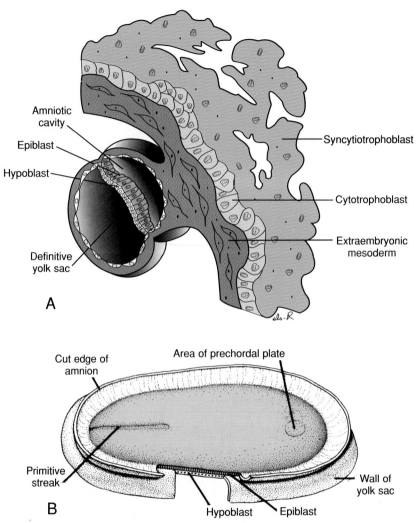

Figure 4.1. **A.** Schematic view of an implantation site at the end of the 2nd week. **B.** Representative view of the germ disc at the end of the 2nd week of development. The amniotic cavity has been opened to permit a view on the dorsal side of the epiblast. Note that the hypoblast and epiblast are in contact with each other and that the primitive streak forms a shallow groove in the caudal region of the embryo.

time, the midline of the embryo consists of two cell layers that form the **notochordal plate** (Fig. 4.3, *B* and *C*). As the hypoblast is replaced by endoderm cells moving in at the streak, **cells** of the notochordal plate proliferate and detach from the endoderm. They then form a solid cord of cells, the **definitive notochord** (Fig. 4.3, *D* and *E*), that underlies the neural tube and serves as the basis for the axial skeleton. Since elongation of the notochord is a dynamic process, the cranial end forms first, and caudal regions are added as the primitive

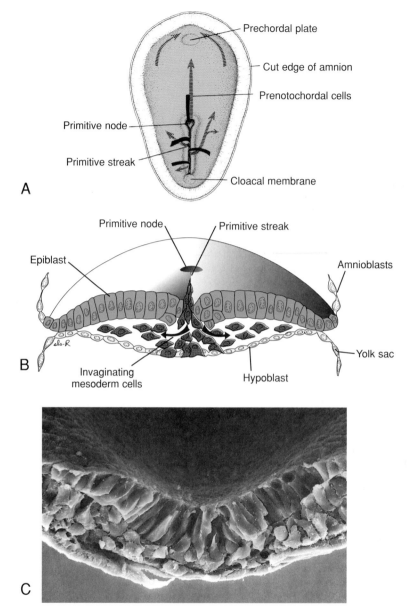

Figure 4.2. **A.** Schematic view of the dorsal side of the germ disc from a 16-day embryo, indicating the movement of surface epiblast cells *(solid black lines)* through the primitive streak and node and the subsequent migration of cells between the hypoblast and epiblast *(broken lines).* **B.** Cross section through the cranial region of the streak at 15 days, showing invagination of epiblast cells. The first cells to move inward displace the hypoblast to create the definitive endoderm. Once definitive endoderm is established, inwardly moving epiblast forms mesoderm. **C.** Scanning electron micrograph through the primitive streak of a mouse embryo, showing migration of epiblast cells.

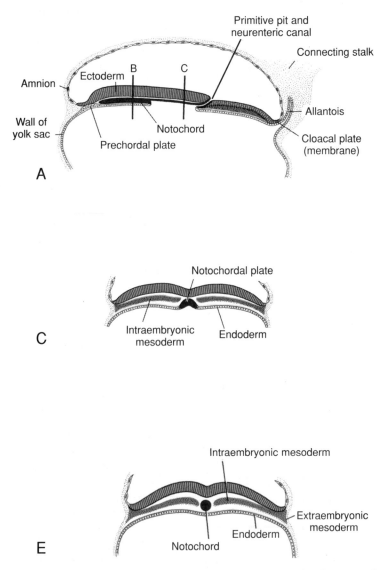

Figure 4.3. Schematic views and scanning electron micrographs illustrating formation of the notochord whereby prenotochordal cells migrate through the primitive streak, become intercalated in the endoderm to form the notochordal plate, and finally detach from the endoderm to form the definitive notochord. Since these events occur in a cranial to caudal sequence, portions of the definitive notochord are established in the head region first. **A.** Drawing of a sagittal section through a 17-day embryo. The most cranial portion of the definitive notochord has formed near the prechordal plate, while prenotochordal cells caudal to this region are intercalated into the endoderm as the notochordal plate. **B.** Scanning electron micrograph of a

---

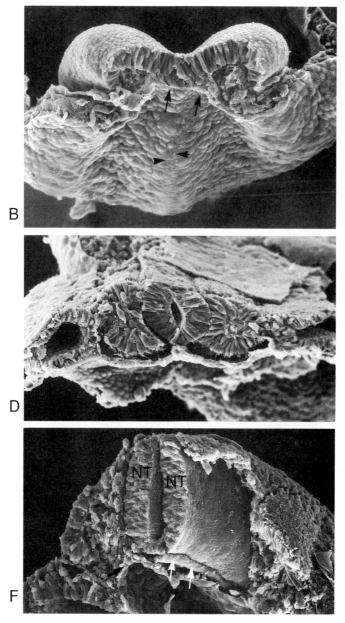

mouse embryo, showing the region of the prechordal plate *(arrows)*. Posterior to this region and extending caudally is the prenotochordal plate *(arrowheads)*. **C.** Schematic cross section through the region of the notochordal plate. Soon, the notochordal plate will detach from the endoderm to form the definitive notochord. **D.** Scanning electron micrograph of a mouse embryo, showing detachment of the notochordal plate from the endoderm. **E.** Schematic view showing the definitive notochord. **F.** Scanning electron micrograph of a mouse embryo, showing the definitive notochord *(arrows)* in close approximation to the neural tube *(NT)*.

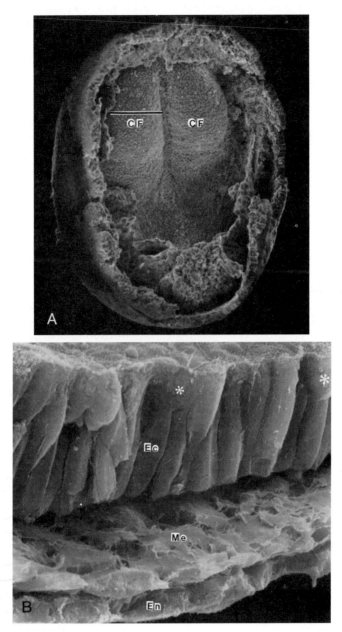

Figure 4.4. A. Scanning electron micrograph (dorsal view) of a mouse embryo (equivalent to approximately 18-day human), showing initial elevation of the cranial neural folds *(CF)*. The primitive streak lies farther caudally and is obscured from view. **B.** Transverse section through the embryo shown in **A** (see line of section). Note three germ layers: pseudostratified columnar cells of the neuroectoderm *(Ec)*, flattened endoderm *(En)*, and mesenchyme *(Me)* sandwiched between these two layers. *Asterisks,* mitotic cells.

streak assumes a more caudal position. The notochord and prenotochordal cells extend cranially to the prechordal plate (future buccopharyngeal membrane) and caudally to the primitive pit. At the point where the pit forms an indentation in the epiblast, a small canal, the **neurenteric canal,** temporarily connects the amniotic and yolk sac cavities (Fig. 4.3*A*).

The cloacal membrane is formed at the caudal end of the embryonic disc (Fig. 4.2*A*). This membrane is similar in structure to the prechordal plate and consists of tightly adherent ectoderm and endoderm cells with no intervening mesoderm. When the cloacal membrane appears, the posterior wall of the yolk sac forms a small diverticulum that extends into the connecting stalk. This diverticulum, the **allantoenteric diverticulum,** or **allantois,** appears at about the 16th day of development (Fig. 4.3*A*). Although in some lower vertebrates the allantois serves as a reservoir for excretion products of the renal system, in humans it remains rudimentary but may be involved in abnormalities of bladder development (see Chapter 15).

Growth of the Germ Disc

The embryonic disc, initially flat and almost round (Fig. 4.2*A*), gradually becomes elongated with a broad cephalic and a narrow caudal end (Figs. 4.4*A* and 4.5, *A* and *B*). Expansion of the embryonic disc occurs mainly in the cephalic region; the region of the primitive streak remains more or less the same size.

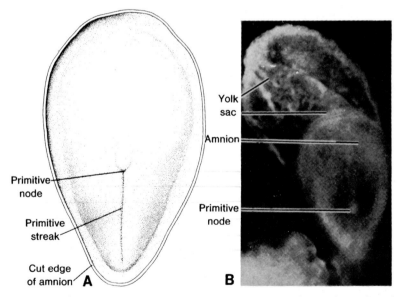

Figure 4.5. **A.** Drawing of the dorsal aspect of an 18-day embryo. The embryo has a pear-shaped appearance and shows the primitive streak and node at its caudal end. **B.** Photograph of an 18-day human embryo, dorsal view. Note the primitive node and, extending forward from it, the notochord. The yolk sac has a somewhat mottled appearance. The length of the embryo is 1.25 mm, and the greatest width is 0.68 mm.

Growth and elongation of the cephalic part of the disc are caused by a continuous migration of cells from the primitive streak region in a cephalic direction. Invagination of surface cells in the primitive streak and their subsequent migration in forward and lateral directions continues until the end of the 4th week. At that stage, the primitive streak shows regressive changes, rapidly diminishes in size, and soon disappears.

That the primitive streak at the caudal end of the disc continues to supply new cells until the end of the 4th week has an important bearing on development of the embryo. In the cephalic part, germ layers begin their specific differentiation by the middle of the 3rd week, whereas in the caudal part, differentiation begins by the end of the 4th week. Thus, gastrulation or formation of the germ layers continues in caudal segments while cranial structures are differentiating and the embryo develops cephalocaudally.

CLINICAL CORRELATES

The beginning of the 3rd week of development, when gastrulation is initiated, is a highly sensitive stage for teratogenic insult. At this time, fate maps can be made for various organ systems, such as the eyes and brain anlage, and these cell populations may be damaged by teratogens. For example, high doses of alcohol at this stage kill cells in the anterior midline of the germ disc, producing a deficiency of the midline in craniofacial structures and resulting in **holoprosencephaly.** In such a child the forebrain is small, the two lateral ventricles often merge into a single ventricle, and the eyes are close together (hypotelorism). Since this stage is reached 2 weeks after fertilization, it is approximately 4 weeks from the last menses. Therefore, the woman may not recognize she is pregnant, having assumed that menstruation is late and will begin shortly. Consequently, she may not take precautions she would normally consider if she knew she was pregnant.

Gastrulation itself may be disrupted by genetic and teratogenic causes. **Caudal dysgenesis (sirenomelia)** is a syndrome in which there is insufficient mesoderm formed in the caudalmost region of the embryo. Since this mesoderm contributes to formation of the lower limbs, urogenital system (intermediate mesoderm), and lumbosacral vertebrae, abnormalities in these structures arise. Affected individuals exhibit a variable spectrum of defects including hypoplasia and fusion of the lower limbs, vertebral abnormalities, renal agenesis, imperforate anus, and anomalies of the genital organs (Fig. 4.6). In humans, the condition is associated with maternal diabetes and other causes. In mice, abnormalities of T, Wnt, and engrailed genes produce a similar phenotype.

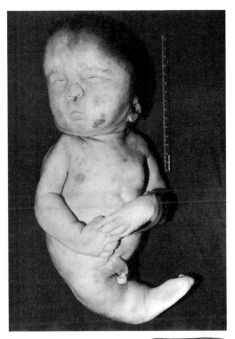

Figure 4.6. Sirenomelia (caudal dysgenesis). Loss of mesoderm in the lumbosacral region has resulted in fusion of the limb buds and other defects.

Sometimes, remnants of the primitive streak persist in the sacrococcygeal region. These clusters of pluripotent cells proliferate and form tumors, known as **sacrococcygeal teratomas,** that often contain tissues derived from all three germ layers (Fig. 4.7). This tumor is the most common tumor in newborns, occurring with a frequency of 1 in 37,000.

Further Development of the Trophoblast

By the beginning of the 3rd week, the trophoblast is characterized by **primary villi** that consist of a cytotrophoblastic core covered by a syncytial layer (Figs. 3.6 and 4.8A). During further development, mesodermal cells penetrate the core of primary villi and grow in the direction of the decidua. The newly formed structure is known as a **secondary villus** (Fig. 4.8B).

By the end of the 3rd week, mesodermal cells in the core of the villus begin to differentiate into blood cells and small blood vessels, thus forming the villous capillary system (Fig. 4.8C). The villus is now known as a **tertiary villus** or **definitive placental villus.** Capillaries in tertiary villi make contact with capillaries developing in mesoderm of the chorionic plate and in the connecting

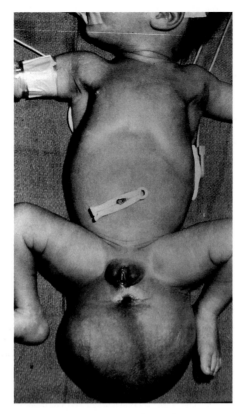

Figure 4.7. Sacrococcygeal teratoma resulting from remnants of the primitive streak. These tumors may become malignant and are more common in females.

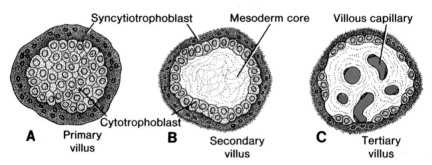

Figure 4.8. Schematic drawings to show development of a villus. **A.** Transverse section of a primary villus, showing a core of cytotrophoblastic cells covered by a layer of syncytium. **B.** Transverse section of a secondary villus with a core of mesoderm covered by a single layer of cytotrophoblastic cells, which, in turn, is covered by syncytium. **C.** Mesoderm of the villus shows a number of capillaries and venules.

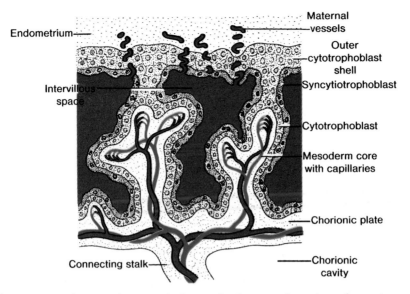

Endometrium

Intervillous space

Maternal vessels

Outer cytotrophoblast shell

Syncytiotrophoblast

Cytotrophoblast

Mesoderm core with capillaries

Chorionic plate

Connecting stalk

Chorionic cavity

Figure 4.9. Schematic drawing of a longitudinal section through a villus at the end of the 3rd week of development. Note that maternal vessels penetrate the cytotrophoblastic shell to enter intervillous spaces, which surround the villi. The capillaries in the villi are in contact with vessels in the chorionic plate and in the connecting stalk, which, in turn, are connected to intraembryonic vessels.

stalk (Figs. 4.9 and 4.10). These vessels, in turn, establish contact with the intraembryonic circulatory system, thereby connecting the placenta and the embryo. Hence, when the heart begins to beat in the 4th week of development, the villous system is ready to supply the embryo proper with essential nutrients and oxygen.

Meanwhile, cytotrophoblastic cells in the villi penetrate progressively into the overlying syncytium until they reach the maternal endometrium. Here they establish contact with similar extensions of neighboring villous stems, thus forming a thin **outer cytotrophoblast shell** (Figs. 4.9 and 4.10). This shell gradually surrounds the trophoblast entirely and attaches the chorionic sac firmly to the maternal endometrial tissue (Fig. 4.10). Villi that extend from the **chorionic plate** to the **decidua basalis (decidual plate)** are called **stem** or **anchoring villi.** Those that branch from the sides of stem villi represent **free (terminal) villi,** through which exchange of nutrients, etc. will occur (Fig. 4.11).

The chorionic cavity, meanwhile, becomes larger, and by the 19th or 20th day the embryo is attached to its trophoblastic shell by only a narrow **connecting stalk** (Fig. 4.10). The connecting stalk later develops into the **umbilical cord,** which forms the connection between placenta and embryo.

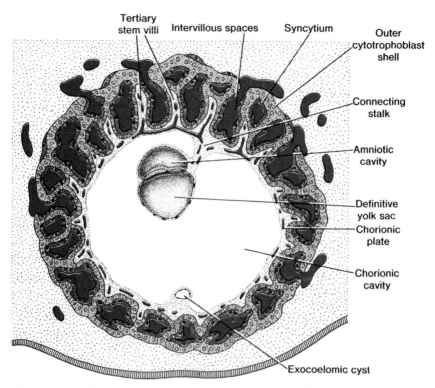

Figure 4.10. Diagram showing a presomite embryo and the trophoblast at the end of the 3rd week. Tertiary and secondary stem villi give the trophoblast a characteristic radial appearance. Intervillous spaces are found throughout the trophoblast and are lined with syncytium. Cytotrophoblastic cells surround the trophoblast entirely and are in direct contact with the endometrium. The embryo is suspended in the chorionic cavity by means of the connecting stalk.

SUMMARY

The most characteristic event occurring during the 3rd week is **gastrulation,** which begins with the appearance of the **primitive streak** having, at its cephalic end, the **primitive node.** In the region of the node and streak, **epiblast** cells move inward **(invaginate)** to form new cell layers: **endoderm** and **mesoderm.** Hence, epiblast gives rise to all three **germ layers** in the embryo. Cells of the **intraembryonic mesodermal germ layer** (Fig. 4.4B) migrate between the two other germ layers until they establish contact with the extraembryonic mesoderm covering the yolk sac and amnion (Figs. 4.2 and 4.3).

Prenotochordal cells invaginating in the primitive pit move forward until they reach the prechordal plate. They intercalate in the endoderm as the **notochordal plate** (Fig. 4.3). With further development, the plate detaches from the endoderm, and a solid cord, the **notochord,** is formed. It forms a midline axis, which will serve as the basis of the axial skeleton (Fig. 4.3).

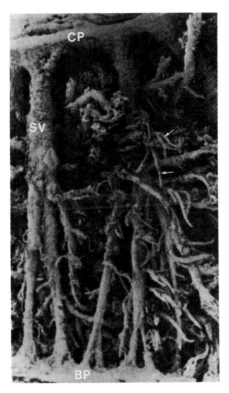

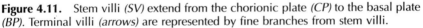

Figure 4.11. Stem villi *(SV)* extend from the chorionic plate *(CP)* to the basal plate *(BP)*. Terminal villi *(arrows)* are represented by fine branches from stem villi.

Hence, by the end of the 3rd week, three basic **germ layers**—consisting of **ectoderm, mesoderm,** and **endoderm**—are established, and tissue and organ differentiation has begun.

In the meantime, the trophoblast has progressed rapidly. **Primary villi** have obtained a mesenchymal core in which small capillaries arise (Fig. 4.10). When these villous capillaries make contact with capillaries in the chorionic plate and connecting stalk, the villous system is ready to supply the embryo with its nutrients and oxygen (Fig. 4.10).

PROBLEMS TO SOLVE

1. A 22-year-old woman consumes large quantities of alcohol at a party and loses consciousness. Three weeks later, she misses her second consecutive period, and a pregnancy test is positive. Should she be concerned about the effects her binge drinking episode might have had on her baby?

2. An ultrasound scan detects a large mass near the sacrum of a 28-week female fetus. What might the origin of such a mass be, and what type of tissue might it contain?

3. On ultrasound examination, it was determined that a fetus had well-developed facial and thoracic regions but caudal structures were abnormal. Kidneys were absent, lumbar and sacral vertebrae were missing, and the hindlimbs were fused. What process may have been disturbed to cause such defects?

SUGGESTED READINGS

Augustine K, Liu ET, Sadler TW: Antisense attenuation of Wnt-1 and Wnt-3a expression in whole embryo culture reveals roles for these genes in craniofacial, spinal cord, and cardiac morphogenesis. *Dev Genet* 14:500, 1993.

Bedding RSP: The origin of the foetal tissues during gastrulation in the rodent. *In* Johnson MH (ed): *Development in Mammals.* New York, Elsevier, 1983;99:1–32.

Bellairs R: The primitive streak. *Anat Embryol* 174:1, 1986.

Herrmann BG: Expression pattern of the brachyuria gene in whole mount TWis/TWis mutant embryos. *Development* 13:913, 1991.

Holzgreve W, Flake AW, Langer JC: The fetus with sacrococcygeal teratoma. *In* Harrison MR, Gollus MS, Filly RA (eds): *The Unborn Patient. Prenatal Diagnosis and Treatment.* Philadelphia, WB Saunders, 1991.

King BF, Mais JJ: Developmental changes in rhesus monkey placental villi and cell columns. *Anat Embryol* 165:361, 1982.

O'Rahilly R: *Developmental Stages in Human Embryos. Part A. Embryos of the First Three Weeks (Stages One to Nine).* Washington, DC, Carnegie Institution of Washington, 1973.

Sulik KK, Lauder JM, Dehart DB: Brain malformations in prenatal mice following acute maternal ethanol administration. *Int J Dev Neurosci* 2:203, 1984.

Tam PPL, Bedding RSP: The formation of mesodermal tissues in the mouse embryo during gastrulation and early organogenesis. *Development* 99:109, 1987.

chapter 5

Embryonic Period 3rd wk
(Third to Eighth Weeks)

During the 3rd to 8th weeks of development, a period known as the **embryonic period** or period of **organogenesis,** each of the three germ layers gives rise to a number of specific tissues and organs. By the end of the embryonic period, the main organ systems have been established. As a result of organ formation, the shape of the embryo changes greatly, and the major features of the external body form are recognizable by the end of the 2nd month.

Derivatives of the Ectodermal Germ Layer

At the beginning of the 3rd week of development, the ectodermal germ layer has the shape of a flat disc that is broader in the cephalic than the caudal region (Fig. 5.1, *A–C*). With appearance of the notochord and under its inductive influence, ectoderm overlying the notochord thickens to form the **neural plate** (Fig. 5.2). Cells of the plate make up the **neuroectoderm,** and their induction represents the initial event in the process of **neurulation.**

The **induction** process is complex, involving stimulation of a responding tissue or group of cells by an inducing tissue, in this case the epiblast by the notochord. It is a process that occurs repeatedly during organogenesis, as, for example, induction of the metanephric tissue by the ureteric bud to form the kidney (see Chapter 15). Signals for these processes and genes that regulate these events are now being identified. Signaling molecules appear to involve members of the **transforming growth factor** β (TGF-β) family, including **activin,** and **fibroblast growth factors** (FGF). However, other signaling molecules are rapidly being identified and may act as **morphogens,** i.e., molecules that are present in concentration gradients to which cells respond in a dose-dependent manner. Examples of molecules with morphogen-like activity are **retinoic acid, neurotransmitters,** and products of the **Wnt genes.** Morphogens trigger a cascade of events in responding cells, and in many cases, the initial process is activation of **homeobox genes.** These genes code for transcription factors that then regulate expression of other genes.

Once induction has occurred, the elongated, slipper-shaped neural plate gradually expands toward the primitive streak (Fig. 5.2, *B* and *C*). By the end of the 3rd week, the lateral edges of the neural plate become more elevated to form **neural folds,** while the depressed midregion forms a groove, the **neural groove** (Figs. 5.2 and 5.3, *A* and *B*). Gradually, the neural folds approach each other in

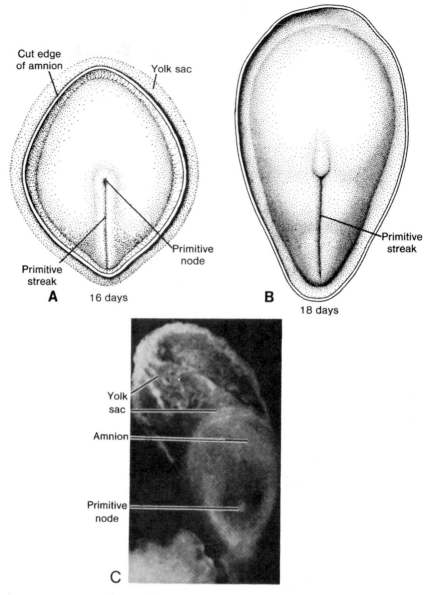

Figure 5.1. **A.** Dorsal view of a 16-day presomite embryo. The primitive streak and node are visible. **B.** Dorsal view of an 18-day presomite embryo. The embryo is pear-shaped with its cephalic region somewhat broader than its caudal end. **C.** Photograph of an 18-day human embryo, dorsal view. Note the primitive node and, extending forward from it, the notochord. The yolk sac has a somewhat mottled appearance. The length of the embryo is 1.25 mm, and the greatest width is 0.68 mm.

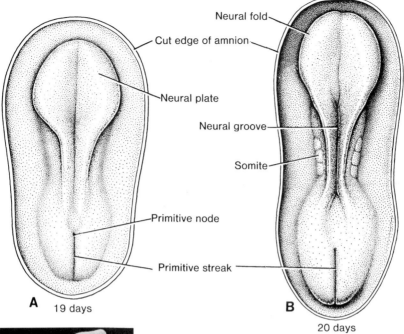

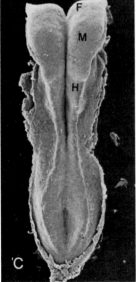

Figure 5.2. **A.** Dorsal view of a late presomite embryo (approximately 19 days). The amnion has been removed. The neural plate is clearly visible. **B.** Dorsal view of a human embryo at approximately 20 days. Note the appearance of somites and formation of the neural groove and neural folds. **C.** Scanning electron micrograph of a mouse embryo (approximately 20-day human) showing the typical appearance of the neural groove stage. Cranial neural folds have segregated themselves into forebrain (*F*, prosencephalon), midbrain (*M*, mesencephalon), and hindbrain (*H*, rhombencephalon) regions.

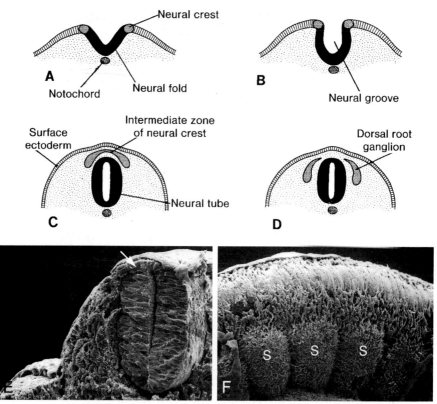

Figure 5.3. Drawings and scanning electron micrographs showing formation and migration of neural crest cells in the spinal cord. **A** and **B.** Crest cells form at the tips of neural folds and do not migrate away from this region until neural tube closure is complete (**C** and **D**). **E.** In scanning electron micrographs of mouse embryos, crest cells at the top of the closed neural tube can be seen migrating away from this area *(arrow).* **F.** In a lateral view with the overlying ectoderm removed, crest cells appear fibroblastic as they move down the sides of the neural tube toward the somites *(S).* Crest cells from the trunk form dorsal root ganglia, ganglia of the sympathetic and parasympathetic systems, melanocytes, and other structures.

the midline, where they fuse (Fig. 5.3*C*). This fusion begins in the region of the future neck (4th somite) and proceeds in cephalic and caudal directions (Figs. 5.5 and 5.6). As a result, the **neural tube** is formed. Until fusion is complete, the cephalic and caudal ends of the neural tube communicate with the amniotic cavity by way of the **cranial** and **caudal neuropores,** respectively (Figs. 5.5, 5.6*A*, and 5.7). Closure of the cranial neuropore occurs approximately at day 25 (18–20-somite stage), whereas the posterior neuropore closes at day 27 (25-somite stage). Neurulation is then complete, and the central nervous system is represented by a closed, tubular structure with a narrow caudal portion, the **spinal cord,** and a much broader cephalic portion characterized by a number of dilations, the **brain vesicles** (see Chapter 20).

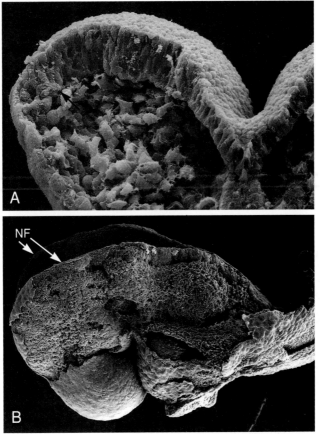

Figure 5.4. **A.** Cross section through the cranial neural folds of a mouse embryo. Neural crest cells at the tip of the folds *(arrow)* migrate and contribute to craniofacial mesenchyme. **B.** Lateral view of the cranial neural folds of a mouse embryo with the surface ectoderm removed. Numerous neural crest cells can be observed leaving the neural folds *(NF)* and migrating beneath the ectoderm that has been removed. Crest cells contribute to many craniofacial structures, including cranial nerve ganglia (V, VII, IX, and X), bones and connective tissue of the face and skull, and the aorticopulmonary septum in the great vessels. Unlike crest cells of the spinal cord, cranial crest exits the neural folds before they fuse.

As the neural folds elevate and fuse, cells at the lateral border or crest of the neuroectoderm begin to dissociate from their neighbors. This cell population is known as the **neural crest** (Figs. 5.3 and 5.4), and it will undergo an epithelial to mesenchymal transition as it leaves the neuroectoderm by active migration and displacement to enter the underlying mesoderm. (**Mesoderm** refers to cells derived from the epiblast and extraembryonic tissues. **Mesenchyme** refers to loosely organized embryonic connective tissue, regardless of origin.) Crest cells then give rise to a heterogeneous array of tissues, including spinal (sensory) and autonomic ganglia; parts of the ganglia of cranial nerves V, VII, IX, and X;

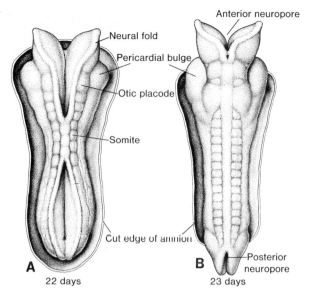

Figure 5.5. **A.** Dorsal view of a human embryo at approximately day 22. Seven distinct somites are visible on each side of the neural tube. **B.** Dorsal view of a human embryo at approximately day 23. Note the pericardial bulge on each side of the midline in the cephalic part of the embryo.

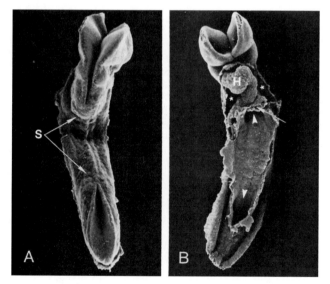

Figure 5.6. Scanning electron micrographs showing dorsal **(A)** and ventral **(B)** views of a mouse embryo (approximately 22-day human). **A.** The neural groove is closing in cranial and caudal directions and is flanked by pairs of somites *(S)*. **B.** Ventral view of the same embryo, showing formation of the gut tube with anterior and posterior intestinal portals *(arrowheads)*, heart *(H)* in the pericardial cavity *(asterisks)*, and the septum transversum *(arrow)* representing the primordium of the diaphragm (see Chapter 11). The neural folds remain open, exposing forebrain and midbrain regions.

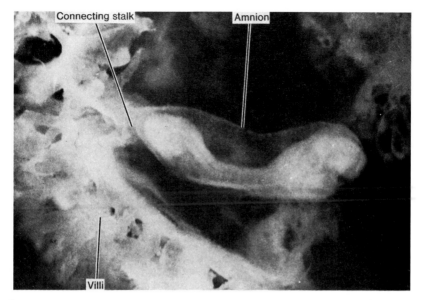

Figure 5.7. Photograph of a 12–13-somite embryo (approximately 23 days). The embryo within its amniotic sac is attached to the chorion by the connecting stalk. Note the well-developed chorionic villi.

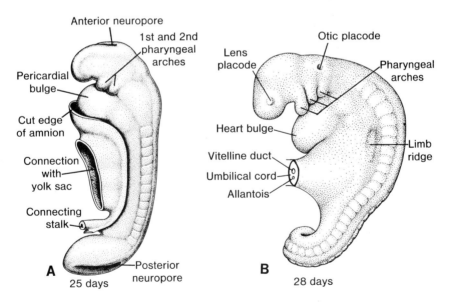

Figure 5.8. **A.** Lateral view of a 14-somite embryo (approximately 25 days). Note the bulging pericardial area and the 1st and 2nd pharyngeal arches. **B.** Schematic drawing showing the left side of a 25-somite embryo approximately 28 days old. The first three pharyngeal arches and lens and otic placodes are visible.

Schwann cells and meninges (pia and arachnoid); melanocytes; medulla of the suprarenal (adrenal) gland; bones and connective tissues of craniofacial structures; and cells of the conotruncal cushions of the heart (see Chapter 12).

By the time the neural tube is closed, two bilateral **ectodermal thickenings, the otic placodes** and the **lens placodes,** become visible in the cephalic region of the embryo (Fig. 5.8*B*). During further development, the otic placodes invaginate and form the **otic vesicles,** which will develop into structures needed for hearing and maintenance of equilibrium (see Chapter 17). At approximately the same time, the **lens placodes** appear. These placodes also invaginate and during the 5th week form the **lenses** of the eyes (see Chapter 18).

In general terms it may be stated that the ectodermal germ layer gives rise to those organs and structures that maintain contact with the outside world: *(a)* the central nervous system; *(b)* the peripheral nervous system; *(c)* the sensory epithelium of the ear, nose, and eye; and *(d)* the epidermis, including the hair and nails. In addition, it gives rise to subcutaneous glands, the mammary gland, the pituitary gland, and the enamel of the teeth.

Derivatives of the Mesodermal Germ Layer

Initially, cells of the mesodermal germ layer form a thin sheet of loosely woven tissue on each side of the midline (Fig. 5.9*A*). By about the 17th day,

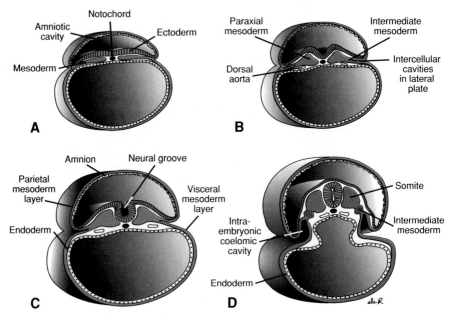

Figure 5.9. Transverse sections showing development of the mesodermal germ layer. **A.** Day 17. **B.** Day 19. **C.** Day 20. **D.** Day 21. The thin mesodermal sheet gives rise to paraxial mesoderm (future somites), intermediate mesoderm (future excretory units), and lateral plate, which is split into parietal and visceral mesoderm layers lining the intraembryonic coelomic cavity.

however, cells close to the midline proliferate and form a thickened plate of tissue known as **paraxial mesoderm** (Fig. 5.9B). More laterally, the mesoderm layer remains thin and is known as the **lateral plate.** With the appearance and coalescence of intercellular cavities in the lateral plate, this tissue is divided into two layers (Fig. 5.9, B and C): (a) a layer continuous with mesoderm covering the amnion, known as the **somatic** or **parietal mesoderm layer;** and (b) a layer continuous with mesoderm covering the yolk sac, known as the **splanchnic** or **visceral mesoderm layer** (Figs. 5.9, C and D, and 5.10). Together, these layers line a newly formed cavity, the **intraembryonic coelomic cavity,** which, on each side of the embryo, is continuous with the extraembryonic coelom. Tissue connecting paraxial and lateral plate mesoderm is known as **intermediate mesoderm** (Figs. 5.9, B and D, and 5.10).

By the beginning of the 3rd week, paraxial mesoderm becomes organized into segments. These segments, known as **somitomeres,** first appear in the cephalic region of the embryo, and their formation proceeds in a cephalocaudal direction. Each somitomere consists of mesodermal cells arranged in concentric whorls around the center of the unit. In the head region, somitomeres form in association with segmentation of the neural plate into **neuromeres,** and contribute the

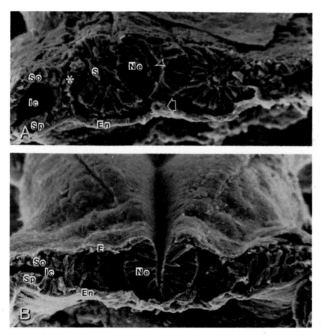

Figure 5.10. Transverse sections through somite regions of mouse embryos (approximately 21-day human) as visualized by scanning electron microscopy. **A.** Section through cervical somites. **B.** Section between somites immediately posterior to the hindbrain. *Arrow,* notochord; *arrowhead,* neural canal; *asterisk,* intermediate mesoderm; E, ectoderm; *En,* endoderm; *Ic,* intraembryonic coelom; *Ne,* neuroectoderm; *S,* Somite; *So,* somatic mesoderm; and *Sp,* splanchic mesoderm.

majority of the head mesenchyme (see Chapter 16). From the occipital region caudally, somitomeres become further organized into somites. The first pair of somites arises in the cervical region of the embryo at approximately the 20th day of development. From here, new somites appear in craniocaudal sequence, at a rate of approximately 3 pairs/day, until at the end of the 5th week, 42–44 pairs are present (Figs. 5.3, 5.5, and 5.8). There are 4 occipital, 7 cervical, 12 thoracic, 5 lumbar, 5 sacral, and 8–10 coccygeal pairs. The 1st occipital and the last 5–7 coccygeal somites later disappear, while the remaining somites form the axial skeleton (see Chapter 9). During this period of development, age of the embryo is expressed in number of somites, and Table 5.1 represents the approximate age of the embryo correlated to the number of somites.

Table 5.1.
Number of Somites Correlated to Approximate Age in Days

Approximate Age (days)	No. of Somites
20	1–4
21	4–7
22	7–10
23	10–13
24	13–17
25	17–20
26	20–23
27	23–26
28	26–29
30	34–35

DIFFERENTIATION OF THE SOMITE

By the beginning of the 4th week, cells forming the ventral and medial walls of the somite lose their compact organization, become polymorphous, and shift their position to surround the notochord (Fig. 5.11, *A* and *B*). These cells, collectively known as the **sclerotome,** form a loosely woven tissue known as **mesenchyme.** They will surround the spinal cord and notochord to form the vertebral column (see Chapter 9).

The remaining dorsal somite wall, now referred to as the **dermomyotome,** gives rise to a new layer of cells (Fig. 5.11*C*) characterized by pale nuclei and darkly stained nucleoli. These cells constitute the **myotome,** and each myotome provides musculature for its own segment (see Chapter 10).

After cells of the dermomyotome have formed the myotome, they lose their epithelial characteristics and spread out under the overlying ectoderm (Fig. 5.11*D*). Here they form **dermis** and subcutaneous tissue of the skin (see Chapter 19). Hence, each somite forms its own **sclerotome** (the cartilage and bone component), its own **myotome** (providing the segmental muscle component), and its own **dermatome,** the segmental skin component. Each myotome and dermatome also has its own segmental nerve component.

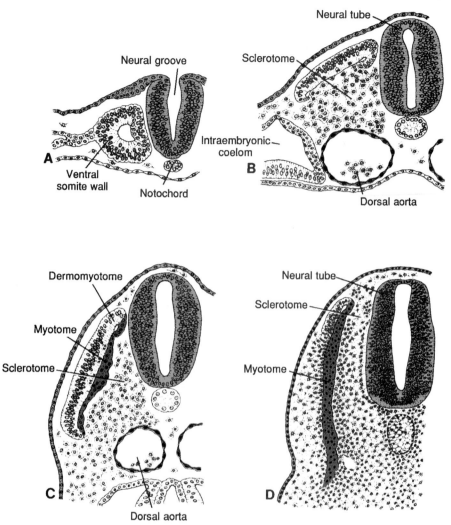

Figure 5.11. Successive stages in development of a somite. **A.** Mesoderm cells are arranged around a small cavity. **B.** Cells of the ventral and medial walls of the somite lose their epithelial arrangement and migrate in direction of the notochord. These cells are collectively referred to as the sclerotome. **C.** The dorsal somite wall gives rise to a new cell layer, the myotome. **D.** After extension of the myotome in a ventral direction, dermatome cells lose their epithelial configuration and spread out under the overlying ectoderm to form dermis.

INTERMEDIATE MESODERM

This tissue, which temporarily connects paraxial mesoderm with the lateral plate (Figs. 5.9*D* and 5.10*A*), differentiates in a manner entirely different from that of the somites. In cervical and upper thoracic regions, it forms segmentally arranged cell clusters (future **nephrotomes**), whereas more caudally it forms an unsegmented mass of tissue known as the **nephrogenic cord.** From this partly segmented, partly unsegmented intermediate mesoderm develop excretory units of the urinary system (see Fig. 15.2) and the gonads.

PARIETAL AND VISCERAL MESODERM LAYERS

The parietal and the visceral mesoderm layer line the intraembryonic coelom (Figs. 5.9, *C* and *D*, 5.10, and 5.12*A*). Parietal mesoderm, together with overlying ectoderm, will form the lateral and ventral body wall. Visceral mesoderm and embryonic endoderm will form the wall of the gut (Fig. 5.12*B*). Cells facing the coelomic cavity will form thin membranes, the **mesothelial** or **serous membranes,** which will line the peritoneal, pleural, and pericardial cavities (Fig. 5.12*B*) (see Chapter 11).

BLOOD AND BLOOD VESSELS

About the beginning of the 3rd week, mesoderm cells located in visceral mesoderm of the wall of the yolk sac differentiate into blood cells and blood vessels. These cells, known as **angioblasts,** form isolated clusters and cords **(angiogenic cell clusters),** which gradually become canalized by confluence of intercellular clefts (Fig. 5.13). Centrally located cells then give rise to primitive blood cells, while those on the periphery flatten and form **endothelial cells** lining **blood islands** (Fig. 5.13, *B* and *C*). Blood islands approach each other rapidly by sprouting of endothelial cells and, after fusion, give rise to small vessels. At the same time, blood cells and capillaries develop in the extraembryonic mesoderm of the villous stems and the connecting stalk (Fig. 5.14). By continuous budding, extraembryonic vessels establish contact with those inside the embryo, thus connecting the embryo and placenta.

Intraembryonic blood cells and blood vessels, including the heart tube, are established in exactly the same manner as described for extraembryonic vessels (see Chapter 12).

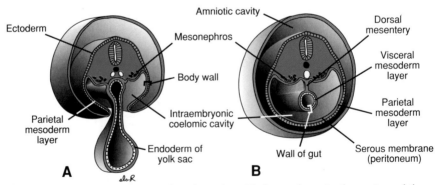

Figure 5.12. **A.** Transverse section through a 21-day embryo in the region of the mesonephros. Note the parietal and visceral mesoderm layers. The intraembryonic coelomic cavities communicate with the extraembryonic coelom (chorionic cavity). **B.** Section at the end of the 4th week. Parietal mesoderm and overlying ectoderm form the ventral and lateral body wall. Note the peritoneal (serous) membrane.

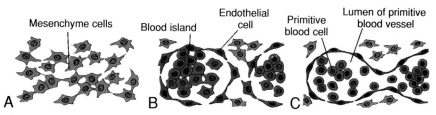

Figure 5.13. Successive stages of blood vessel formation. **A.** Undifferentiated mesenchyme cells. **B.** Blood island formation. **C.** Primitive capillary. Note the differentiation of mesenchymal cells into primitive blood cells and endothelial cells.

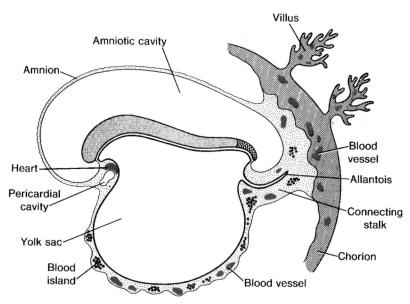

Figure 5.14. Extraembryonic blood vessel formation in the villi, chorion, connecting stalk, and wall of the yolk sac in a presomite embryo of approximately 19 days.

In summary, the following tissues and organs are considered to be of mesodermal origin: *(a)* supporting tissues such as connective tissue, cartilage, and bone; *(b)* striated and smooth musculature; *(c)* blood and lymph cells and the walls of the heart, blood, and lymph vessels; *(d)* kidneys, gonads, and their corresponding ducts; *(e)* the cortical portion of the suprarenal gland; and *(f)* the spleen.

Derivatives of the Endodermal Germ Layer

The gastrointestinal tract is the main organ system derived from the endodermal germ layer. Its formation is greatly dependent on **cephalocaudal** and **lateral folding** of the embryo. **Cephalocaudal folding is caused mainly by the rapid, longitudinal growth of the central nervous system, whereas transverse or**

lateral folding is produced by formation of rapidly growing somites. Hence, formation of the tube-like gut is a passive event and consists of the inversion and incorporation of part of the endoderm-lined yolk sac into the body cavity. As an additional result of the folding movements, the initial wide communication between the embryo and the yolk sac becomes constricted until only a narrow, long duct, the **vitelline duct,** remains.

The endodermal germ layer covers the ventral surface of the embryo and forms the roof of the yolk sac (Fig. 5.15*A*). With development and growth of the brain vesicles, however, the embryonic disc begins to bulge into the amniotic cavity and to fold in a cephalocaudal direction. This folding is most pronounced in the regions of the head and tail, where the **head fold** and **tail fold** are formed (Fig. 5.15).

As a result of cephalocaudal folding, a continuously larger portion of the endoderm-lined cavity is incorporated into the body of the embryo proper (Fig. 5.15*C*). In the anterior part, the endoderm forms the **foregut;** in the tail region, it forms the **hindgut.** The part between foregut and hindgut is known as the

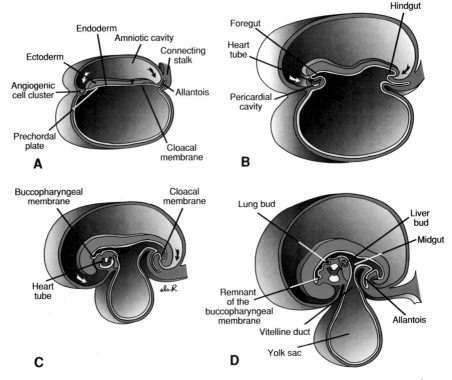

Figure 5.15. Drawings of sagittal midline sections of embryos at various stages of development to demonstrate cephalocaudal folding and its effect on position of the endoderm-lined cavity. **A.** Presomite embryo. **B.** Seven-somite embryo. **C.** Fourteen-somite embryo. **D.** At the end of the 1st month. Note the angiogenic cell clusters in relation to the prechordal (buccopharyngeal membrane) plate.

midgut. Temporarily, the midgut communicates with the yolk sac by way of a broad stalk, the **omphalomesenteric** or **vitelline duct** (Fig. 5.15*D*). This duct is wide initially, but with further growth of the embryo it becomes narrow and much longer (Fig. 5.20).

At its cephalic end, the foregut is temporarily bounded by the prechordal plate, an ectodermal-endodermal membrane that is now called the **buccopharyngeal membrane** (Fig. 5.15, *A* and *C*). At the end of the 3rd week, the buccopharyngeal membrane ruptures, thus establishing an open connection between the amniotic cavity and the primitive gut (Fig. 5.15*D*). The hindgut also terminates temporarily at an ectodermal-endodermal membrane known as the **cloacal membrane** (Fig. 5.15*C*).

As a result of rapid growth of the somites, the initial flat embryonic disc begins to fold in a lateral direction, and the embryo obtains a round appearance (Fig. 5.16). Simultaneously, the ventral body wall of the embryo is established, except for a small part in the ventral abdominal region where the yolk sac stalk is attached.

While the foregut and hindgut are established, as a result of the formation of the head fold and tail fold, respectively, the midgut remains in communication with the yolk sac. Initially, this connection is wide (Fig. 5.16*A*), but as a result of lateral folding it gradually becomes long and narrow, to form the **vitelline duct** (Figs. 5.16*B* and 5.17). Only much later, when the vitelline duct is obliterated, does the midgut lose its connection with the original endoderm-lined cavity and obtain its free position in the abdominal cavity (Fig. 5.16*C*).

Another important result of cephalocaudal and lateral folding is partial incorporation of the allantois into the body of the embryo, where it forms the **cloaca** (Fig. 5.17*A*). The distal portion of the allantois remains in the connecting stalk. By the 5th week, the yolk sac stalk and connecting stalk merge to form the umbilical cord (Figs. 5.17 and 7.9).

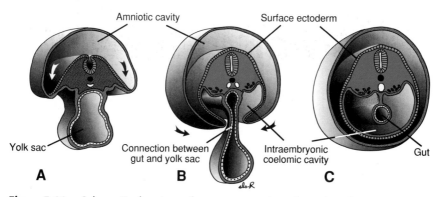

Figure 5.16. Schematic drawings of transverse sections through embryos at various stages of development to show the effect of lateral folding on the endoderm-lined cavity. **A.** Folding is initiated. **B.** Transverse section through the midgut to show the connection between the gut and yolk sac. **C.** Section just below the midgut to show the closed ventral abdominal wall and gut suspended from the dorsal abdominal wall by its mesentery.

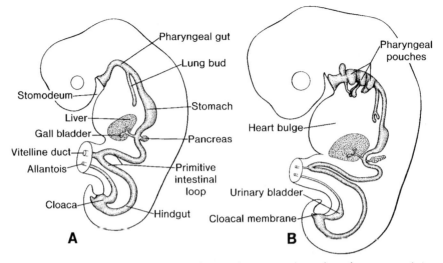

Figure 5.17. Schematic drawings of sagittal sections through embryos at various stages of development to show derivatives of the endodermal germ layer. Note the pharyngeal pouches and epithelial lining of the lung buds and trachea. Note the liver, gallbladder, and pancreas. The urinary bladder is derived from the cloaca and, at this stage of development, is in open connection with the allantois.

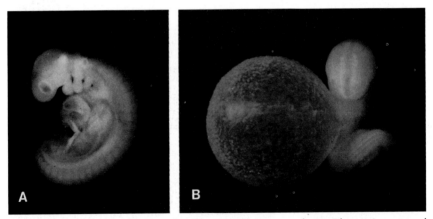

Figure 5.18. **A.** Lateral view of a 28-somite human embryo. The main external features are the pharyngeal arches and somites. Note the pericardial-liver bulge. Limb buds are not visible. **B.** Photograph of the same embryo but taken from a different angle to demonstrate the size of the yolk sac.

In humans, the yolk sac is vestigial and in all probability has a nutritive role only in early stages of development (Fig. 5.18). In the 2nd month of development, it is found in the chorionic cavity (Fig. 5.21).

Hence, the endodermal germ layer initially forms the epithelial lining of the primitive gut and the intraembryonic portions of the allantois and vitelline duct

(Fig. 5.17*A*). During further development, it gives rise to *(a)* the epithelial lining of the respiratory tract; *(b)* the **parenchyma** of the thyroid, parathyroids, liver, and pancreas (see Chapters 14 and 16); *(c)* the reticular stroma of the tonsils and thymus; *(d)* the epithelial lining of the urinary bladder and urethra (see Chapter 15); and *(e)* the epithelial lining of the tympanic cavity and auditory tube (see Chapter 17).

External Appearance During the Second Month

At the end of the 4th week, when the embryo has approximately 28 somites, the main external features are the somites and pharyngeal arches (Figs. 5.18 and 5.19). The age of the embryo is, therefore, usually expressed in somites (Table 5.1). Since counting the number of somites becomes difficult during the 2nd month of development, the age of the embryo is then indicated as the **crown-rump length (CRL)** and expressed in millimeters (Table 5.2).

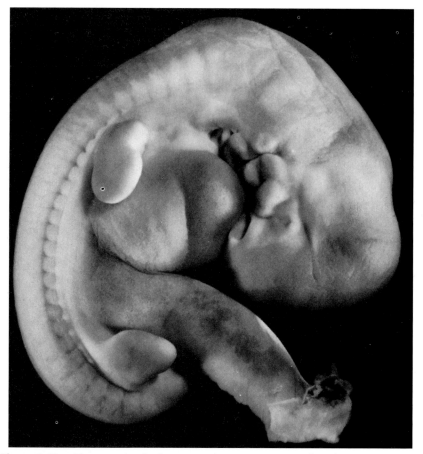

Figure 5.19. Photograph of a human embryo (crown-rump length (CRL) 9.8 mm, 5th week) (×29.9). Note that the forelimbs have a paddle-shaped appearance.

Table 5.2.
Crown-Rump Length (CRL) Correlated to Approximate Age in Weeks

CRL (mm)	Approximate Age (weeks)
5–8	5
10–14	6
17–22	7
28–30	8

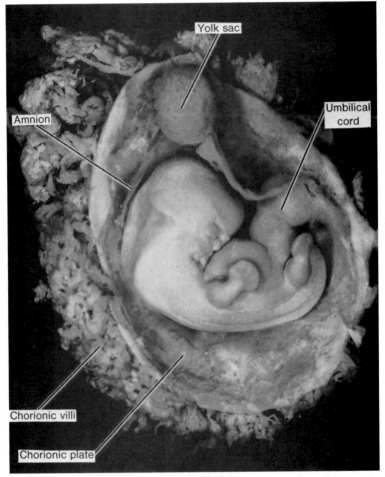

Figure 5.20. Photograph of a human embryo (CRL 13 mm, 6th week). Note that the yolk sac is visible in the chorionic cavity.

CRL is the measurement from the vertex of the skull to the midpoint between the apices of the buttocks. Owing to considerable variation in the degree of flexure from one embryo to another, it is understandable that measurements given in Table 5.2 are only approximate indications of the real age of the embryo.

During the 2nd month, the external appearance of the embryo is changed greatly by the enormous size of the head and formation of the limbs, face, ears, nose, and eyes. By the beginning of the 5th week, forelimbs and hindlimbs appear as paddle-shaped buds (Fig. 5.19). The former are located dorsal to the pericardial swelling at the level of the 4th cervical to the 1st thoracic somites, thus explaining their innervation by the brachial plexus. Hindlimb buds appear slightly later just caudal to attachment of the umbilical stalk at the level of the lumbar and upper sacral somites. With further growth, the terminal portion of the buds flattens and becomes separated from the proximal, more cylindrically shaped segment by a circular constriction (Fig. 5.20). Soon, four radial grooves separating five slightly thicker areas appear on the distal portion of the buds, foreshadowing formation of the digits (Fig. 5.20).

These grooves, known as **rays,** appear in the hand region first and shortly afterward in the foot, as the arm is slightly more advanced in development than the leg. While fingers and toes are being formed (Fig. 5.21), a second constriction

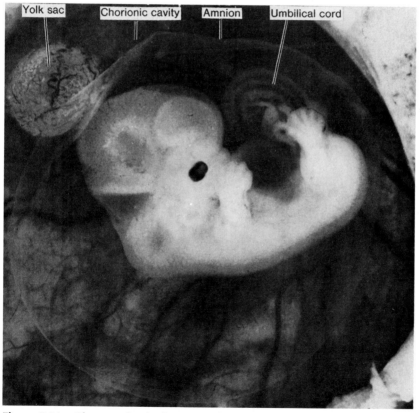

Figure 5.21. Photograph of a human embryo (CRL 21 mm, 7th week) (×4). The chorionic sac is open to show the embryo in its amniotic sac. The yolk sac, umbilical cord, and vessels in the chorionic plate of the placenta are clearly visible. Note the enormous size of the head in comparison to the remaining part of the body.

divides the proximal portion of the buds into two segments, and the three parts characteristic of the adult extremities can be recognized (Fig. 5.22).

CLINICAL CORRELATES

It is evident from the above account that most major organs and organ systems are formed during the period from the 3rd to 8th week. This period is, therefore, also called the **period of organogenesis** and is critical for normal development. Stem cell populations are establishing each of the organ primordia, and these interactions are sensitive to insult from genetic and environmental influences. Thus, this period is when most gross structural birth defects are induced. Unfortunately, the mother may not realize she is pregnant during this critical time, especially during the 3rd and 4th weeks that are

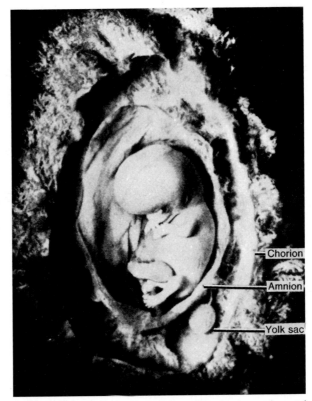

Figure 5.22. Photograph of a human embryo (CRL 25 mm, 7th to 8th week). The chorion and the amnion have been opened. Note the size of the head, the eye, the auricle of the ear, the well-formed toes, the swelling in the umbilical cord caused by intestinal loops, and the yolk sac in the chorionic cavity.

particularly vulnerable. Consequently, she may not avoid pote
harmful influences, such as cigarette smoking and alcohol.

Being familiar with the main events of organogenesis is
assistance in identifying the time that a particular defect was ...
If presented with a child having a closure defect of the anterior
neuropore, such as anencephaly, one can quickly calculate that the
abnormality must have been initiated on the 23rd to 25th days of
development when the neuropore normally closes. Similarly, in a child
without upper limbs, the insult must have affected the limb buds in the
5th week of gestation.

SUMMARY

The **embryonic period** extends from the 3rd to the 8th week of development and is the period during which each of the three germ layers gives rise
to its own tissues and organ systems. As a result of organ formation, major
features of body form are established (Table 5.3).

The **ectodermal germ layer** gives rise to those organs and structures that
maintain contact with the outside world: (a) **central nervous system;** (b)
peripheral nervous system; (c) **sensory epithelium of ear, nose, and eye;** (d)
skin, including hair and nails; and (e) **pituitary, mammary, and sweat glands**
and **enamel of the teeth.** Each of these systems is discussed in a separate
chapter.

Important components of the **mesodermal germ layer** are **paraxial, intermediate,** and **lateral plate** mesoderm. Paraxial mesoderm forms **somitomeres**
that give rise to mesenchyme of the head and organize into **somites** in
occipital and caudal segments. Somites give rise to the **myotome** (muscle
tissue), **sclerotome** (cartilage and bone), and **dermatome** (subcutaneous tissue
of the skin), which are **all supporting tissues of the body.** Mesoderm also gives
rise to the **vascular system,** i.e., the heart, arteries, veins, lymph vessels, and
all blood and lymph cells. Furthermore, it gives rise to the **urogenital system:**
kidneys, gonads, and their ducts (but not the bladder). Finally, the **spleen** and
cortex of the suprarenal glands are mesodermal derivatives.

The **endodermal germ layer** provides the epithelial lining of the **gastrointestinal tract, respiratory tract,** and **urinary bladder.** It also forms the
parenchyma of the **thyroid, parathyroids, liver,** and **pancreas.** Finally, the
epithelial lining of the **tympanic cavity** and **auditory tube** are lined by
epithelium of endodermal origin.

As a result of formation of organ systems and rapid growth of the central
nervous system, the initial flat embryonic disc begins to fold in a **cephalocaudal direction,** thus establishing the **head and tail folds.** The disc also
folds in a **transverse direction (lateral folds),** thus establishing the **rounded
body form.** Connection with the yolk sac and placenta is maintained
through the **vitelline duct** and umbilical cord, respectively.

.able 5.3.

Summary of Key Events During the Embryonic Period

Days	Somites	Length (*mm*)	Figure	Characteristic Features
14–15	0	0.2	5.1*A*	Appearance of primitive streak
16–18	0	0.4	5.1*B*	Notochordal process appears; hemopoietic cells present in yolk sac
19–20	0	1–20	5.2*A*	Intraembryonic mesoderm spread under entire ectoderm; primitive streak complete; umbilical vessels and cranial neural folds beginning to form
20–21	1–4	2.0–3.0	5.2, *B* and *C*	Cranial neural folds elevated, and deep neural groove established; embryo beginning to bend
22–23	5–12	3.0–3.5	5.5, *A* and *B*, 5.6, 5.7	Fusion of neural folds begins in cervical region; cranial and caudal neuropores open widely; visceral arches 1 and 2 present; heart tube beginning to fold
24–25	13–20	3.0–4.5	5.8*A*	Cephalocaudal folding under way; cranial neuropore closing or closed; optic vesicles formed; otic placodes appear
26–27	21–29	3.5–5.0	5.8*B*, 5.18, *A* and *B*	Caudal neuropore closing or closed; upper limb buds appear; 3 pairs of visceral arches present
28–30	30–35	4.0–6.0	5.8*B*	Fourth visceral arch formed; hindlimb buds appear; otic vesicle and lens placode present
31–35		7.0–10.0	5.19	Forelimbs, paddle-shaped; nasal pits formed; embryo tightly C-shaped
36–42		9.0–14.0	5.20	Digital rays present in hand and footplates; brain vesicles prominent; external auricle forming from auricular hillocks; umbilical herniation initiated
43–49		13.0–22.0	5.21	Pigmentation of retina visible; digital rays separating; nipples and eyelids formed; maxillary swellings fuse with medial nasal swellings as upper lip forms; prominent umbilical herniation
50–56		21.0–31.0	5.22	Limbs long and bent at elbows and knees; fingers and toes free; face more human-like; tail disappears; umbilical herniation persists until the end of the third month

PROBLEMS TO SOLVE

1. Why are the 3rd to 8th weeks of embryogenesis so critical for normal development and also the most sensitive for induction of structural defects?

SUGGESTED READINGS

Eichele G: Retinoids and vertebrate limb pattern formation. *Trends Genet* 5:226, 1990.
Jessell TM, Melton DA: Diffusible factors in vertebrate embryonic induction. *Cell* 68:257, 1992.

Lauder JM: Neurotransmitters as growth regulatory signals: role of receptors and second ⌐
  Trends Neurosci 16:236, 1993.
Meier T, Tam PPL: Metameric pattern development in the embryonic axis of th⌐
  Differentiation of the cranial segments. *Differentiation* 21:95, 1982.
Muller F, O'Rahilly R: The development of the human brain, the closure of the cranial ⌐
  the beginning of secondary neurulation at stage 12. *Anat Embryol* 176:413, 1987.
O'Rahilly R, Muller F: Bidirectional closure of the rostral neuropore. *Am J Anat* 184:259, ⌐⌐
O'Rahilly R, Muller F: *Developmental Stages in Human Embryos*. Washington, DC, Carnegie
  Institution of Washington, 1987.
Schoenwolf G, Bortier H, Vakaet L: Fate mapping the avian neural plate with quail-chick chimeras:
  origin of prospective median wedge cells. *J Exp Zool* 249:271, 1989.
Slack JM: Embryonic induction. *Mech Dev* 41:91, 1993.
Streeter GL: Developmental horizons in human embryos: age group XI, 13–20 somites, and age
  group XII, 21–29 somites. *Contrib Embryol* 30:211, 1942.
Streeter GL: Developmental horizons in human embryos: age group XIII, embryos 4 or 5 mm. long,
  and age group XIV, indentation of lens vesicle. *Contrib Embryol* 31:26, 1945.
Tam PPL, Beddington RSP: The formation of mesodermal tissues in the mouse embryo during
  gastrulation and early organogenesis. *Development* 99:109, 1987.
Tam PPL, Meier S, Jacobson AG: Differentiation of the metameric pattern in the embryonic axis of
  the mouse. II. Somitomeric organization of the presomitic mesoderm. *Differentiation* 21:109, 1982.

chapter 6

Fetal Period
(Third Month to Birth)

Development of the Fetus

The period from the beginning of the 3rd month to the end of intrauterine life is known as the **fetal period.** It is characterized by maturation of tissues and organs and rapid growth of the body. Few malformations arise during this period, although deformations caused by mechanical forces, such as intrauterine compression, may occur (see Chapter 8). Also, insults to the central nervous system may result in postnatal behavioral disturbances and lowered intelligence.

The length of the fetus is usually indicated as the **crown-rump length (CRL)** (sitting height) or as the **crown-heel length (CHL),** the measurement from the vertex of the skull to the heel (standing height). These measurements, expressed in centimeters, are then correlated with the age of the fetus expressed in weeks or months (Table 6.1). Growth in length is particularly striking during the 3rd, 4th, and 5th months, while increase in weight is most striking during the last 2 months of gestation. In general, **the length of pregnancy is considered to be 280 days or 40 weeks after the onset of the last normal menstrual period (LNMP) or, more accurately, 266 days or 38 weeks after fertilization.** For the purposes of the following discussion, age is calculated from the time of fertilization and is expressed in weeks or calendar months.

Monthly Changes

One of the most striking changes taking place during fetal life is the relative slowdown in growth of the head compared with the rest of the body. At the beginning of the 3rd month, the head constitutes approximately one-half CRL (Fig. 6.1). By the beginning of the 5th month, the size of the head is about one-third CHL, and at birth, it is approximately one-fourth CHL (Fig. 6.2). Hence, with time, growth of the body accelerates, but that of the head slows down.

During the **3rd month,** the face becomes more human-looking (Figs. 6.3 and 6.4). The eyes, initially directed laterally, become located on the ventral aspect of the face, and the ears come to lie close to their definitive position at the side of the head (Fig. 6.3). The limbs reach their relative length in comparison to the rest of the body, although the lower limbs are still a little shorter and less developed than the upper extremities. **Primary ossification centers** are present in the long bones and skull by the 12th week. Also by the 12th week, external genitalia

Table 6.1.
Growth in Length and Weight During the Fetal Period

Age (weeks)	CRL (cm)	Weight (gm)
9–12	5–8	10–45
13–16	9–14	60–200
17–20	15–19	250–450
21–24	20–23	500–820
25–28	24–27	900–1300
29–32	28–30	1400–2100
33–36	31–34	2200–2900
37–38	35–36	3000–3400

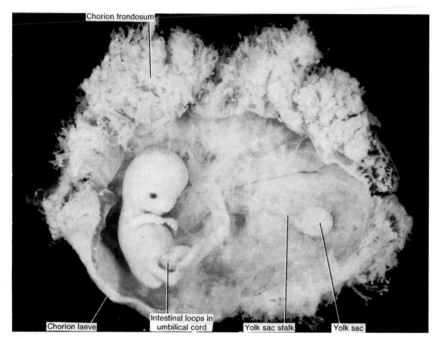

Figure 6.1. Photograph of a 9-week fetus. Note the large size of the head compared with that of the remaining part of the body. The yolk sac and long vitelline duct are visible in the chorionic cavity. Note the umbilical cord and herniation of intestinal loops. One side of the chorion has many villi (chorion frondosum), while the other side is almost smooth (chorion laeve),

develop to such a degree that the sex of the fetus can be determined by external examination (ultrasound). During the 6th week **intestinal loops cause a large swelling in the umbilical cord,** but by the 12th week they withdraw into the abdominal cavity. At the end of the 3rd month, reflex activity can be evoked in aborted fetuses, indicating muscular activity. These movements are so small, however, that they are not noticed by the mother.

During the **4th** and **5th months,** the fetus lengthens rapidly (Fig. 6.5 and Table 6.1), and at the end of the first half of intrauterine life its CRL is approximately

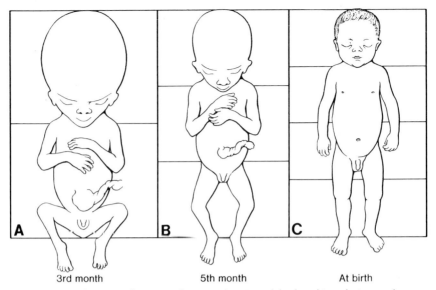

| 3rd month | 5th month | At birth |

Figure 6.2. Schematic drawings showing the size of the head in relation to the rest of the body at various stages of development.

15 cm, i.e., about half the total length of the newborn. The weight of the fetus, however, increases little during this period and by the end of the 5th month is still less than 500 gm.

The fetus is covered with fine hair, called **lanugo hair;** eyebrows and head hair are also visible. **During the 5th month, movements of the fetus are usually clearly recognized by the mother.**

During the **second half of intrauterine life,** weight increases considerably, particularly during the last 2½ months, when 50% of the full-term weight (approximately 3200 gm) is added. During the **6th month,** the skin of the fetus is reddish and has a wrinkled appearance because of the lack of underlying connective tissue. A fetus born during the 6th month or the first half of the 7th month has great difficulty surviving. Although several organ systems are able to function, the respiratory system and the central nervous system have not differentiated sufficiently, and coordination between the two systems is not yet well established.

During the last 2 months, the fetus obtains well-rounded contours as the result of deposition of subcutaneous fat (Fig. 6.6). By the end of intrauterine life, the skin is covered by a whitish, fatty substance **(vernix caseosa),** composed of secretory products from sebaceous glands. When the fetus is 28 weeks old, it is able to survive, although with great difficulty.

At the end of the **9th month,** the skull has the largest circumference of all parts of the body, an important fact with regard to its passage through the birth canal. At the time of birth, the weight of a normal fetus is 3000–3400 gm; its CRL, about 36 cm; and its CHL, about 50 cm. Sexual characteristics are pronounced, and the testes should be in the scrotum.

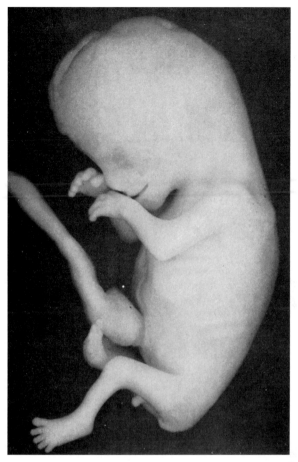

Figure 6.3. Photograph of an 11-week fetus. The umbilical cord still shows a swelling at its base, caused by herniated intestinal loops. Toes are developed, and the sex of the fetus can be recognized. The skull of this fetus lacks the normal smooth contours.

Time of Birth

The date of birth is most accurately indicated as 266 days or 38 weeks after fertilization. The oocyte is usually fertilized within 12 hours after ovulation, and coitus must have occurred within 24 hours preceding fertilization. A pregnant woman usually will see her obstetrician when two successive menstrual bleeds have failed to occur. By that time, her recollection about coitus is usually vague, and it is readily understandable that the day of fertilization is difficult to determine.

The obstetrician calculates the date of birth as 280 days or 40 weeks from the first day of the **last normal menstrual period (LNMP).** In women with regular 28-day menstrual periods, the method is rather accurate, but when cycles are irregular, substantial miscalculations may be made. It must be remembered that the time between ovulation and the succeeding menstrual bleeding is constant (14 days 1 day), but the time between ovulation and the preceding menses is highly variable. An additional complication occurs when the woman has some bleeding about 14 days after fertilization as a result of erosive activity by the implanting blastocyst (see Chapter 3). Hence, it is evident that the day of delivery is not always easy to determine. In general, most fetuses are born within 10–14 days of the calculated delivery date. If they are born much earlier, they are categorized as **premature;** if born later, they are considered **postmature.**

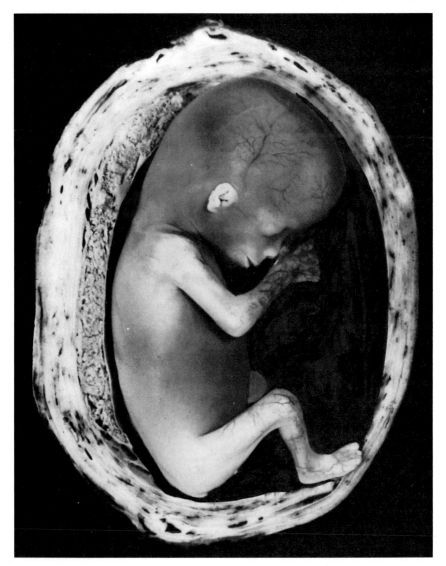

Figure 6.4. Photograph of a 12-week fetus in utero. Note the extremely thin skin and underlying blood vessels. The face has all the human characteristics, but the ears are still primitive. Movements begin at this time but are usually not felt by the mother.

Occasionally, the age of an embryo or small fetus will have to be determined. By combining data on the onset of the last menstrual period with fetal length, weight, and other morphological characteristics typical for a given month of development, a reasonable estimate of the age of the fetus can be formulated. A valuable tool for assisting in this determination is **ultrasound,** which can provide an accurate (1–2 days) measurement of CRL during the 7th to 14th weeks. Measurements commonly used in the 16th to 30th weeks are **biparietal diameter (BPD),** head and abdominal circumference, and femur length. An accurate determination of fetal size and age is important for managing pregnancy, especially in cases where the mother may have a small pelvis or the baby has a birth defect.

CLINICAL CORRELATES

Considerable variability exists in fetal length and weight, and sometimes these values do not correspond with the calculated age of the fetus in months or weeks. Most factors influencing length and weight are genetically determined, but it is now known that environmental factors also play an important role.

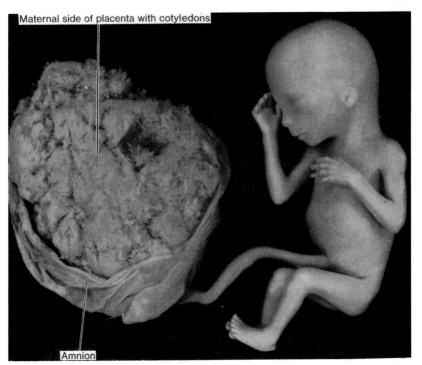

Maternal side of placenta with cotyledons

Amnion

Figure 6.5. Photograph of an 18-week-old fetus connected to the placenta by its umbilical cord. The skin of the fetus is thin as a result of the absence of subcutaneous fat. Note the placenta with its cotyledons and the amnion.

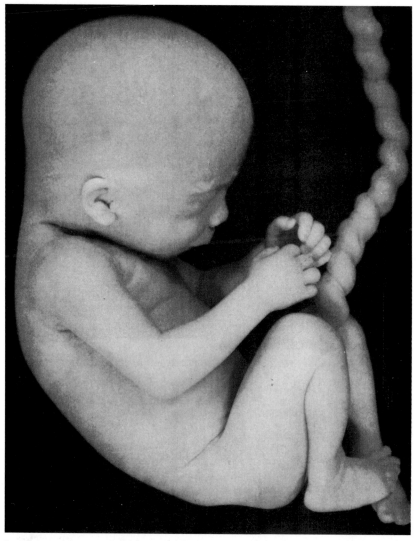

Figure 6.6. Photograph of a 7-month-old fetus. This fetus would possibly be able to survive. It now has well-rounded contours as a result of deposition of subcutaneous fat. Note the spiral twisting of the umbilical cord.

Intrauterine growth retardation (IUGR) is a term applied to infants who are at or below the 10th percentile for their expected birth weight at a given gestational age. Sometimes, these infants have been described as small for dates, **small for gestational age (SGA),** fetally malnourished, or dysmature. Approximately 1 in 10 babies will suffer IUGR and will, therefore, have an increased risk for neurological deficiencies, congenital malformations, meconium aspiration, hypoglycemia, hypocalcemia, and respiratory distress syndrome (RDS). Factors that cause such babies include chromosomal abnormalities (10%); teratogens; congenital infections (rubella, cytomegalovirus, toxoplasmosis, and syphilis); poor maternal health (hypertension and renal and cardiac disease); the mother's nutritional status and socioeconomic level; her use of cigarettes, alcohol, and other drugs; placental insufficiency; and multiple births (twins, triplets, etc.). Small fetuses that weigh less than 500 gm seldom survive, while those that weigh 500–1000 gm may live if provided with expert care. Infants may be small because of IUGR, but full term. However, they may also be small if they are born prematurely before term.

Several approaches are now available to the perinatologist for assessing growth and development of the fetus in utero. In combination, these techniques are designed to detect malformations, chromosomal abnormalities, and overall growth of the fetus. The least traumatic of these procedures is ultrasonography, which employs ultrasound to produce images of the placenta and offspring. Ultrasonic scans can determine placental and fetal size and position, multiple births, and malformations such as neural tube, cardiac, and abdominal wall defects (Fig. 6.7, A and B).

Another approach involves withdrawing amniotic fluid and is termed amniocentesis. A needle is inserted through the mother's abdominal wall and uterus into the amniotic cavity. Approximately 20–30 mL of fluid are withdrawn, and therefore, the procedure is usually not performed prior to the 14th week of gestation due to insufficient quantities of fluid prior to this time. The fluid itself is analyzed for α-fetoprotein (AFP). This substance is a fetal protein that is present in high concentrations in the amniotic fluid of offspring with open neural tube defects, such as spina bifida and anencephaly, and abdominal malformations, such as gastroschisis and omphalocele (see Chapter 8). (This protein is also present in maternal serum and can be measured, but with less reliability than assays of amniotic fluid.) Fetal cells, which are present in amniotic fluid, are grown in culture and analyzed for chromosomal abnormalities. In this manner, major chromosomal alterations such as translocations, breaks, trisomies, and monosomies can be identified. With use of special stains, such as Giemsa, banding patterns unique for each chromosome can be determined (see Chapter 8). Furthermore, as more and more of the human genome is sequenced, Southern blotting can be performed to provide more detailed analysis of DNA structure.

Another technique involves obtaining a small piece of chorionic villus tissue (chorionic villus sampling (CVS). This tissue contains

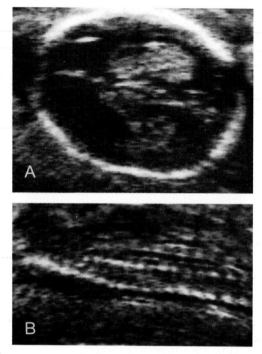

Figure 6.7. Ultrasonograms of a normal child's head **(A)** and vertebral column **(B)** at 7 months gestation. Use of this technique can provide an estimate of fetal age and detect some malformations such as neural tube defects (see Figs. 9.14 and 20.30).

numerous rapidly dividing fetal cells that are available for immediate analysis of chromosomal and biochemical defects, such as inborn errors of metabolism. The approach offers the advantages of being able to be performed early in pregnancy (8 weeks) and of immediate cell analysis without waiting for cell cultures. Early detection of abnormalities is desirable from the standpoint of the decision to terminate pregnancy. A disadvantage of the technique is the inability to determine AFP levels.

Generally, these prenatal diagnostic techniques are not used on a routine basis (although ultrasonography is approaching routine use), being reserved instead for high-risk pregnancies. Indications for employing the tests include *(a)* advanced maternal age, i.e., 35 years or older; *(b)* history of neural tube defects in the family; *(c)* birth of a previous child with a chromosome abnormality, i.e., Down syndrome; *(d)* chromosome abnormalities in either parent; and *(e)* a mother who is a carrier of X-linked recessive disorders. Risks from the tests themselves are small. There is approximately 0.5% fetal loss with amniocentesis and 0.8% fetal loss with chorionic villus sampling (CVS).

SUMMARY

The **fetal period extends from the 9th week of gestation until birth** and is characterized by rapid growth of the body and maturation of organ systems. Growth in length is particularly striking during the 3rd, 4th, and 5th months (approximately 5 cm/month), while increase in weight is most striking during the last 2 months of gestation (approximately 700 gm/month) (Table 6.1).

A striking change is the relative slowdown in the growth of the head. In the 3rd month, it is about one-half CRL. By the 5th month, the size of the head is about one-third CHL, and at birth, it is one-fourth CHL (Fig. 6.2).

During the 5th month, fetal movements are clearly recognized by the mother, and the fetus is covered with fine, small hair.

A fetus born during the 6th or the beginning of the 7th month has difficulty surviving, mainly because the respiratory and central nervous systems have not differentiated sufficiently.

In general, the **length of pregnancy** for a full-term fetus is considered to be **280 days** or **40 weeks** after onset of the last menstruation or, **more accurately, 266 days or 38 weeks after fertilization.**

A variety of prenatal screening techniques are available, including **ultrasonography, amniocentesis,** and **chorionic villus sampling (CVS).** These procedures are used for determining placental and fetal growth, congenital malformations, and chromosomal abnormalities. They are generally reserved for high-risk pregnancies.

PROBLEMS TO SOLVE

1. Amniocentesis reveals an elevated α-fetoprotein level. What would be included in a differential diagnosis, and how would a definitive one be made?

2. A 40-year-old woman is approximately 8 weeks pregnant. What tests are available to determine whether or not her unborn child has Down syndrome? What are the advantages of each technique, and what are the risks?

3. Why is it important to determine the status of an infant prenatally? What maternal or family factors might raise your concern about the well-being of an unborn infant?

SUGGESTED READINGS

Barnea ER, Hustin J, Jauniaux E (eds): *The First Twelve Weeks of Gestation.* Berlin, Springer-Verlag, 1992.

Benson CB, Doubilet PM: Sonographic prediction of gestational age '91—accuracy of second-trimester and third-trimester fetal measurements. *AJR* 157:1275, 1991.

Boehm CE, Kazazian HH Jr: Prenatal diagnosis by DNA analysis. *In* Harrison MR, Golbus MS, Filly RA (eds): *The Unborn Patient: Prenatal Diagnosis and Treatment.* 2nd ed. Philadelphia, WB Saunders, 1991.

Brock DJH: Prenatal diagnosis—chemical methods. *Br Med J* 32:16, 1976.

Creasy RK, Resnik R: Intrauterine growth retardation. *In* Creasy RK, Resnik R (eds): *Maternal-Fetal Medicine: Principles and Practice.* 2nd ed. Philadelphia, WB Saunders, 1989.

Filly RA: Sonographic anatomy of the normal fetus. *In* Harrison MR, Golbus MS, Filly RA (eds): *The Unborn Patient: Prenatal Diagnosis and Treatment.* 2nd ed. Philadelphia, WB Saunders, 1991.

Haddow JE: α-Fetoprotein. *In* Harrison MR, Golbus MS, Filly RA (eds): *The Unborn Patient: Prenatal Diagnosis and Treatment.* 2nd ed. Philadelphia, WB Saunders, 1991.

Harrison MR, Golbus MS, Filly RA (eds): *The Unborn Patient: Prenatal Diagnosis and Treatment.* 2nd ed. Philadelphia, WB Saunders, 1991.

Holtzman NA: Prenatal screening for neural tube defects. *Pediatrics* 71:658, 1983.

Jones M, Battaglia F: Intrauterine growth retardation. *Am J Obstet Gynecol* 127:540–549, 1977.

Kolata G: First trimester prenatal diagnosis. *Science* 221:1031, 1983.

Kurtz AB, Needleman L: Ultrasound assessment of fetal age. *In* Callen PW (ed): *Ultrasonography in Obstetrics and Gynecology.* Philadelphia, WB Saunders, 1988.

Modanlon HE, et al: Macrosomia—maternal, fetal, and neonatal implications. *Obstet Gynecol* 55:420, 1980.

Nash JE, Persaud TVN: Embryopathic risks of cigarette smoking. *Exp Pathol* 33:65, 1988.

O'Rahilly R, Muller F: *Developmental Stages in Human Embryos.* Washington, DC, Carnegie Institution of Washington, 1987.

Seeds JW: Impaired fetal growth: definition and clinical diagnosis. *Obstet Gynecol* 64:303–310, 1984.

Spirt BA, Fordon LP, Oliphant M: *Prenatal Ultrasound: A Color Atlas With Anatomic and Pathologic Correlation.* New York, Churchill Livingstone, 1987.

Thompson MW, McInnes RR, Willard HF: *Thompson and Thompson: Genetics in Medicine.* 5th ed. Philadelphia, WB Saunders, 1991.

Weaver DD: Inborn errors of metabolism. *In* Weaver DD (ed): *Catalogue of Prenatally Diagnosed Conditions.* Baltimore, Johns Hopkins University Press, 1989.

Wilson RD: How to perform genetic amniocentesis. *J SOGC* 13:61, 1991.

chapter 7

Fetal Membranes and Placenta

By the beginning of the 2nd month, the **trophoblast** is characterized by a great number of secondary and tertiary villi that give it a radial appearance (Fig. 7.1). The villi are anchored in the mesoderm of the **chorionic plate** and are attached peripherally to the maternal decidua by way of the outer **cytotrophoblast shell.** The surface of the villi is formed by the syncytium, resting on a layer of cytotrophoblastic cells that, in turn, cover a core of vascular mesoderm (Fig. 7.2, *A* and *C*). The capillary system developing in the core of the villous stems soon comes in contact with capillaries of the chorionic plate and connecting stalk, thus giving rise to the extraembryonic vascular system (see Fig. 4.9).

During the following months, numerous small extensions sprout from existing villous stems into the surrounding **lacunar** or **intervillous spaces.** Initially, these newly formed villi are primitive (Fig. 7.2*C*), but by the beginning of the 4th month, cytotrophoblastic cells as well as some connective tissue cells disappear. The syncytium and endothelial wall of the blood vessels are then the only layers that separate the maternal and fetal circulations (Fig. 7.2, *B* and *D*). Frequently, the syncytium becomes very thin, and large pieces containing several nuclei may break off and drop into the intervillous blood lakes. These pieces, known as **syncytial knots,** enter the maternal circulation and usually degenerate without causing any symptoms. Disappearance of cytotrophoblastic cells progresses from the smaller to larger villi, and although some always persist in large villi, they do not participate in the exchange between the two circulations.

Chorion Frondosum and Decidua Basalis

In the early weeks of development, villi cover the entire surface of the chorion (Fig. 7.1). As pregnancy advances, villi on the embryonic pole continue to grow and expand, thus giving rise to the **chorion frondosum** (bushy chorion). Villi on the abembryonic pole degenerate, and by the 3rd month this side of the chorion is smooth and is known as the **chorion laeve** (Figs. 7.3 and 7.4*A*).

The difference in embryonic and abembryonic poles of the chorion is also reflected in the structure of the **decidua,** which is the functional layer of the endometrium and is shed during parturition. The decidua over the chorion frondosum, the **decidua basalis,** consists of a compact layer of large cells, **decidual cells,** with abundant amounts of lipids and glycogen. This layer, the

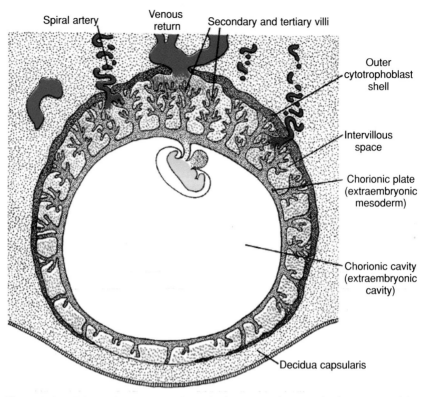

Spiral artery

Venous return

Secondary and tertiary villi

Outer cytotrophoblast shell

Intervillous space

Chorionic plate (extraembryonic mesoderm)

Chorionic cavity (extraembryonic cavity)

Decidua capsularis

Figure 7.1. Schematic representation of a human embryo at the beginning of the 2nd month of development. At the embryonic pole, villi are numerous and well formed; at the abembryonic pole, they are few in number and poorly developed.

decidual plate, is tightly connected to the chorion. The decidual layer over the abembryonic pole is known as the **decidua capsularis** (Fig. 7.4A). With increase in the size of the chorionic vesicle, this layer becomes stretched and degenerates. Subsequently, the chorion laeve comes into contact with the uterine wall **(decidua parietalis)** on the opposite side of the uterus, and the two fuse (Figs. 7.4–7.6), thereby obliterating the uterine lumen. Hence, the only portion of the chorion participating in the exchange process is the chorion frondosum, which, together with the decidua basalis, makes up the **placenta.** Similarly, fusion of the amnion and chorion to form the **amniochorionic membrane** obliterates the chorionic cavity (Fig. 7.4, *A* and *B*). It is this membrane that ruptures during labor (breaking of the water).

Structure of the Placenta

By the beginning of the 4th month, the placenta has two components: *(a)* a **fetal portion,** formed by the chorion frondosum; and *(b)* a **maternal portion,** formed by the decidua basalis (Fig. 7.4B). On the fetal side, the placenta is

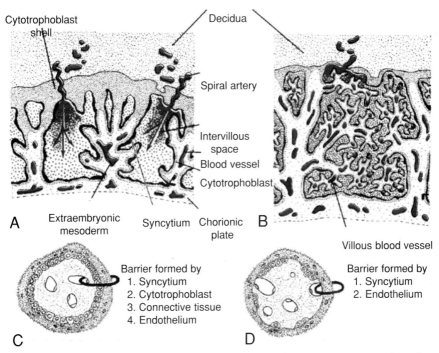

Figure 7.2. Structure of villi at various stages of development. **A.** During the 4th week. Note how the extraembryonic mesoderm penetrates the stem villi in the direction of the decidual plate. **B.** During the 4th month. In many small villi the wall of the capillaries is in direct contact with the syncytium. **C** and **D.** Enlargement of the villus as shown in **A** and **B,** respectively.

bordered by the **chorionic plate** (Fig. 7.7); on its maternal side, it is bordered by the decidua basalis, of which the **decidual plate** is most intimately incorporated into the placenta. In the **junctional zone,** trophoblast and decidua cells intermingle. This zone is characterized by decidual and syncytial giant cells and is rich in amorphous extracellular material. By this time, most cytotrophoblast cells have degenerated. Between the chorionic and decidual plates are the intervillous spaces that are filled with maternal blood. They are derived from lacunae in the syncytiotrophoblast and are lined with syncytium of fetal origin. The villous trees grow into the intervillous blood lakes (Figs. 7.1 and 7.7).

During the 4th and 5th months, the decidua forms a number of septa, the **decidual septa,** which project into intervillous spaces but do not reach the chorionic plate (Fig. 7.7). These septa have a core of maternal tissue, but their surface is covered by a layer of syncytial cells, so that at all times a syncytial layer separates maternal blood in intervillous lakes from fetal tissue of the villi. As a result of this septum formation, the placenta is divided into a number of compartments or **cotyledons** (Fig. 7.8). Since the decidual septa do not reach the chorionic plate, contact between intervillous spaces in the various cotyledons is maintained.

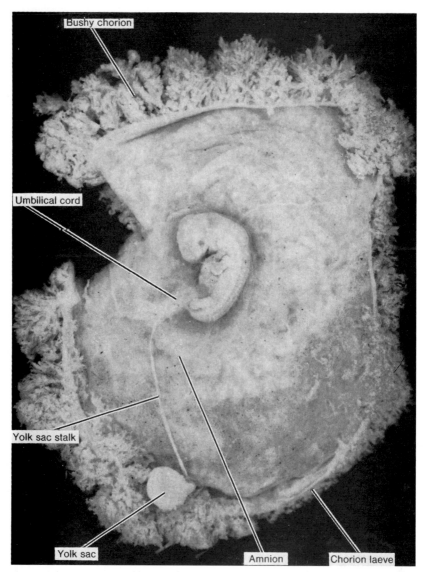

Figure 7.3. Photograph of a 6-week embryo. The amniotic sac and chorionic cavity have been opened to expose the embryo. Note the bushy appearance of the trophoblast at the embryonic pole in contrast to small villi at the abembryonic pole. Note also the connecting stalk and yolk sac with its extremely long duct.

As a result of the continuous growth of the fetus and expansion of the uterus, the placenta also enlarges. Its increase in surface area roughly parallels that of the expanding uterus, and throughout pregnancy it covers approximately 15–30% of the internal surface of the uterus. The increase in thickness of the placenta results from arborization of existing villi and is not caused by further penetration into maternal tissues.

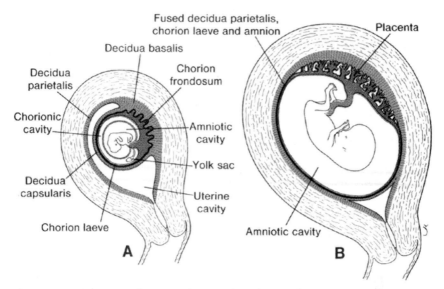

Decidua
parietalis

Decidua basalis

Fused decidua parietalis,
chorion laeve and amnion

Placenta

Chorion
frondosum

Chorionic
cavity

Amniotic
cavity

Yolk sac

Decidua
capsularis

Uterine
cavity

Chorion laeve

Amniotic cavity

A

B

Figure 7.4. Schematic drawings showing the relation of fetal membranes and wall of the uterus. **A.** End of the 2nd month. Note the yolk sac in the chorionic cavity between the amnion and chorion. At the abembryonic pole, villi have disappeared (chorion laeve). **B.** End of the 3rd month. The amnion and chorion have fused, and the uterine cavity is obliterated by fusion of the chorion laeve and the decidua parietalis.

Full-Term Placenta

At full term, the placenta has a discoid shape, a diameter of 15–25 cm, is approximately 3 cm thick, and has a weight of about 500–600 gm. At birth, it is torn from the uterine wall and, approximately 30 minutes after birth of the child, is expelled from the uterine cavity. When, after birth, the placenta is viewed from the **maternal side,** 15–20 slightly bulging areas, the **cotyledons,** covered by a thin layer of decidua basalis are clearly recognizable (Fig. 7.8*B*). Grooves between the cotyledons are formed by decidual septa. Much of the decidua remains temporarily in the uterus and is expelled with subsequent uterine bleeds.

The **fetal surface** of the placenta is covered entirely by the chorionic plate. A number of large arteries and veins, the **chorionic vessels,** converge toward the umbilical cord (Fig. 7.8*A*). The chorion, in turn, is covered by the amnion. Attachment of the umbilical cord is usually eccentric and occasionally even marginal. Rarely, however, does it insert into the chorionic membranes outside the placenta **(velamentous insertion).**

Circulation of the Placenta

Cotyledons receive their blood through 80–100 spiral arteries that pierce the decidual plate and enter the intervillous spaces at more or less regular intervals (Fig. 7.7). The lumen of the spiral artery is narrow, resulting in an increased

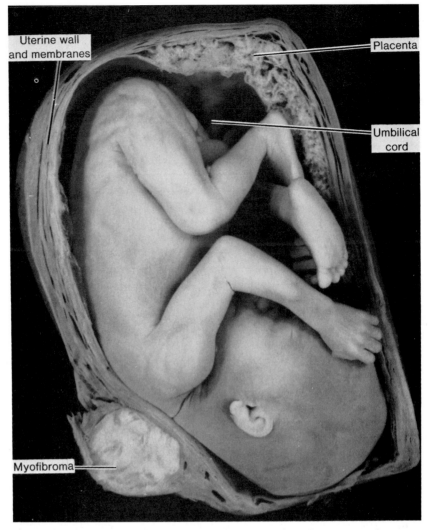

Figure 7.5. Photograph of a 19-week-old fetus in its natural position in the uterus. Note the umbilical cord and placenta. The lumen of the uterus is obliterated. In the wall of the uterus is a large growth, known as a myofibroma.

blood pressure when entering the intervillous space. This pressure forces the blood deep into the intervillous spaces and bathes the numerous small villi of the villous tree in oxygenated blood. As the pressure decreases, blood flows back from the chorionic plate toward the decidua, where it enters the endometrial veins (Fig. 7.7). Hence, blood from the intervillous lakes drains back into the maternal circulation through the endometrial veins.

Collectively, the intervillous spaces of a mature placenta contain approximately 150 mL of blood, which is replenished about 3 or 4 times/minute. This blood

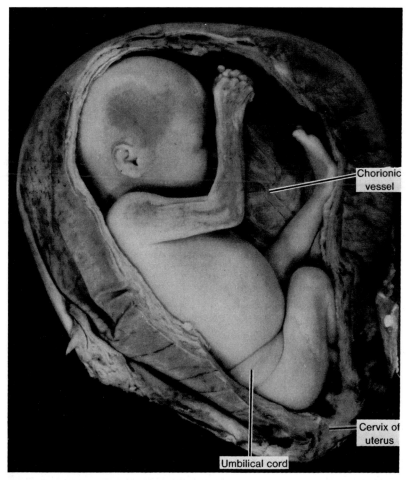

Figure 7.6. Photograph of a 23-week-old fetus in the uterus. Portions of the wall of the uterus and the amnion have been removed to show the fetus. In the background are placental vessels converging toward the umbilical cord. Note that the umbilical cord is tightly wound around the abdomen, possibly causing abnormal fetal position in the uterus (breech position).

The image is labeled: Chorionic vessel, Cervix of uterus, Umbilical cord.

moves along the chorionic villi, which have a surface area varying from 4 to 14 m². It must be remembered, however, that placental exchange does not take place in all villi, only in those in which fetal vessels are in intimate contact with the covering syncytial membrane. In these villi, the syncytium often has a brush border consisting of numerous microvilli, thus greatly increasing the surface area and, consequently, the exchange rate between maternal and fetal circulations (Fig. 7.2D). The **placental membrane** separates maternal and fetal blood and is initially composed of four layers: (a) the endothelial lining of fetal vessels; (b) the connective tissue in the villus core; (c) the cytotrophoblastic layer; and (d) the syncytium (Fig. 7.2C). From the 4th month on, however, the placental membrane

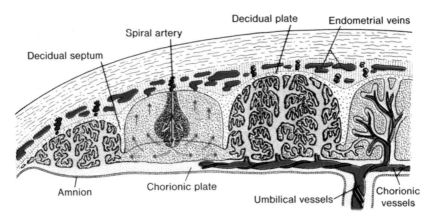

Figure 7.7. Composite drawing of the placenta in the second half of pregnancy. The cotyledons are partially separated from each other by the decidual (maternal) septa. Note that most of the intervillous blood returns to the maternal circulation by way of the endometrial veins. A small portion enters neighboring cotyledons. The intervillous spaces are lined by syncytium.

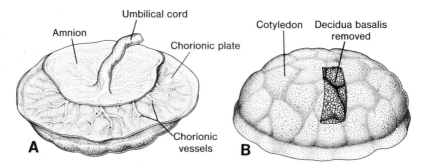

Figure 7.8. Drawing of a full-term placenta. **A.** As seen from the fetal side. Note that the chorionic plate and umbilical cord are covered by amnion. **B.** As seen from the maternal side. Note the cotyledons. In one area, the decidua has been removed. The maternal side of the placenta is always carefully inspected at birth, and frequently, one or more cotyledons with a whitish appearance are present due to excessive fibrinoid formation and infarction of a group of intervillous lakes.

becomes much thinner, since the endothelial lining of the vessels comes in intimate contact with the syncytial membrane, thus greatly increasing the rate of exchange (Fig. 7.2D). Sometimes called the **placental barrier,** the placental membrane is not a true barrier, since many substances pass through it freely. Since the maternal blood in the intervillous spaces is separated from the fetal blood by a chorionic derivative, the human placenta is considered to be of the **hemochorial** type.

Function of the Placenta

Main functions of the placenta are *(a)* **exchange of metabolic and gaseous products** between maternal and fetal bloodstreams and *(b)* **production of hormones.**

EXCHANGE OF GASES

Exchange of gases, such as oxygen, carbon dioxide, and carbon monoxide, is accomplished by simple diffusion. At term, the fetus extracts 20–30 mL of oxygen per minute from the maternal circulation, and it is understandable that even a short-term interruption of the oxygen supply will be fatal for the fetus. Placental blood flow is critical to oxygen supply, since the amount of oxygen reaching the fetus is primarily dependent on delivery and not diffusion.

EXCHANGE OF NUTRIENTS AND ELECTROLYTES

Exchange of nutrients and electrolytes, such as amino acids, free fatty acids, carbohydrates, and vitamins, is rapid and increases as pregnancy advances.

TRANSMISSION OF MATERNAL ANTIBODIES

Maternal antibodies are taken up by pinocytosis by the syncytiotrophoblast and subsequently transported to fetal capillaries. In this manner, the fetus acquires maternal antibodies of the immunoglobulin G (IgG) (7S) class against various infectious diseases and obtains passive immunity against diphtheria, smallpox, measles, and others but not against chickenpox and whooping cough. Passive immunity is important because the fetus has little capacity to produce its own antibodies until after birth.

CLINICAL CORRELATES

Of great importance is **Rh incompatibility,** which is related to erythrocyte antigens. If the fetus is Rh-positive and the mother Rh-negative, fetal red blood cells invading the maternal bloodstream may elicit an antibody response in the mother. Maternal antibodies against fetal antigens then return to the fetus and cause a breakdown of red blood cells. Small bleeds at the surface of the villi are probably responsible for this antigen-antibody interaction between fetus and mother. Breakdown of fetal red blood cells, known as **erythroblastosis fetalis** or **hemolytic disease of the newborn (HDN)** may lead to intrauterine death. Spectrophotometric analysis of amniotic fluid may provide an indication about the extent of the disease, and intrauterine blood transfusions into the fetus or exchange transfusions after birth may prevent death. **Rh immunoglobulin** given to the mother prevents the disease and has significantly lowered its occurrence and the requirement for fetal transfusion.

HORMONE PRODUCTION

By the end of the 4th month, the placenta produces **progesterone** in sufficient amounts to maintain pregnancy in case the corpus luteum is removed or fails to function properly. In all probability, all hormones are synthesized in the syncytial trophoblast. In addition to progesterone, the placenta produces increasing amounts of **estrogenic hormones (predominately estriol)** until just before the end of pregnancy, when a maximum level is reached. These high levels of estrogens stimulate uterine growth and development of the mammary gland.

The syncytiotrophoblast also produces **gonadotropins (human chorionic gonadotropin or hCG),** which have an effect similar to that of luteinizing hormones of the anterior lobe of the pituitary. These hormones are excreted by the mother in the urine, and in the early stages of gestation, their presence is used as an indicator of pregnancy. Another hormone produced by the placenta is **somatomammotropin** (formerly **placental lactogen**). It is a growth hormone-like substance that gives the fetus priority on maternal blood glucose and makes the mother somewhat diabetogenic.

CLINICAL CORRELATES

Most maternal hormones do not cross the placenta. Those hormones that do cross, such as thyroxine, do so only at a slow rate. Of great danger are some synthetic progestins that cross the placenta at a rapid rate and may cause masculinization in female fetuses. Even more dangerous has been the use of the synthetic estrogen **diethylstilbestrol,** which easily crosses the placenta. This compound produces carcinoma of the vagina and abnormalities of the testes in individuals who were exposed to it during their intrauterine life (see Chapter 8).

Although the placental barrier is frequently considered to act as a protective mechanism against damaging factors, many viruses, such as rubella, cytomegalovirus, Coxsackie, variola, varicella, measles, and poliomyelitis virus, traverse the placenta without difficulty. Once in the fetus, some viruses cause infections, which, in turn, may result in cell death and birth defects (see Chapter 8).

Unfortunately, most drugs and drug metabolites traverse the placenta without difficulty and many cause serious damage to the embryo (see Chapter 8). In addition, fetal drug addiction can occur after maternal use of heroin and cocaine.

Amnion and Umbilical Cord

The line of reflection between the amnion and embryonic ectoderm (**amnio-ectodermal junction**) is oval and is known as the **primitive umbilical ring.** At the 5th week of development, the following structures pass through the ring (Fig. 7.9, *A* and *C*): (*a*) the **connecting stalk,** containing the allantois and the umbilical vessels consisting of two arteries and one vein; (*b*) the **yolk stalk (vitelline duct)** accompanied by the vitelline vessels; and (*c*) the **canal connecting the intraembryonic and extraembryonic coelomic cavities** (Fig. 7.9*C*). The yolk sac proper occupies a space in the **chorionic cavity,** i.e. , the space between the amnion and chorionic plate (Fig. 7.9*B*).

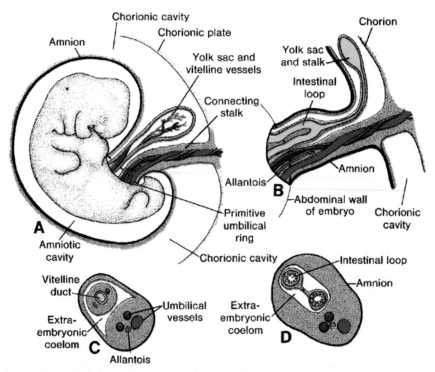

Figure 7.9. **A.** Schematic drawing of a 5-week embryo to show structures passing through the primitive umbilical ring. **B.** Schematic drawing of the primitive umbilical cord of a 10-week embryo. **C.** Transverse section through the structures at the level of the umbilical ring. **D.** Transverse section through the primitive umbilical cord, showing intestinal loops protruding in the cord.

During further development, the amniotic cavity enlarges rapidly at the expense of the chorionic cavity, and the amnion begins to envelop the connecting and yolk sac stalks, thereby crowding them together and causing formation of the **primitive umbilical cord** (Fig. 7.9B). Distally, the cord then contains the yolk sac stalk and umbilical vessels. More proximally, it contains some intestinal loops and the remnant of the allantois (Fig. 7.9, B and D). The yolk sac is found in the chorionic cavity and is connected to the umbilical cord by its stalk. At the end of the 3rd month, the amnion has expanded to such an extent that it comes in contact with the chorion, thereby obliterating the chorionic cavity (Fig. 7.4B). The yolk sac then usually shrinks and is gradually obliterated.

The abdominal cavity is temporarily too small for the rapidly developing intestinal loops, and some of them are pushed into the extraembryonic coelomic space in the umbilical cord. These extruding intestinal loops form a **physiological umbilical hernia** (see Chapter 14). At about the end of the 3rd month, the loops are withdrawn into the body of the embryo, and the coelomic cavity in the cord is obliterated. When, in addition, the allantois and the vitelline duct and its vessels are obliterated, all that remains in the cord are the umbilical vessels surrounded by the **jelly of Wharton.** This tissue is rich in proteoglycans and functions as a protective layer for the blood vessels. The walls of the arteries are muscular and contain many elastic fibers, which contribute to a rapid constriction and contraction of the umbilical vessels after the cord is tied off.

CLINICAL CORRELATES

Normally, there are two arteries and one vein in the umbilical cord. In 1 in 200 newborns, however, only one artery is present, and these babies have an approximately 20% chance of having cardiac and other vascular defects. The missing artery either fails to form (agenesis) or degenerates early in development.

Occasionally, tears in the amnion result in **amniotic bands** that may encircle part of the fetus, particularly the limbs and digits. Amputations, **ring constrictions,** and other abnormalities may result, including craniofacial deformations (Fig. 7.10). Origin of the bands is probably from infections or toxic insults that involve either the fetus, fetal membranes, or both. Bands then form from the amnion, like scar tissue, constricting fetal structures.

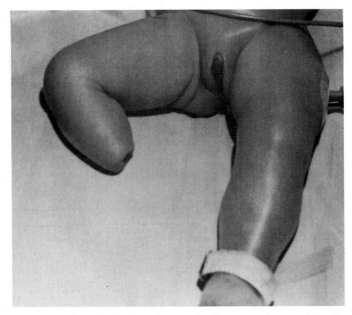

Figure 7.10. Photograph of infant showing limb amputation resulting from amniotic bands.

PLACENTAL CHANGES AT THE END OF PREGNANCY

At the end of pregnancy, a number of changes occur in the placenta that may be indications of reduced exchange between the two circulations. These changes include *(a)* an increase in fibrous tissue in the core of the villus, *(b)* an increase in thickness of basement membranes in fetal capillaries, *(c)* obliterative changes in small capillaries of the villi, and *(d)* deposition of fibrinoid on the surface of the villi in the junctional zone and in the chorionic plate. Excessive fibrinoid formation frequently causes infarction of an intervillous lake or sometimes of an entire cotyledon. The cotyledon then assumes a whitish appearance.

At birth, the umbilical cord is approximately 2 cm in diameter and 50–60 cm long. It is tortuous, causing **false knots.** An extremely long cord may encircle the neck of the fetus, usually without increased risk, whereas a short one may cause difficulties during delivery by pulling the placenta from its attachment in the uterus.

AMNIOTIC FLUID

The amniotic cavity is filled with a clear, watery fluid that is produced, in part, by amniotic cells but is derived primarily from maternal blood. The amount of fluid increases from approximately 30 mL at 10 weeks gestation, to 350 mL at 20 weeks, to 800–1000 mL at 37 weeks. During the early months of pregnancy, the embryo is suspended by its umbilical cord in this fluid, which serves as a protective cushion. The fluid *(a)* absorbs jolts, *(b)* prevents adherence of the embryo to the amnion, and *(c)* allows for fetal movements. The volume of amniotic fluid is replaced every 3 hours. From the beginning of the 5th month, the fetus swallows its own amniotic fluid, and it is estimated that it drinks about 400 mL/day, which is about half of the total amount. Fetal urine is added daily to the amniotic fluid in the 5th month, but this urine is mostly water, since the placenta is functioning as an exchange for metabolic wastes. During childbirth, the amniochorionic membrane forms a hydrostatic wedge that helps to dilate the cervical canal.

CLINICAL CORRELATES

Premature rupture of the amnion occurs in 10% of pregnancies and represents the most common cause of preterm labor. Furthermore, clubfoot and lung hypoplasia may be caused by **oligohydramnios** following amnion rupture. Causes for rupture are largely unknown, but in some cases, trauma plays a role.

Hydramnios or **polyhydramnios** is the term used to describe an excess of amniotic fluid (1500–2000 mL), whereas **oligohydramnios** refers to a decreased amount (less than 400 mL). Both conditions are associated with an increased incidence of birth defects. Primary causes of hydramnios include idiopathic causes (35%), maternal diabetes (25%), and congenital malformations, including central nervous system disorders (e.g., anencephaly) and gastrointestinal defects (atresias, e.g., esophageal) that prevent the infant from swallowing the fluid. Oligohydramnios is a rare occurrence that may result from renal agenesis.

Fetal Membranes in Twins

Arrangement of fetal membranes in twins varies considerably and is dependent on the type of twins as well as on the time of separation of **monozygotic twins.**

DIZYGOTIC TWINS

Approximately two-thirds of twins are dizygotic or fraternal, and their incidence of 7–11/1000 births increases with increasing maternal age. They result from simultaneous shedding of two oocytes and fertilization by two different spermatozoa. Since both zygotes have a totally different genetic constitution, the twins have no more resemblance than brothers or sisters. They may or may not be of different sex. Both zygotes implant individually in the uterus, and each develops its own placenta, its own amnion, and its own chorionic sac (Fig. 7.11A). Sometimes, however, the two placentas are located so close together that fusion occurs. Similarly, the walls of the chorionic sacs may also come into close apposition and fuse (Fig. 7.11B). Occasionally, each member of dizygotic twins possesses red blood cells of two different types **(erythrocyte mosaicism),** indicating that fusion of the two placentas was so intimate that red cells were exchanged.

MONOZYGOTIC TWINS

The second type of twins develops from a single fertilized ovum and is known as **monozygotic** or **identical twins.** The twinning rate for monozygotic twins is 3–4/1000. They result from splitting of the zygote at various stages of development. The earliest separation is believed to occur at the two-cell stage, in which case two separate zygotes develop. Both blastocysts implant separately, and each embryo has its own placenta and chorionic sac (Fig. 7.12A). Although the arrangement of the membranes of these twins resembles that of dizygotic twins, the two can be recognized as partners of a monozygotic pair by their strong resemblance in blood groups, fingerprints, sex, and external appearance, such as eye and hair color.

In most cases, splitting of the zygote occurs at the early blastocyst stage. The inner cell mass splits into two separate groups of cells within the same blastocyst cavity (Fig. 7.12B). The two embryos have a common placenta and a common chorionic cavity but have separate amniotic cavities (Fig. 7.12B). In rare cases, the separation occurs at the bilaminar germ disc stage just before the appearance of the primitive streak (Fig. 7.12C). This method of splitting results in formation of two partners with a single placenta and a common chorionic and amnion sac. Although the twins have a common placenta, blood supply to each of the partners is usually well balanced.

Although the occurrence of triplets is not uncommon (1 in about 7600 pregnancies), birth of quadruplets, quintuplets, and so forth is rare. In recent years, multiple births, such as sextuplets, have occurred more frequently in mothers given gonadotropins (fertility drugs) for ovulatory failure.

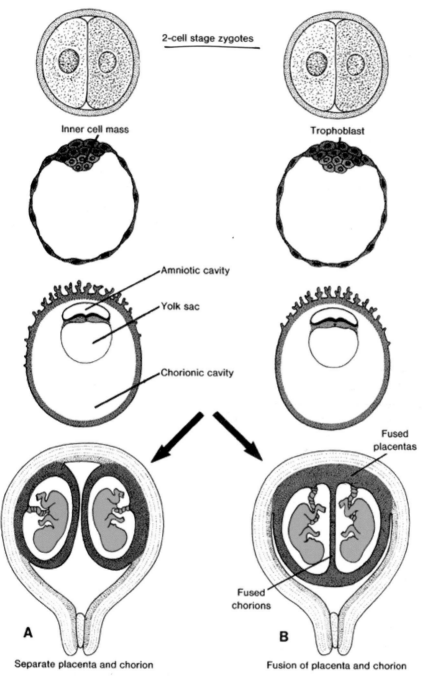

2-cell stage zygotes

Inner cell mass

Trophoblast

Amniotic cavity

Yolk sac

Chorionic cavity

Fused placentas

Fused chorions

A

B

Separate placenta and chorion

Fusion of placenta and chorion

Figure 7.11. Schematic drawings showing development of dizygotic twins. Normally, each embryo has its own amnion, chorion, and placenta **(A)**, but sometimes the placentas are fused **(B).** Each embryo usually receives the appropriate amount of blood, but on occasion, more blood is shunted to one of the partners through large anastomoses.

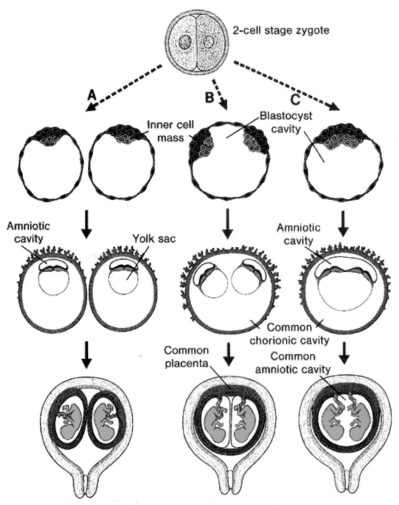

Figure 7.12. Schematic diagrams showing the possible relations of fetal membranes in monozygotic twins. **A.** Splitting occurs at the two-cell stage, and each embryo has its own placenta, amniotic cavity, and chorionic cavity. **B.** Splitting of the inner cell mass into two completely separated groups. The two embryos have a common placenta and a common chorionic sac but have separate amniotic cavities. **C.** Splitting of the inner cell mass at a late stage of development. The embryos have a common placenta, a common amniotic cavity, and a common chorionic cavity.

CLINICAL CORRELATES

Twin pregnancies have a higher incidence of perinatal mortality and morbidity and a tendency toward preterm delivery. Approximately 12% of premature infants result from twin pregnancies, and twins are usually smaller at birth. Low birth weight and prematurity place infants of twin pregnancies at great risk, and approximately 10–20% of them will die compared with only 2% of infants from single pregnancies.

The incidence of twinning may be much higher, since twins are conceived more often than they are born. Many twins die before birth, and some studies indicate that only 29% of women pregnant with twins actually give birth to two infants. The term **vanishing twin** refers to the death of one fetus. This disappearance occurs in the 1st trimester or early 2nd trimester and may result from resorption or formation of a **fetus papyraceus** (Fig. 7.13).

Another problem leading to increased mortality among twins is the **twin transfusion syndrome**, which occurs in 5–15% of monochorionic monozygotic pregnancies. In this condition, placental vascular anastomoses, which occur in a balanced arrangement in most monochorionic placentas, are formed such that one twin receives most of the blood flow while the other is compromised. As a result, one twin is larger than the other (Fig. 7.14). The outcome is poor, with the death of both twins occurring in 60–100% of cases.

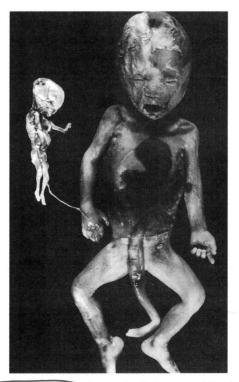

Figure 7.13. Fetus papyraceus. One twin is larger, while the other has been compressed and mummified, hence the term papyraceus.

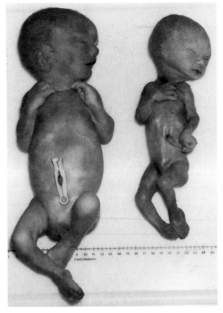

Figure 7.14. Monozygotic twins with twin transfusion syndrome. Placental vascular anastomoses produced unbalanced blood flow to the two fetuses.

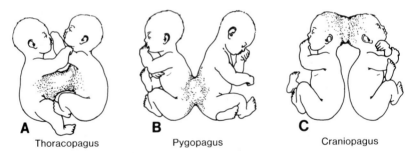

A	B	C
Thoracopagus	Pygopagus	Craniopagus

Figure 7.15. Schematic drawings of thoracopagus, pygopagus, and craniopagus twins. Conjoined twins can be separated only if they have no vital parts in common.

Splitting of the zygote during later stages of development may result in an abnormal or incomplete splitting of the axial area of the germ disc. Such incompletely separated discs lead to formation of **conjoined (Siamese) twins.** According to the nature and degree of the union, they are classified as **thoracopagus** (*pagos,* fastened), **pygopagus,** and **craniopagus** (Figs. 7.15 and 7.16). Occasionally, partners of monozygotic twins are connected to each other only by a common skin bridge or by a common liver bridge. Several conjoined twins have successfully been separated by surgical procedures.

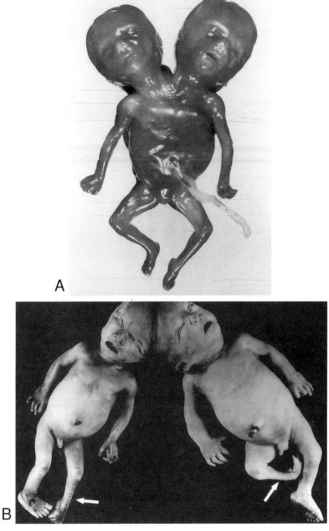

Figure 7.16. Examples of conjoined twins. **A.** Twins with two heads, a broad thorax, two spines, two partially fused hearts, four lungs, and a duplicated gut down to the ileum. **B.** Twins joined at the head (craniopagus) with multiple deformations of the limbs.

SUMMARY

The **placenta** consists of two components: *(a)* a fetal portion, derived from the **chorion frondosum** or **villous chorion,** and *(b)* a maternal portion, derived from the **decidua basalis.** The space between the chorionic and decidual plates is filled with **intervillous lakes** of maternal blood. **Villous trees** (fetal tissue) grow into the maternal blood lakes and are bathed in them. The fetal circulation is at all times separated from the maternal circulation by *(a)* a syncytial membrane (a chorion derivative) and *(b)* endothelial cells from fetal capillaries. Hence, the human placenta is of the **hemochorial** type.

Intervillous lakes of the fully grown placenta contain approximately 150 mL of maternal blood, which is renewed 3 or 4 times/minute. The villous area varies from 4 to 14 m^2, thus facilitating exchange between mother and child.

Main functions of the placenta are *(a)* exchange of gases; *(b)* exchange of nutrients and electrolytes; *(c)* transmission of maternal antibodies, providing the fetus with passive immunity; *(d)* production of hormones, such as progesterone, estradiol, and estrogen (in addition, it produces chorionic gonadotropin [hCG] and somatomammotropin); and *(e)* detoxification of some drugs.

The **amnion** provides a large sac containing amniotic fluid in which the fetus is suspended by its umbilical cord. The fluid *(a)* absorbs jolts, *(b)* allows for fetal movements, and *(c)* prevents adherency of the embryo to surrounding tissues. The fetus swallows amniotic fluid, which is absorbed through its gut and cleared by the placenta. The fetus adds urine to the amniotic fluid, but this is mostly water. An increased amount of amniotic fluid (hydramnios) is associated with anencephaly and esophageal atresia, whereas a decreased amount (oligohydramnios) is related to renal agenesis.

The **umbilical cord** is surrounded by the amnion and contains *(a)* two umbilical arteries, *(b)* one umbilical vein, and *(c)* Wharton's jelly, which serves as a protective cushion for the vessels.

Fetal membranes in twins vary according to their origin and time of formation. Two-thirds of twins are **dizygotic** or **fraternal twins** and have two amnions, two chorions, and two placentas, which sometimes are fused. **Monozygotic twins** usually have two amnions, one chorion, and one placenta. In cases of **conjoined twins,** in which the fetuses are not entirely split from each other, there is one amnion, one chorion, and one placenta.

PROBLEMS TO SOLVE

1. An ultrasound at 7 months of gestation shows too much space (fluid accumulation) in the amniotic cavity. What is this condition called, and what are its causes?

2. Later in her pregnancy, a woman realizes that she was probably exposed to toluene in the workplace during the 3rd week of gestation but tells a fellow worker that she is not concerned about her baby because the placenta protects her infant from toxic factors by acting as a barrier. Is she correct?

SUGGESTED READINGS

Bassett JM: Current perspectives on placental development and its integration with fetal growth. *Proc Nutr Soc* 50:311, 1991.
Benirschke K: Implantation, placental development and uteroplacental blood flow. *In* Reid DE, Ryan KJ, Benirschke K (eds): *Principles and Management of Human Reproduction.* Philadelphia, WB Saunders, 1972.

Benirschke K, Kaufman P: *The Pathology of the Human Placenta.* Berlin, Springer-Verlag, 1990.

Bergsma D (ed): Conjoined twins. *Birth Defects* III(1):1–147, 1967.

Bisonnette J: Placental and fetal physiology. *In* Gabbe SG, Neibyl JR, Simpson JL (eds): *Obstetrics, Normal and Problem Pregnancies.* New York, Churchill Livingstone, 1986.

Bulmer MJ: *The Biology of Twinning in Man.* Oxford, Clarendon Press, 1970.

Chamberlain G, Wilkinson A (eds): *Placental Transfer.* Baltimore, University Park Press, 1979.

Gadd RL: The liquor amnii. *In* Philipp EE, Barnes J, Newton M (eds): *Scientific Foundations of Obstetrics and Gynecology.* Philadelphia, FA Davis, 1970.

Hay WW: In vivo measurements of placental transport and metabolism. *Proc Nutr Soc* 50:355, 1991.

Levi S: Ultrasonic assessment of the high rate of human multiple pregnancy in the first trimester. *J Clin Ultrasound* 4:3, 1976.

Naeye RL: *Disorders of the Placenta, Fetus, and Neonate.* St Louis, Mosby-Year Book, 1992.

Neubert D, Merker HJ, Nau H, Langman J: *Role of Pharmacokinetics in Prenatal and Perinatal Toxicology.* Stuttgart, Georg Thieme, 1978.

Nyberg DA, Callan PW: Ultrasound evaluation of the placenta. *In* Callen PW (ed): *Ultrasonography in Obstetrics and Gynecology.* 2nd ed. Philadelphia, WB Saunders, 1988.

Peipert JF, Donnenfeld AE: Oligohydramnios: a review. *Obstet Gynecol* 46:325, 1991.

Petraglia F, Angioni S, Coukos G, Uccelli E, Diodmenica P, Deramundo BM, Genazzani AD, Garuti GC, Segre A: Neuroendocrine mechanisms regulating placental hormone production. *Contrib Gynecol Obstet* 18:147, 1991.

Schnaufer L: Conjoined twins. *In* Raffensperger JG (ed): *Swenson's Pediatric Surgery.* 5th ed. Norwalk, CT, Appleton & Lange, 1990.

Spencer R: Conjoined twins: theoretical embryologic basis. *Teratology* 45:591, 1992.

Wallenburg HCS, Wladimiroff JW: The amniotic fluid: II. Polyhydramnios and oligohydramnios. *J Perinat Med* 6:233, 1977.

chapter 8

Congenital Malformations

Congenital malformations, congenital anomalies, and **birth defects** are synonymous terms used to describe structural, behavioral, functional, and metabolic disorders present at birth. The science that studies the causes of these disorders is **teratology** (Gr. *teratos*, monster). Major structural anomalies occur in 2–3% of liveborn infants, and an additional 2–3% are recognized in children by age 5 years for a total of 4–6%. Birth defects are the leading cause of infant mortality (Fig. 8.1), accounting for approximately 21% of all infant deaths. They are the 5th leading cause of years of potential life lost (Fig. 8.2) prior to age 65 and a major contributor to disabilities. They are also nondiscriminatory, such that mortality rates produced by birth defects are the same for Asians, African Americans, Latin Americans, Caucasians, and Native Americans.

In 40–60% of all birth defects, the cause is unknown. Genetic factors, such as chromosome abnormalities and mutant genes, account for approximately 15%; environmental factors produce approximately 10%; a combination of genetic and environmental influences (multifactorial inheritance) produces 20–25%; and twinning causes 0.5–1%.

Minor anomalies occur in approximately 15% of newborns. These structural abnormalities, such as microtia (small ears), pigmented spots, and short palpebral fissures, are not detrimental to the health of the individual but in some cases are associated with major defects. For example, infants with one minor anomaly have a 3% chance of having a major malformation; those with two minor anomalies have a 10% chance; and those with three or more minor anomalies have a 20% chance. Therefore, minor anomalies serve as clues for diagnosing more serious underlying defects.

There are several types of anomalies:

① **Malformations** occur during formation of structures, e.g., during organo-genesis. They may result in complete or partial absence of a structure or in alterations of its normal configuration. Malformations are caused by environmental and/or genetic factors acting independently or in concert. Most malformations have their origin during the **3rd to 8th weeks of gestation.**

② **Disruptions** result in morphological alterations of structures after their formation and are due to destructive processes. Vascular accidents leading to bowel atresias (see Chapter 12) and defects produced by amniotic bands (see Chapter 9) are examples of destructive factors that produce disruptions.

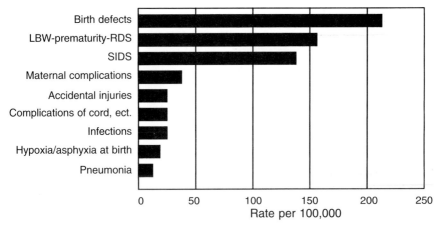

Figure 8.1. Graph showing that birth defects are the leading cause of infant mortality in the United States in 1988. *LBW,* low birth weight; *RDS,* respiratory distress syndrome; and *SIDS,* sudden infant death syndrome.

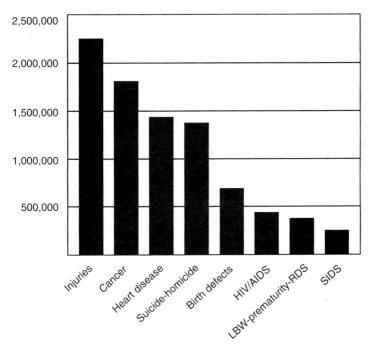

Figure 8.2. Graph showing that birth defects are the 5th leading cause of years of potential life lost before age 65 in the United States in 1988.

③ **Deformations** are due to mechanical forces that mold a part of the fetus over a prolonged period of time. Clubfeet, due to compression in the amniotic cavity, are an example. Deformations often involve the musculoskeletal system and may be reversible postnatally.

④ **Syndrome** refers to a group of anomalies occurring together that have a specific, common etiology. This term indicates that a diagnosis has been made and that the risk of recurrence is known. In contrast, **association** refers to the nonrandom appearance of two or more anomalies that occur together more frequently than by chance alone but for which the etiology has not been determined. Examples include **CHARGE** (**c**olobomas, **h**eart defects, **a**tresia of the choanae, **r**etarded growth, **g**enital anomalies, and **e**ar abnormalities) and **VACTERL** (**v**ertebral, **a**nal, **c**ardiac, **t**racheoesophageal, **r**enal, and **l**imb anomalies). Associations are important because, although they do not constitute a diagnosis, recognition of one or more of the components promotes the search for others in the group.

Environmental Factors

Until the early 1940's, it was assumed that congenital defects were caused primarily by hereditary factors. With the discovery by Gregg that German measles affecting a mother during early pregnancy caused abnormalities in the embryo, it suddenly became evident that congenital malformations in humans could also be caused by environmental factors.

Observations by Lenz, linking limb defects to the sedative **thalidomide** in 1961, made it clear that drugs could cross the placenta and produce birth defects. Since that time, many agents have been identified as **teratogens** (factors that cause anomalies) (see Table 8.1, page 139).

INFECTIOUS AGENTS

Rubella or German Measles

Gregg was the first to suggest that German measles affecting pregnant women in the early stages of gestation could lead to congenital malformations in the offspring. At present, it is well established that **rubella virus** can cause malformations of the eye (cataract and microphthalmia); internal ear (congenital deafness due to destruction of the organ of Corti); heart (persistence of the ductus arteriosus as well as atrial and ventricular septal defects); and, occasionally, teeth (enamel layer). The virus may also be responsible for some cases of brain abnormalities and mental retardation. More recently, it has become evident that the virus also causes intrauterine growth retardation, myocardial damage, and vascular abnormalities.

The type of malformation is determined by the stage of embryonic development at which infection occurs. For example, cataracts result from infection during the 6th week of pregnancy and deafness from infection during the 9th week. Cardiac defects follow infection in the 5th to 10th weeks, and dental deformities follow infection between the 6th and 9th weeks. Abnormalities of the central nervous system follow infection in the 2nd trimester.

It is extremely difficult to determine the exact incidence of malformation in the offspring of infected mothers, since German measles may be mild and thus escape detection or may be accompanied by unusual clinical features and remain unrecognized. Furthermore, as pointed out above, some birth defects are not recognized until the child is 2–4 years of age. On the other hand, rashes caused by other viruses may be incorrectly attributed to rubella.

In a prospective study on the effect of rubella virus, the risk of malformations in infants examined immediately after birth was estimated at 47% when the infection occurred during the first 4 weeks of pregnancy; 22% following infection in the 5th to 8th weeks; 7% following infection in the 9th to 12th weeks; and 6% following infection in the 13th to 16th weeks. Prematurity and fetal death may also follow infection in the first 8 weeks.

If abnormalities such as mental retardation and dental defects, which do not become evident until later in life, were to be considered, it is likely that the above percentages would be higher (65% of congenital deafness due to rubella is not discovered until the 4th year).

In the past decade, two important advances have been made. Laboratory tests are now available that permit detection of the virus in specimens from patients and determination of antibody levels in the serum of patients. An important application of this test is to determine if a patient is immune and, therefore, need not fear the occurrence of rubella during pregnancy. An epidemiological study of 600 women has shown that 85% were immune. A second important advance was the discovery that the virus infects the fetus by way of the placenta and that the infection of the child may persist after birth for a number of months or years. These children, who usually show no sign of infection, can transmit the virus to hospital personnel, such as nurses, doctors, and other hospital attendants. Safe and effective vaccines for rubella have recently been developed and administered.

Cytomegalovirus

Cytomegalovirus has been positively identified as causing malformations and chronic fetal infection, which persists after birth. The congenital cytomegalic inclusion disease is, in all probability, the result of a human cytomegalovirus infection acquired in utero from an asymptomatically infected mother. Principal findings of the infection are microcephaly, cerebral calcifications, blindness and chorioretinitis, and hepatosplenomegaly. Some infants have kernicterus and multiple petechiae of the skin. Initially, the disease was recognized only at autopsy and was based on the presence of enlarged cells, with large nuclei containing giant inclusion bodies. The inclusion bodies are most common in cells lining the renal tubules and may be present in the urine. The disease is often fatal when affecting the embryo or fetus, but in case of survival, meningoencephalitis may cause mental retardation. Since the disease is usually unrecognized in pregnant women, it is not known what the difference is between an early and a late infection during development. It seems likely that when the embryo is affected at an early stage of development, the damage is so severe that it is unable to survive. Those cases that come to our attention are probably fetuses that have been infected only late in pregnancy.

Herpes Simplex Virus

There are a few reports in the literature that show that intrauterine infection of the fetus with **herpes simplex** occasionally occurs. Usually, the infection is transmitted close to the time of delivery, and the abnormalities reported are microcephaly, microphthalmos, retinal dysplasia, hepatosplenomegaly, and mental retardation. In most cases, however, the child acquires the infection from the mother at birth as a venereal disease, and symptoms of the disease then develop during the first 3 weeks of age. These symptoms are characterized by inflammatory reactions.

Varicella (Chickenpox)

There is approximately a 20% chance of congenital anomalies occurring following maternal **varicella** infection in the 1st trimester. Defects include limb hypoplasia, mental retardation, and muscle atrophy.

Human Immunodeficiency Virus (HIV)

This virus causes **acquired immunodeficiency disease (AIDS)** and may be transmitted to the fetus. The virus does not appear to be a major teratogen, although microcephaly, growth retardation, and abnormal facies have been attributed to its effects.

Other Viral Infections and Hyperthermia

Malformations following maternal infection with measles, mumps, hepatitis, poliomyelitis, ECHO virus, Coxsackie virus, and influenza virus have been described. Prospective studies indicate, however, that the malformation rate following exposure to these agents is low if not nonexistent.

A complicating factor introduced by these and other infectious agents is that most are **pyrogenic** and increased body temperature (**hyperthermia**) is teratogenic. In one report, 7 of 63 (11%) anencephalic infants were born to mothers with a history of hyperthermia at the time that, in the embryo, the neural folds are closing. Interestingly, in two of these cases the episode of hyperthermia appeared to be related to sauna bathing and not to infection.

Toxoplasmosis

Maternal infection with the protozoan parasite *Toxoplasma gondii,* acquired from poorly cooked meat, domestic animals (cats), or soil contaminated with feces, has been shown to produce congenital malformations. The affected child may have cerebral calcification, hydrocephalus, or mental retardation. Chorioretinitis, microphthalmos, and other ocular defects have also been reported. It is impossible to give precise figures on the incidence of malformations caused by toxoplasmosis, since, as in the case of cytomegalovirus, the disease is usually unrecognized in pregnant women.

Syphilis

Syphilis is increasing in incidence and may lead to congenital deafness and mental retardation in the offspring. In addition, many other organs, such as the lungs and liver, are characterized by diffuse fibrosis.

RADIATION

The teratogenic effect of **ionizing radiation** has been known for many years, and it is well recognized that microcephaly, skull defects, spina bifida, blindness, cleft palate, and defects of the extremities may result from treating pregnant women with large doses of x-rays or radium. Although the maximum safe dose for the human fetus is not known, in mice the fetus can be damaged with a dose as small as 5 rad. It must be realized that the nature of the malformation depends on the dose of radiation and the stage of development at which the radiation is given.

Studies of the offspring of Japanese women pregnant at the time of the atomic bomb explosions over Hiroshima and Nagasaki revealed that among the survivors, 28% aborted, 25% gave birth to children who died in their 1st year of life, and 25% of the surviving children had abnormalities of the central nervous system, such as microcephaly and mental retardation.

In addition to the effect of direct radiation on the embryo, indirect effects on germ cells must be considered. Indeed, relatively small doses of radiation in mice have been shown to cause mutations that subsequently led to the occurrence of congenital malformations in succeeding generations.

CHEMICAL AGENTS

The role of chemical agents and pharmaceutical drugs in the production of abnormalities in humans is difficult to assess for two reasons: *(a)* most studies are retrospective, relying on the mother's memory for a history of exposure; and *(b)* there is such a large number of pharmaceutical drugs employed by pregnant women. A National Institutes of Health study discovered that among pregnant women, 900 different drugs were taken, for an average of 4/woman. Only 20% of pregnant women used no drugs during their pregnancy. Even with this widespread use of chemical agents, relatively few of the many drugs used during pregnancy have been positively identified as being teratogenic. One example is **thalidomide,** an antinauseant and sleeping pill. In 1961, it was noted in West Germany that the frequency of **amelia** and **meromelia** (total or partial absence of the extremities), a rare hereditary abnormality, had suddenly increased (Fig. 8.3). This observation led to examination of the prenatal histories of affected children, resulting in the discovery that many mothers had taken thalidomide early in pregnancy. The causal relationship between thalidomide and meromelia was discovered only because the drug produced such an unusual type of abnormality. If the defect had been of a more common type, such as cleft lip or

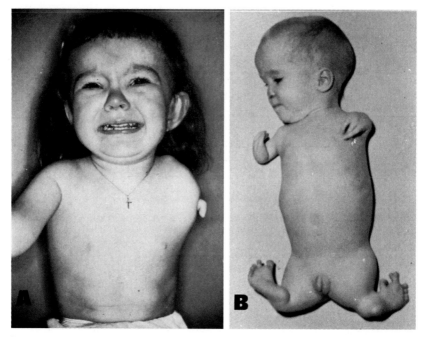

Figure 8.3. A. Photograph of a child with unilateral amelia. **B.** Patient with meromelia. The hand is attached to the trunk by an irregularly shaped bone. Both infants were born to mothers who took thalidomide.

heart malformations, the association with the drug might easily have been overlooked.

Defects produced by thalidomide are absence or gross deformities of the long bones, intestinal atresia, and cardiac abnormalities. As a result of the discovery that thalidomide was directly related to meromelia, the drug was immediately removed from the market. The incidence of meromelia has since been reduced dramatically.

Another dangerous drug is **aminopterin.** This compound belongs to the antimetabolites, is an **antagonist of folic acid,** and has been used as an **antineoplastic** agent. Defects produced by aminopterin include anencephaly, meningocele, hydrocephalus, and cleft lip and palate. Since many **antineoplastic** agents inhibit mitosis, it is not surprising that they are potent teratogens.

Other drugs also have teratogenic potential, including the anticonvulsants **diphenylhydantoin (phenytoin), valproic acid,** and **trimethadione,** which are used by **epileptic women.** In a retrospective study on 427 pregnancies in 186 epileptic women, the frequency of major malformations such as heart abnormalities, facial clefts, and microcephaly was twice as high as expected. Specifically, diphenylhydantoin produces a broad spectrum of abnormalities, including craniofacial defects, nail and digital hypoplasia, growth abnormalities, and mental deficiency. These defects constitute a distinct pattern of dysmorphogenesis known as the **"fetal hydantoin syndrome."**

Valproic acid produces neural tube defects and heart, craniofacial, and limb anomalies. **Trimethadione,** used in the treatment of petit mal seizures, produces a characteristic pattern of abnormalities, including malformed ears, cleft palate, cardiac defects, and urogenital and skeletal anomalies, that, collectively, are referred to as the **"trimethadione syndrome."** As with diphenylhydantoin, delayed physical and mental development are also components of the syndrome.

Antipsychotic and **antianxiety agents** (major and minor tranquilizers, respectively) are suspected producers of congenital malformations. The antipsychotics **phenothiazine** and **lithium** have been implicated as teratogens. Although evidence for the teratogenicity of phenothiazines is conflicting, that concerning lithium has been better documented. In any case, it has been strongly suggested that use of these agents during pregnancy carries a high risk.

Similar observations have been made for the antianxiety agents **meprobamate, chlordiazepoxide,** and **diazepam (Valium).** In a prospective study it was observed that severe anomalies occurred in 12% of infants from mothers exposed to meprobamate and 11% in those exposed to chlordiazepoxide, compared with 2.6% of controls. Likewise, retrospective studies with diazepam have demonstrated up to a fourfold increase in cleft lip with or without cleft palate in offspring from mothers taking the drug during pregnancy.

The **anticoagulant, warfarin,** is teratogenic, whereas **heparin** does not appear to be. Warfarin causes hypoplasia of the nasal cartilage, chondrodysplasia, central nervous system defects, including mental retardation, and atrophy of the optic nerves.

Antihypertensive agents that inhibit **angiotensin-converting enzyme (ACE inhibitors)** produce growth retardation, renal dysfunction, fetal death, and oligohydramnios.

In addition to the drugs discussed in some detail, caution has been expressed regarding a number of other compounds that might be damaging to the embryo or fetus. The most prominent among these are propylthiouracil and potassium iodide (goiter and mental retardation), streptomycin (deafness), sulfonamides (kernicterus), the antidepressant imipramine (limb deformities), tetracyclines (bone and tooth anomalies), amphetamines (oral clefts and cardiovascular abnormalities), and quinine (deafness). Finally, there is increasing evidence that aspirin (salicylates), the most commonly ingested drug during pregnancy, is potentially harmful to the developing offspring when used in large doses.

One of the increasing problems in today's society is the effect of social drugs such as LSD (lysergic acid diethylamide), PCP (phencyclidine, "angel dust"), marijuana, alcohol, and cocaine. In the case of LSD, limb abnormalities and malformations of the central nervous system have been reported. A comprehensive review of more than 100 publications, however, led to the conclusion that pure LSD used in moderate doses is not teratogenic and does not cause genetic damage.

A similar lack of conclusive evidence for teratogenicity has been described for marijuana and PCP. A case report of malformations and behavioral abnormalities in an infant whose mother used PCP throughout her pregnancy suggests a possible relationship between the drug and the infant's defects.

Cocaine has been reported to cause spontaneous abortion, growth retardation, microcephaly, neurobehavioral problems, urogenital anomalies, and gastroschisis. Many abnormalities produced by cocaine may be due to its action as a vasoconstrictor that causes hypoxia.

A well-documented association exists between maternal alcohol ingestion and congenital abnormalities. Defects include craniofacial abnormalities (short palpebral fissures and hypoplasia of the maxilla), limb deformities (altered joint mobility and position), and cardiovascular defects (ventricular septal abnormalities). These malformations, together with mental retardation and growth deficiency, make up the "fetal alcohol syndrome" (Fig. 8.4). Even moderate alcohol consumption during pregnancy may be detrimental to embryonic development.

Cigarette smoking has not been linked to major birth defects. Smoking does contribute to intrauterine growth retardation and premature delivery, however. There is also evidence that it causes behavioral disturbances.

Recently, **isotretinoin (13-*cis*-retinoic acid),** an analogue of **vitamin A,** has been shown to cause a characteristic pattern of malformations known as the **isotretinoin or vitamin A embryopathy.** The drug is prescribed for the treatment of cystic acne and other chronic dermatoses but is highly teratogenic. Associated features of the embryopathy include reduced and abnormal ear development, a flat nasal bridge, mandibular hypoplasia, cleft palate, hydrocephaly, neural tube defects, and heart anomalies involving the conotruncal region.

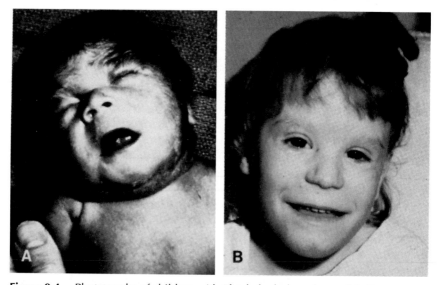

Figure 8.4. Photographs of children with "fetal alcohol syndrome." **A.** Severe case. **B.** Slightly affected child. Note in both children the short palpebral fissures and hypoplasia of the maxilla. Usually, the defect includes other craniofacial abnormalities. Cardiovascular defects and limb deformities are also common.

HORMONES

Androgenic Agents

Synthetic progestins were frequently used during pregnancy to prevent abortion. The progestins ethisterone and norethisterone have considerable androgenic activity, and many cases of masculinization of the genitalia in female embryos have been reported. The abnormalities consisted of an enlarged clitoris associated with varying degrees of fusion of the labioscrotal folds.

Diethylstilbestrol

Diethylstilbestrol, a synthetic estrogen, was commonly used in the 1940's and 1950's to prevent abortion. This practice was contraindicated in 1971 when it was determined that young women aged 16–22 years had an increased incidence of carcinomas of the vagina and cervix following exposure to the drug in utero. Furthermore, a high percentage of these exposed women suffered from reproductive dysfunction that appears to be due, in part, to congenital malformations of the uterus, uterine tubes, and upper vagina. Male embryos exposed in utero can also be affected, as evidenced by an increase in malformations of the testes and abnormal sperm analysis among these individuals. In contrast to females, however, males do not demonstrate an increased risk of developing carcinomas of the genital system.

Oral Contraceptives

Birth control pills containing estrogens and progestogens, appear to have a low teratogenic potential. Since other hormones, such as diethylstilbestrol, produce abnormalities, however, use of oral contraceptives should be discontinued if pregnancy is suspected.

Cortisone

Experimental work has repeatedly shown that cortisone injected into mice and rabbits at certain stages of pregnancy causes a high percentage of cleft palates in the offspring. However, it has been impossible to implicate cortisone as an environmental factor causing cleft palate in humans.

MATERNAL DISEASE

Disturbances in carbohydrate metabolism during pregnancy in diabetic mothers cause a high incidence of stillbirths, neonatal deaths, abnormally large infants, and congenital malformations. The risk of congenital anomalies in children of diabetic mothers is 3–4 times that for the offspring of nondiabetic mothers and has been reported to be as high as 80% in the offspring from diabetics with long-standing disease. A variety of malformations have been observed, including cardiac, skeletal, and central nervous system anomalies. Caudal dysgenesis also can occur in these offspring and consists of partial or complete agenesis of sacral vertebrae in conjunction with hindlimb hypoplasia.

Factors responsible for these deformities have not been delineated, although evidence suggests that altered glucose levels play a role and that **insulin** is not teratogenic. In this respect, a significant correlation exists between the severity and duration of the mother's disease and the incidence of malformations. Also, strict control of maternal metabolism with aggressive **insulin therapy** reduces the occurrence of malformations. Such therapy, however, increases the frequency and severity of **hypoglycemic episodes.** Numerous animal studies have shown that during gastrulation and neurulation stages, mammalian embryos are dependent on glucose as an energy source, such that even brief episodes of lowered blood glucose are teratogenic. Therefore, caution must be exercised in managing the pregnant diabetic woman, and therapy should be initiated prior to conception.

In the case of non-insulin-dependent diabetes, **oral hypoglycemic agents** may be employed. These agents include the sulfonylureas and biguanides. Both classes of agents have been implicated as teratogens, such that they must be employed with caution.

Phenylketonuria (PKU)

Mothers with **phenylketonuria (PKU),** in which the enzyme phenylalanine hydroxylase is deficient, resulting in increased serum concentrations of phenylalanine, are at risk for having infants with mental retardation, microcephaly, and cardiac defects. Women with the disease who maintain their low phenylalanine diet prior to conception reduce the risk to the infants to background rates.

NUTRITIONAL DEFICIENCIES

Although many nutritional deficiencies, particularly vitamin deficiencies, have been proven to be teratogenic in experimental work, there is no definite evidence that they are teratogenic in humans. Thus, with the exception of **endemic cretinism,** which is related to maternal **iodine deficiency,** no analogies to animal experiments have been found in humans.

HYPOXIA

Hypoxia induces congenital malformations in a great variety of experimental animals. Whether the same is valid for humans remains to be seen. Although children born at relatively high altitudes are usually lighter in weight and smaller than those born near or at sea level, an increase in the incidence of congenital malformations has not been noted. In addition, women with cyanotic cardiovascular disease often give birth to small infants, but usually without gross congenital malformations.

ENVIRONMENTAL CHEMICALS

A few years ago, it was noted in Japan that a number of mothers with diets consisting mainly of fish had given birth to children with multiple neurological symptoms resembling cerebral palsy. Further examination revealed that the fish contained an abnormally high level of **organic mercury,** which was spewed into Minamata Bay and other coastal waters of Japan by large industries. Many of the mothers did not show any symptoms themselves, indicating that the fetus was more sensitive to mercury than the mother. In the United States, similar observations were made when seed corn sprayed with a mercury-containing fungicide was fed to hogs and the meat was subsequently eaten by a pregnant woman. Similarly in Iraq, several thousand babies were affected after mothers ate grain treated with mercury-containing fungicides.

Lead has been associated with increased abortions, growth retardation, and neurological disorders.

Among the pesticides, the defoliant 2,4,5-T (**Agent Orange**) has been implicated as a teratogen. When an exhaustive review of the effects of 2,4,5-T on mammalian reproduction was made, however, no evidence could be found that the herbicide was teratogenic in humans.

PRINCIPLES OF TERATOLOGY

As a result of laboratory studies and observations by clinical scientists, factors determining the capacity of an agent to produce birth defects have been defined. These **principles of teratology** were first formulated by Wilson in 1959 and have stood the test of time. They include

1. Susceptibility to teratogenesis depends on the genotype of the conceptus and the manner in which this genetic composition interacts with the environment. The maternal genome is also important with respect to drug metabolism, resistance to infection, and other biochemical and molecular processes that will impact on the conceptus.
2. Susceptibility to teratogens varies with the developmental stage at the time of exposure. The most sensitive period for inducing birth defects is the **3rd to 8th weeks** of gestation , the period of embryogenesis. Each organ system may have one or more stages of susceptibility. For example, cleft palate can be induced at the blastocyst stage (day 6), during gastrulation (day 14), at the early limb bud stage (5th week), or when the palatal shelves are forming (7th week). Furthermore, while most abnormalities are produced during the period of embryogenesis, defects may also be induced prior to or after this period, such that no stage of development is completely safe.
3. Manifestations of abnormal development depend on dose and duration of exposure to a teratogen.
4. Teratogens act in specific ways (**mechanisms**) on developing cells and tissues to initiate abnormal embryogenesis (**pathogenesis**).
5. The manifestations of abnormal development are death, malformation, growth retardation, and functional disorders.

CLINICAL CORRELATES

It is important to remember that many birth defects can be prevented. For example, supplementation of salt or water supplies with iodine eliminates mental retardation and bone deformities resulting from **cretinism.** Placing diabetic and phenylketonuric women under strict metabolic control prior to conception reduces the incidence of birth defects in their offspring. **Folate supplementation** lowers the incidence of neural tube defects, such as spina bifida and anencephaly. Avoidance of alcohol and other drugs during **all** stages of pregnancy reduces the incidence of birth defects.

As physicians, it is important, when prescribing drugs to women of childbearing age, to consider the possibility of pregnancy and the potential teratogenicity of the compounds. Recently, hundreds of children have been born with severe craniofacial, cardiac, and neural tube defects produced by **retinoids (vitamin A embryopathy).** These compounds are used for the treatment of cystic acne (isotretinoin, 13-*cis*-retinoic acid) but are also effective topically **(Retin-A)** for common acne and reducing wrinkles. Oral preparations are highly teratogenic, and recent evidence suggests that topical applications may also cause abnormalities. Since patients with acne are usually young and may be sexually active, these agents must be used cautiously.

Chromosomal and Genetic Factors

Chromosomal abnormalities may be **numerical** or **structural** and are important causes of congenital malformations and spontaneous abortions. It is estimated that 50% of all conceptions end in spontaneous abortion and that 50% of these abortuses have major chromosome abnormalities. Thus, approximately 25% of all conceptuses have a major chromosomal defect. The most common chromosome abnormalities in abortuses are 45,X (Turner syndrome), triploidy, and trisomy 16. Chromosome abnormalities also account for 7% of major birth defects, while gene mutations account for an additional 7%.

NUMERICAL ABNORMALITIES

The normal human somatic cell contains 46 chromosomes; the normal gamete contains 23. Normal somatic cells are **diploid** or $2n$; normal gametes are **haploid** or **n.** **Euploid** refers to any exact multiple of **n,** e.g., diploid or triploid. **Aneuploid** refers to any chromosome number that is noneuploid and is usually applied when an extra chromosome is present **(trisomy)** or when one is missing **(monosomy).** Aneuploidy results from **nondisjunction** during meiosis or mitosis (see Chapter 1) and may involve the autosomes or sex chromosomes.

Trisomy 21 (Down Syndrome)

Down syndrome is usually caused by the presence of an extra copy of **chromosome 21 (trisomy 21).** Clinically, features of children with Down syndrome include growth retardation; varying degrees of mental retardation;

craniofacial abnormalities, including upward slanting eyes, epicanthal folds (extra skin folds at the medial corners of the eyes), flattened facies, and small ears; cardiac defects; and hypotonia (Fig. 8.5). In 95% of cases, the syndrome is caused by trisomy 21 due to meiotic nondisjunction, and in 75% of these instances, nondisjunction occurs during oocyte formation. Furthermore, women over 35 years have a greater risk of having an affected child.

In approximately 4% of cases of Down syndrome there is an unbalanced translocation between chromosome 21 and either of chromosomes 13, 14, or 15. The final 1% are due to mosaicism resulting from mitotic nondisjunction (see Chapter 1). These individuals have some cells with a normal chromosome number and some that are aneuploid. They may exhibit few or many of the characteristics of Down syndrome, depending on the numbers of abnormal cells and their location.

Trisomy 18

Patients with this chromosomal arrangement show the following features: mental retardation, congenital heart defects, low-set ears, and flexion of fingers and hands (Fig. 8.6). In addition, patients frequently show micrognathia, renal anomalies, syndactyly, and malformations of the skeletal system. The incidence of this condition is about 1 in 5000 newborns. The infants usually die by age 2 months.

Trisomy 13

The main abnormalities of this syndrome are mental retardation, holoprosencephaly, congenital heart defects, deafness, cleft lip and palate, and eye defects

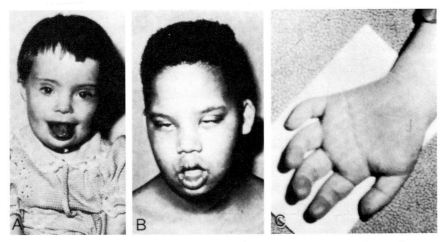

Figure 8.5. **A** and **B.** Photographs of children with Down syndrome. The syndrome is characterized by the following features: a flat, broad face; oblique palpebral fissures; epicanthus; furrowed lower lip; and a broad hand with single transverse or simian crease **(C).** The children with Down syndrome are frequently mentally retarded and have congenital heart abnormalities.

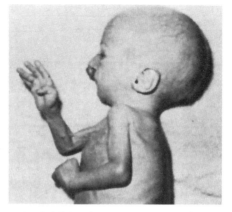

Figure 8.6. Photograph of child with trisomy 18. Note the prominent occiput, cleft lip, micrognathia, low-set ears, and one or more flexed fingers.

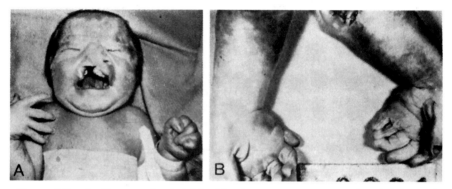

Figure 8.7. **A.** Photograph of child with trisomies 13–15. Note the cleft lip and palate, the sloping forehead, and microphthalmia. **B.** Frequently, the syndrome is accompanied by polydactyly.

such as microphthalmia, anophthalmia, and coloboma (Fig. 8.7). The incidence of this abnormality is about 1 in 15,000 live births. Most of the infants die by age 3 months.

Klinefelter Syndrome

The clinical features of Klinefelter syndrome, found only in males and usually detected at puberty, are sterility, testicular atrophy, hyalinization of the seminiferous tubules, and in most cases gynecomastia. The cells have 47 chromosomes with a sex chromosomal complement of the XXY type, and a sex chromatin body is found in 80% of cases. The incidence is about 1 in 500 males. Nondisjunction of the XX homologues is the most common causative event. Occasionally, patients with Klinefelter syndrome have 48 chromosomes, i.e., 44 autosomes and 4 sex chromosomes (XXXY). Although mental retardation is not generally part of the syndrome, the more X chromosomes there are, the more likely there will be some degree of mental impairment.

Turner Syndrome

Turner syndrome, found in women with an unmistakably female appearance (Fig. 8.8), is characterized by the absence of ovaries (**gonadal dysgenesis**) and short stature. Other abnormalities frequently found are webbed neck, lymphedema of the extremities, skeletal deformities, and a broad chest with widely spaced nipples. Approximately 55% of affected individuals will be monosomic for the X and chromatin negative due to nondisjunction. In 75% of these cases, nondisjunction in the male gamete is the cause. In the remainder of the cases, however, structural abnormalities of the X chromosome (15%) or mosaicism (30%) cause the syndrome.

Triple X Syndrome

Patients with triple X syndrome are infantile, with scanty menses and some degree of mental retardation. They have two sex chromatin bodies in their cells.

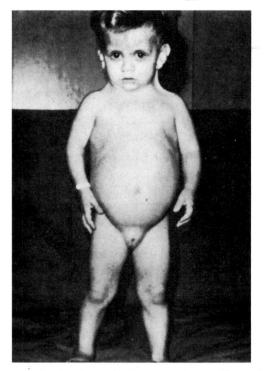

Figure 8.8. Photograph of patient with Turner syndrome. The main characteristics are webbed neck, short stature, broad chest, and absence of sexual maturation.

STRUCTURAL ABNORMALITIES

Structural chromosome abnormalities involve one or more chromosomes and usually result from chromosome breakage. Breaks are caused by environmental factors such as viruses, radiation, and drugs. The result of breakage depends on what happens to the broken pieces. In some cases, the broken piece of a chromosome is lost, and the infant with partial **deletion** of a chromosome is abnormal. A well-known syndrome caused by partial deletion of the short arm of chromosome 5 is the **cri-du-chat syndrome.** The children have a cat-like cry, microcephaly, mental retardation, and congenital heart disease. Many other relatively rare syndromes are known to result from a partial chromosome loss.

Microdeletions, spanning only a few **contiguous genes,** also occur. Sites where these deletions occur are called **contiguous gene complexes** and can be identified by **high-resolution chromosome banding techniques** (see Chapter 1). An example of a microdeletion involves the long arm of chromosome 15 (15q11–15q13). Inheriting the deletion on the maternal chromosome results in **Angelman syndrome,** and the children are mentally retarded, cannot speak, exhibit poor motor development, and are prone to unprovoked and prolonged periods of laughter (Fig. 8.9). If the defect is inherited on the paternal chromosome, the **Prader-Willi syndrome** is produced, and affected individuals are characterized by hypotonia, obesity, mental retardation, hypogonadism, and cryptorchidism (Fig. 8.10). Cases that exhibit differential expression, depending on whether the genetic material is inherited from the mother or the father, represent **genomic imprinting** (see Chapter 3).

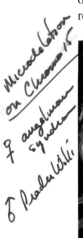

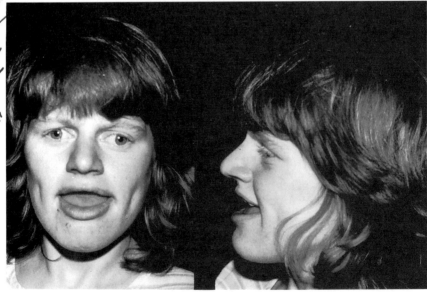

Figure 8.9. Photograph of a patient with Angelman syndrome resulting from a microdeletion on maternal chromosome 15. If the defect is inherited on the paternal chromosome, Prader-Willi syndrome occurs (see Fig. 8.10).

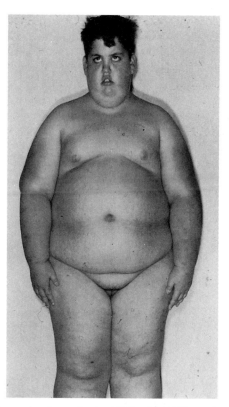

Figure 8.10. Photograph of a patient with Prader-Willi syndrome resulting from a microdeletion on paternal chromosome 15. If the defect is inherited on the maternal chromosome, Angelman syndrome occurs (see Fig. 8.9).

Fragile sites are regions of chromosomes that demonstrate a propensity to separate or break under certain cell manipulations. For example, fragile sites can be enhanced by culturing lymphocytes in folate-deficient medium. Although numerous fragile sites have been defined, only the site located on the long arm of the X chromosome (X q27) has been correlated with an altered phenotype and is called the **fragile X syndrome.** The syndrome is characterized by mental retardation, large ears, prominent jaw, and pale blue irides. Males are affected more often than females (4/2000 versus 1/2000), which may account for the preponderance of males among the mentally retarded. The syndrome is second only to Down syndrome as a cause of chromosomally derived mental retardation.

MUTANT GENES

Many congenital malformations in humans are inherited, and some show a clear mendelian pattern of inheritance. In many cases, the abnormality is directly attributable to a change in the structure or function of a single gene, hence the name **single gene mutation.** It is estimated that this type of defect makes up approximately 8% of all human malformations.

With exception of the X and Y chromosomes in the male, genes exist as pairs or **alleles,** such that there are two doses for each genetic determinant, one from the mother and one from the father. If a mutant gene produces an abnormality in a single dose, despite the presence of a normal allele, it is a **dominant mutation.** If both alleles must be abnormal (double dosage) or if the mutation that occurs is X-linked in the male, it is a **recessive mutation.** Gradations in the effects of mutant genes may occur due to modifying factors.

In addition to causing congenital malformations, defective gene action causes a large number of inborn errors of metabolism. These diseases, among which phenylketonuria, homocystinuria, and galactosemia are the best known, are frequently accompanied by or cause various degrees of mental retardation.

As mapping of the human genome continues, the association of specific genes with their normal functions and the abnormalities they cause will become more precise. Already, new molecular techniques such as **fluorescence in situ hybridization (FISH),** which uses specific DNA probes for identifying deletions of genetic material, have improved our ability to detect gene and chromosome abnormalities.

SUMMARY

Many factors may interact with the differentiating and growing embryo. The result, however, is not necessarily a **gross malformation.** In some instances, the teratogenic agent may be so toxic or may affect a vital organ system of the embryo or fetus so severely that **death** results. In other cases, the environmental influence may be so mild that the embryo or fetus is able to survive but some of its organ systems are affected. This may result in partial or total **growth retardation** or a **functional impairment** such as mental retardation.

A variety of agents (Table 8.1) are known to produce congenital malformations in approximately 2–3% of all liveborn infants. These agents include viruses, such as rubella and cytomegalovirus; radiation; drugs, such as thalidomide, aminopterin, anticonvulsants, antipsychotics, and antianxiety compounds; social drugs, such as PCP, cigarettes, and alcohol; hormones, such as diethylstilbestrol; maternal diabetes; and chromosomal abnormalities, such as trisomy 21 (Down syndrome). Effects of teratogens are dependent on the **maternal and fetal genotype,** the **stage of development** when exposure occurs, and the **dose and duration of exposure** of the agent. Most major malformations are produced during the **period of embryogenesis (teratogenic period),** but in stages prior to and after this time the fetus is also susceptible, such that no period of gestation is completely free of risk. **Prevention** of many birth defects is possible but is dependent on an awareness by physicians and by women of childbearing age of the risks involved.

Table 8.1.
Teratogens Associated With Human Malformations

Teratogen	Congenital Malformation
Infectious agents	
Rubella virus	Cataracts, glaucoma, heart defects, deafness
Cytomegalovirus	Microcephaly, blindness, mental retardation
Herpes simplex virus	Microphthalmia, microcephaly, retinal dysplasia
Varicella virus	Limb hypoplasia, mental retardation, muscle atrophy
HIV	Microcephaly, growth retardation
Toxoplasmosis	Hydrocephalus, cerebral calcifications, microphthalmia
Syphilis	Mental retardation, deafness
Physical agents	
X-rays	Microcephaly, spina bifida, cleft palate, limb defects
Hyperthermia	Anencephaly
Chemical agents	
Thalidomide	Limb defects, heart malformations
Aminopterin	Anencephaly, hydrocephaly, cleft lip and palate
Diphenylhydantoin (phenytoin)	Fetal hydantoin syndrome: facial defects, mental retardation
Valproic acid	Neural tube defects, heart, craniofacial, and limb anomalies
Trimethadione	Cleft palate, heart defects, urogenital and skeletal abnormalities
Lithium	Heart malformations
Amphetamines	Cleft lip and palate, heart defects
Warfarin	Chondrodysplasia, microcephaly
ACE inhibitors	Growth retardation, fetal death
LSD	Limb and central nervous system defects
Cocaine	Growth retardation, microcephaly, behavioral abnormalities, gastroschisis
Alcohol	Fetal alcohol syndrome, short palpebral fissures, maxillary hypoplasia, heart defects, mental retardation
Isotretinoin (vitamin A)	Vitamin A embryopathy: small abnormally shaped ears, mandibular hypoplasia, cleft plate, heart defects
Organic mercury	Multiple neurological symptoms: similar to cerebral palsy
Lead	Growth retardation, neurological disorders
Hormones	
Androgenic agents (ethisterone, norethisterone)	Masculinization of female genitalia: fused labia, clitoral hypertrophy
Diethylstilbestrol (DES)	Malformation of the uterus, uterine tubes, and upper vagina; vaginal cancer; malformed testes
Maternal diabetes	Variety of malformations; heart and neural tube defects most common

PROBLEMS TO SOLVE

1. What are the factors that influence the action of a teratogen?

2. A young woman in only the 3rd week of her pregnancy develops a fever of 104° but refuses to take any medication because she is afraid that drugs will harm her baby. Is she correct?

3. Are women over age 35 years at greater risk for having a child with a congenital defect? What test(s) would you recommend for prenatal diagnosis in such a patient?

4. A young insulin-dependent diabetic woman is planning a family and is concerned about the potentially harmful effects of her disease on her unborn child. Are her concerns valid, and what would you recommend?

SUGGESTED READINGS

Bill WB, Schumacher GFV, Bibbo M: Pathological semen and anatomical abnormalities of the genital tract in human male subjects exposed to diethylstilbestrol in utero. *J Urol* 117:477, 1977.

Brent RL, Beckman DA: Angiotensin-converting enzyme inhibitors, an embryopathic class of drugs with unique properties: information for clinical teratology counselors. *Teratology* 43:543, 1991.

Brent RL, Holmes LB: Clinical and basic science from the thalidomide tragedy: what have we learned about the causes of limb defects? *Teratology* 38:241, 1988.

Carr DH: Chromosome studies in spontaneous abortions. *Obstet Gynecol* 26:308, 1965.

Centers for Disease Control. *MMWR Morb Mortal Wkly Rep* 38(37):633, 1989.

Corby DG: Aspirin in pregnancy: maternal and fetal effects. *Pediatrics* 62:930, 1978.

Dansky LV, Finnell RH: Parental epilepsy, anticonvulsant drugs, and reproductive outcome—epidemiologic and experimental findings spanning 3 decades. Two human studies. *Reprod Toxicol* 5:301, 1991.

Eibs HG, Spielmann H, Hagele M: Teratogenic effects of cyproterone acetate and medroxyprogesterone treatment during the pre- and postimplantation period of mouse embryos. *Teratology* 25:27, 1982.

Gelehrter TD, Collins FS: *Principles of Medical Genetics.* Baltimore, Williams & Wilkins, 1990.

Generoso WM, Rutledge JC, Cain KT, Hughes LA, Downing DJ: Mutagen induced fetal anomalies and death following treatment of females within hours after mating. *Mutat Res* 199:175, 1988.

Gorlin RJ, Cohen MM, Levin LS (eds): *Syndromes of the Head and Neck.* 3rd ed. New York, Oxford University Press, 1990.

Gregg NM: Congenital cataract following German measles in mothers. *Trans Ophthalmol Soc Aust* 3:35, 1941.

Jones KL (ed): *Smith's Recognizable Patterns of Human Malformation.* 4th ed. Philadelphia, WB Saunders, 1988.

Jones KL, Smith DW, Ulleland CN, et al: Pattern of malformation in offspring of chronic alcoholic mothers. *Lancet* 1:1267, 1973.

Kaufman RH, Binder GS, Gray PM, Adam E: Upper genital tract changes associated with exposure in utero to diethylstilbestrol. *Am J Obstet Gynecol* 128:51, 1977.

Knoll JHM, Nicholls RD, Magenis RE, Graham JM Jr, Lalande M, Latt SA: Angelman and Prader-Willi syndrome share a common chromosome 15 deletion but differ in parental origin of the deletion. *Am J Med Genet* 32:285, 1989.

Lammer EJ, et al: Retinoic acid embryopathy. *N Engl J Med* 313:837–841, 1985.

Lenke RR, Levy HL: Maternal phenylketonuria and hyperphenylalaninemia. An international survey of untreated and treated pregnancies. *N Engl J Med* 303:1202, 1980.

Lenz W: A short history of thalidomide embryopathy. *Teratology* 38:203, 1988.

Lenz W: Thalidomide and congenital abnormalities. *Lancet* 1:1219, 1962.

Lockwood C, Ghidni A, Romero R, Hobbins JC: Amniotic band syndrome: reevaluation of its pathogenesis. *Am J Obstet Gynecol* 160:1030, 1989.

Miller P, Smith DW, Shepard TH: Maternal hyperthermia as a possible cause of anencephaly. *Lancet* 1:519, 1978.

Mills JL, et al: Lack of relationship of increased malformation rates in infants of diabetic mothers to glycemic control during organogenesis. *N Engl J Med* 318:671, 1988.

Sadler TW, Denno KM, Hunter ES III: Effects of altered maternal metabolism during gastrulation and neurulation stages of development. *Ann N Y Acad Sci* 678:48, 1993.

Shenefelt RE: Morphogenesis of malformations in hamsters caused by retinoic acid: relation to dose and stage of development. *Teratology* 5:103, 1972.

Shepard TH: *Catalog of Teratogenic Agents.* 7th ed. Baltimore, Johns Hopkins University Press, 1992.

Stevenson RE, Hall JG, Goodman RM (eds): *Human Malformations and Related Anomalies.* New York, Oxford University Press, 1993, vols I and II. Wald N: Folic acid and prevention of neural tube defects. *Ann N Y Acad Sci* 678:112, 1993.

Warkany J, Kalter H: Congenital malformations. *N Engl J Med* 265:993, 1961.

Werler MM, Prober BR, Holmes LB: Smoking and pregnancy. *In* Sever JL, Brent RL (eds): *Teratogen Update: Environmentally Induced Birth Defect Risks.* New York, Alan R Liss, 1986.

Wilkins L, Jones HW Jr, Holman GH, Stempfel RS Jr: Masculinization of the female fetus associated with administration of oral and intramuscular progestins during gestation; nonadrenal female pseudohermaphroditism. *J Clin Endocrinol Metab* 18:559, 1958.

Wilson JG, Fraser FC: *Handbook of Teratology.* New York, Plenum Press, 1977, vols 1–3.

PART II

Special Embryology

chapter 9

Skeletal System
(Skull, Limbs, Vertebral Column, Ribs and Sternum)

The skeletal system develops from **paraxial** and **lateral plate (somatic layer) mesoderm** and from **neural crest.** Paraxial mesoderm forms a segmented series of tissue blocks on each side of the neural tube, known as **somitomeres** in the head region and **somites** from the occipital region caudally. Somites differentiate into a ventromedial part, the **sclerotome,** and a dorsolateral part, the **dermomyotome.** At the end of the 4th week, sclerotome cells become polymorphous and form a loosely woven tissue known as **mesenchyme** or embryonic connective tissue (Fig. 9.1). It is characteristic for mesenchymal cells to migrate and to differentiate in many different ways. They may become fibroblasts, chondroblasts, or **osteoblasts (bone-forming cells).**

The bone-forming capacity of mesenchyme is not restricted to cells of the sclerotome but occurs also in the somatic mesoderm layer of the body wall, which contributes mesoderm cells for formation of the pelvic and shoulder girdles and the long bones of the limbs. It has also been shown that neural crest cells in the head region differentiate into mesenchyme and participate in formation of bones of the face and skull. Occipital somites and somitomeres also contribute to formation of the cranial vault and base of the skull. In some bones, such as the flat bones of the skull, mesenchyme differentiates directly into bone, a process known as **membranous ossification** (Fig. 9.2). In most bones, however, mesenchymal cells first give rise to **hyaline cartilage models,** which, in turn, become ossified by **endochondral ossification** (Figs. 9.4 and 9.10). In the following paragraphs, development of the most important bony structures and some of their abnormalities are discussed.

Skull

The skull can be divided into two parts: the **neurocranium,** which forms a protective case around the brain; and the **viscerocranium,** which forms the skeleton of the face.

NEUROCRANIUM

The neurocranium is most conveniently divided into two portions: *(a)* the membranous part consisting of **flat bones,** which surround the brain as a vault;

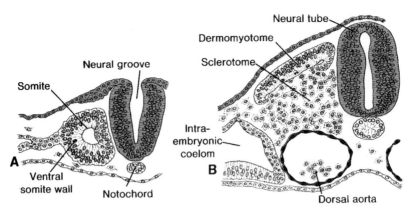

Figure 9.1. Development of the somite. **A.** Paraxial mesoderm cells are arranged around a small cavity. **B.** As a result of further differentiation, cells in the ventromedial wall lose their epithelial arrangement and become mesenchymal. They are collectively referred to as the sclerotome. Cells in the dorsolateral wall of the somite form the dermomyotome.

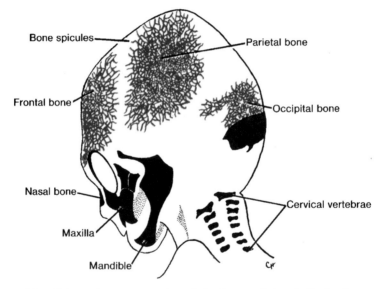

Figure 9.2. Schematic representation of the bones of the skull of a 3-month-old fetus. Note the spread of bone spicules from primary ossification centers in the flat bones of the skull.

and *(b)* the **cartilaginous part** or **chondrocranium,** which forms bones of the base of the skull.

Membranous Neurocranium

The roof and most of the sides of the skull develop from neural crest cells, with only the occipital region and posterior parts of the otic capsule arising from paraxial mesoderm (Fig. 9.6). Mesenchyme from these two sources invests the brain and undergoes **membranous ossification.** As a result, a number of flat, membranous bones are formed that are characterized by the presence of needle-like **bone spicules.** These spicules progressively radiate from primary ossification centers toward the periphery (Fig. 9.2). With further growth during fetal and postnatal life, membranous bones enlarge by apposition of new layers on the outer surface and by simultaneous osteoclastic resorption from the inside.

Newborn Skull

At birth, the flat bones of the skull are separated from each other by narrow seams of connective tissue, the **sutures,** which are also derived from neural crest. At points where more than two bones meet, sutures are wide and known as **fontanelles** (Fig. 9.3). The most prominent of these is the **anterior fontanelle,** which is found where the two parietal and two frontal bones meet. Sutures and fontanelles allow the bones of the skull to overlap each other (a process called **molding**) during the birth process. Soon after birth, membranous bones move back to their original positions and give the skull a large, round appearance. In fact, the size of the vault is strikingly large compared with the small facial region (Fig. 9.3*B*).

Several sutures and fontanelles remain membranous for a considerable time after birth. Growth of the bones of the vault continues after birth and is caused mainly by growth of the brain. Although a 5–7-year-old child has nearly all of its cranial capacity, some sutures remain open until adulthood. In the first few years

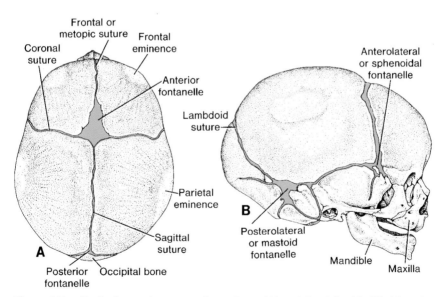

Figure 9.3. Skull of a newborn, seen from above **(A)** and the right side **(B).** Note the anterior and posterior fontanelles and sutures. The posterior fontanelle closes about 3 months after birth; the anterior fontanelle, about the middle of the 2nd year. Many of the sutures disappear during adult life.

after birth, palpation of the anterior fontanelle may give valuable information as to whether ossification of the skull is proceeding normally and whether intracranial pressure is normal.

Cartilaginous Neurocranium or Chondrocranium

The cartilaginous neurocranium or chondrocranium of the skull consists initially of a number of separate cartilages. Those that lie in front of the rostral limit of the notochord, which ends at the level of the pituitary gland in the center of the sella turcica, are derived from neural crest cells and form the **prechordal chondrocranium.** Those that lie posterior to this limit arise from paraxial mesoderm and form the **chordal chondrocranium.** When these cartilages fuse and ossify by endochondral ossification, the base of the skull is formed.

The base of the occipital bone is formed by the **parachordal cartilage** and the bodies of three **occipital sclerotomes** (Fig. 9.4). Rostral to the occipital baseplate

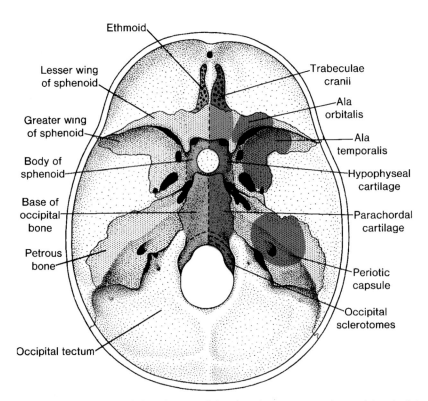

Figure 9.4. Schematized dorsal view of the chondrocranium or base of the skull in the adult. On the right side in blue are the various embryonic components participating in formation of the median part of the chondrocranium; in red are components for the lateral part. On the left are the names of the adult structures. Bones that form rostral to the rostral half of the sella turcica arise from neural crest and constitute the prechordal (in front of the notochord) chondrocranium. Those forming posterior to this landmark arise from paraxial mesoderm (chordal chondrocranium).

are the **hypophyseal cartilages** and **trabeculae cranii.** These cartilages soon fuse to form the body of the **sphenoid** and **ethmoid,** respectively. In this manner, an elongated median plate of cartilage extending from the nasal region to the anterior border of the **foramen magnum** is formed.

A number of other mesenchymal condensations arise on either side of the median plate. The most rostral, the **ala orbitalis,** forms the lesser wing of the sphenoid bone. Caudally, it is followed by the **ala temporalis,** which gives rise to the greater wing of the sphenoid. A third component, the **periotic capsule,** gives rise to the petrous and mastoid parts of the temporal bone. These components later fuse with the median plate and with each other, except for openings through which cranial nerves leave the skull (Fig. 9.4).

VISCEROCRANIUM

The viscerocranium consists of the bones of the face and is formed mainly from the first two pharyngeal arches (see Chapter 16). The 1st arch gives rise to a dorsal portion, the **maxillary process,** which extends forward beneath the region of the eye and gives rise to the **maxilla, the zygomatic bone,** and **part of the temporal bone** (Fig. 9.5). The ventral portion is known as the **mandibular process** and contains **Meckel's cartilage.** Mesenchyme around Meckel's cartilage condenses and ossifies by membranous ossification to give rise to the **mandible.** Meckel's cartilage disappears except in the **sphenomandibular** ligament. The dorsal tip of the mandibular process, along with that of the 2nd

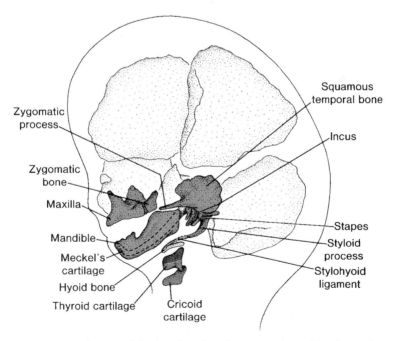

Figure 9.5. Lateral view of the head and neck region of an older fetus, showing derivatives of the arch cartilages participating in formation of bones of the face.

pharyngeal arch, later gives rise to the **incus,** the **malleus,** and the **stapes** (Fig. 9.5). Ossification of the three ossicles begins in the 4th month, thus making these the first bones to become fully ossified. Mesenchyme for formation of the bones of the face is derived from neural crest cells, including the nasal and lacrimal bones (Fig. 9.6).

At first, the face is small in comparison with the neurocranium. This appearance is caused by *(a)* virtual absence of the paranasal air sinuses and *(b)* the small size of the bones, particularly the jaws. With the appearance of teeth and development of the air sinuses, the face obtains its human characteristics.

CLINICAL CORRELATES

It should be noted that neural crest cells originating in the neuro-ectoderm form the facial skeleton and most of the skull. These cells also represent a vulnerable population as they leave the neuroecto-derm and are often a target for teratogens. Therefore, it is not surprising that craniofacial abnormalities are common birth defects (see also Chapter 16).

In some cases, the cranial vault fails to form (cranioschisis), and brain tissue exposed to amniotic fluid degenerates, resulting in anen-cephaly. The defect is due to failure of the cranial neuropore to close (Fig. 9.7A). Children with such severe skull and brain defects are not viable. Children with relatively small defects in the skull through which brain tissue and/or meninges herniate (**encephalocele** or **cranial**

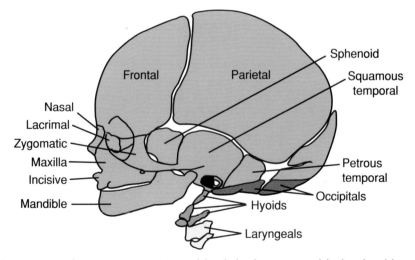

Figure 9.6. Schematic representation of the skeletal structures of the head and face. Mesenchyme for these structures is derived from neural crest *(blue),* lateral plate mesoderm *(yellow),* and paraxial mesoderm (somites and somitomeres) *(red).*

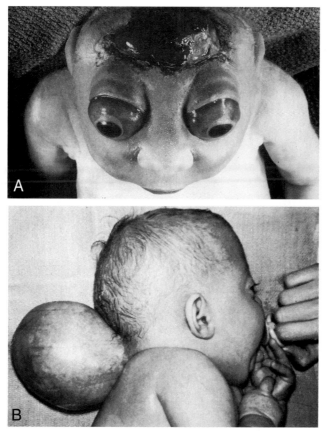

Figure 9.7. **A.** Photograph of a child with anencephaly. Cranial neural folds that fail to elevate fuse, leaving the cranial neuropore open. The skull never forms, and brain tissues degenerate. **B.** Photograph of a patient with meningocele. This is a rather common abnormality, which frequently can be successfully repaired.

meningocele) are, however, observed frequently (Fig. 9.7*B*) and may be treated successfully. In such cases, the extent of neurological deficits depends on the amount of damage to brain tissue.

Another important category of cranial abnormalities is caused by premature closure of one or more sutures. These abnormalities are collectively known as **craniosynostosis.** The shape of the skull depends on which of the sutures closed prematurely. Early closure of the sagittal suture results in frontal and occipital expansion, and the skull becomes long and narrow **(scaphocephaly)** (Fig. 9.8*A*). Premature closure of the coronal suture results in a short, high skull, known as **acrocephaly** or **tower skull** (Fig. 9.8*B*). If the coronal and lambdoid sutures close

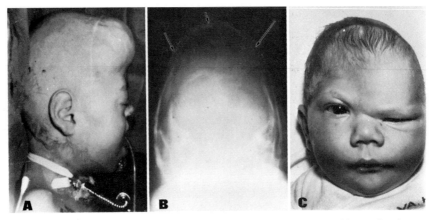

Figure 9.8. A. Photograph of a child with scaphocephaly caused by early closure of the sagittal suture. Note the frontal and occipital bossing. **B.** X-ray of a child with acrocephaly caused by early closure of the coronal suture. **C.** Photograph of a child with plagiocephaly resulting from early closure of coronal and lambdoid sutures on one side of the skull (see also Fig. 9.3**B**).

prematurely on one side only, asymmetric craniosynostosis, known as **plagiocephaly,** results (Fig. 9.8*C*).

A great handicap in operating on patients with craniosynostosis is the tendency of the bones to reunite after the prematurely closed sutures have been opened. Consequently, the skull is removed and broken into pieces, and the fragments are replaced with large intervening spaces. Spaces are filled by bone growth at the edges of the pieces until a complete skull is formed.

Microcephaly is usually an abnormality in which the brain fails to grow and, consequently, the skull fails to expand. Children with microcephaly are often severely retarded.

Limbs

Limb buds become visible as outpocketings from the ventrolateral body wall at the end of the 4th week of development (Fig. 9.9*A*). Initially, they consist of a mesenchymal core, derived from the somatic layer of lateral plate mesoderm that will form the bones and connective tissues of the limb, covered by a layer of cuboidal ectoderm. Mesenchyme signals ectoderm at the limb tip to thicken and form the **apical ectodermal ridge (AER)** (Fig. 9.10*A*). In return, the ridge exerts an inductive influence on the underlying mesenchyme. Thus, mesenchyme adjacent to the AER remains as a population of undifferentiated, rapidly proliferating cells, whereas cells located farther away from the influence of the AER begin to differentiate into cartilage and muscle. In this manner, development of the limb proceeds in a proximodistal direction.

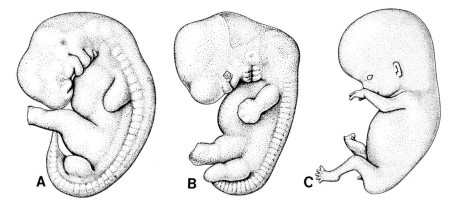

Figure 9.9. Schematic drawings of human embryos to demonstrate development of the limb buds. **A.** At 5 weeks. **B.** At 6 weeks. **C.** At 8 weeks. Note that the hindlimb buds are somewhat behind in development, compared with those of the forelimbs.

In 6-week-old embryos, the terminal portion of the limb buds becomes flattened to form the **handplates** and **footplates** and is separated from the proximal segment by a circular constriction (Fig. 9.9*B*). Later, a second constriction divides the proximal portion into two segments, and the main parts of the extremities can be recognized (Fig. 9.9*C*). Fingers and toes are formed when **cell death** in the AER separates this ridge into five parts (Fig. 9.11*A*). Further formation of the digits is dependent on their continued outgrowth under the influence of the five segments of ridge ectoderm, condensation of the mesenchyme to form cartilaginous digital rays, and the death of intervening tissue between the rays (Fig. 9.11, *B* and *C*). Patterning of the digits is dependent on a group of cells located at the base of the limbs on their posterior border, known as the **zone of polarizing activity (ZPA).** These cells establish a morphogen gradient that appears to involve **retinoic acid (vitamin A)** and a series of **homeobox genes** to produce the normal sequence of digits.

Development of the upper and lower limbs is similar, except that morphogenesis of the lower limb is approximately 1–2 days behind that of the upper limb. Also, during the 7th week of gestation, the limbs rotate in opposite directions. The upper limb rotates 90° laterally, so that the extensor muscles lie on the lateral and posterior surface and the thumbs lie laterally, whereas the lower limb rotates approximately 90° medially, placing the extensor muscles on the anterior surface and the big toe medially.

While the external shape is being established, mesenchyme in the buds begins to condense, and by the 6th week of development, the first **hyaline cartilage models,** foreshadowing the bones of the extremities, can be recognized (Fig. 9.10). Ossification of the bones of the extremities, **endochondral ossification,** begins by the end of the embryonic period. Primary **ossification centers** are present in all long bones of the limbs by the 12th week of development. From the primary center in the shaft or **diaphysis** of the bone, endochondral ossification progresses gradually toward the ends of the cartilaginous "model."

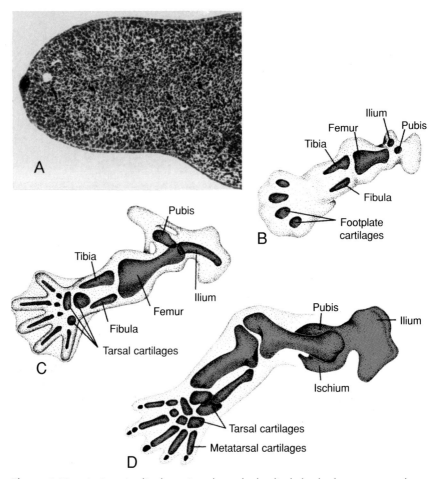

Figure 9.10. **A.** Longitudinal section through the limb bud of a mouse embryo, showing a core of mesenchyme covered by a layer of ectoderm that thickens at the limb tip to form the apical ectodermal ridge (AER). In humans, this occurs during the 5th week of development. **B.** Schematic drawing of the lower extremity of an early 6-week embryo, illustrating the first hyaline cartilage models. **C** and **D.** Similar drawings showing the complete set of cartilage models at the end of the 6th and the beginning of the 8th week, respectively.

At birth, the diaphysis of the bone is usually completely ossified, but the two extremities, known as the **epiphyses,** are still cartilaginous. Shortly thereafter, however, ossification centers arise in the epiphyses. Temporarily, a cartilage plate remains between the diaphyseal and epiphyseal ossification centers. This plate, known as the **epiphyseal plate,** plays an important role in growth in the length of the bones. On both sides of the plate, endochondral ossification proceeds. When the bone has acquired its full length, the epiphyseal plates disappear, and the epiphyses unite with the shaft of the bone.

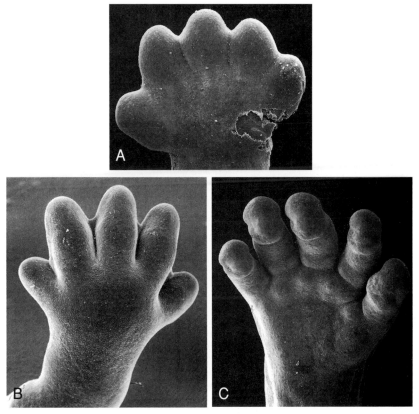

Figure 9.11. Scanning electron micrographs of human hands. **A.** At 48 days. Cell death in the apical ectodermal ridge creates a separate ridge for each digit. **B.** At 51 days. Cell death in the interdigital spaces produces separation of the digits. **C.** At 56 days. Digit separation is complete. Note the finger pads that will create patterns for fingerprints.

In long bones, an epiphyseal plate is found on each extremity; in smaller bones, such as the phalanges, it is found only at one extremity; and in irregular bones, such as the vertebrae, one or more primary centers of ossification and usually several secondary centers are present.

CLINICAL CORRELATES

Knowledge about the appearance of various ossification centers is used by radiologists to determine whether a child has reached his or her proper maturation age. Useful information of "bone age" is obtained from ossification studies in the hands and wrists of children. Prenatal analysis of fetal bones by ultrasonography provides information about fetal growth and gestational age.

Abnormalities of the limbs vary greatly and may be represented by partial **(meromelia)** or complete absence **(amelia)** of one or more of the extremities. Sometimes, the long bones may be absent, and rudimentary hands and feet are attached to the trunk by small, irregularly shaped bones **(phocomelia, a form of meromelia)** (Fig. 9.12, *A* and *B*). Sometimes, all segments of the extremities are present but are abnormally short **(micromelia).**

Although these abnormalities are rare and mainly of a hereditary nature, cases of teratogen-induced limb defects have been documented. For example, a high incidence of children with limb malformations was born between 1957 and 1962. It was noted that many mothers of these infants had taken **thalidomide,** a drug widely used as a sleeping pill and antinauseant. Subsequently, it was established that this drug causes a characteristic syndrome of malformations consisting of absence or gross deformities of the long bones, intestinal atresia, and cardiac anomalies. Studies indicate that the most sensitive period for teratogen-induced limb malformations is the **4th and 5th weeks** of development.

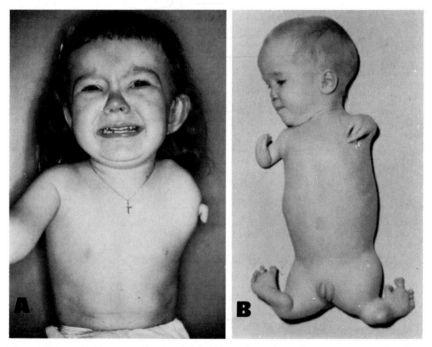

Figure 9.12. **A.** Photograph of a child with unilateral amelia. **B.** Patient with a form of meromelia called phocomelia. The hands and feet are attached to the trunk by irregularly shaped bones.

A different category of limb abnormalities consists of the presence of extra fingers or toes **(polydactyly)** (Fig. 9.13A). The extra digit frequently lacks proper muscular connections. Abnormalities with an excessive number of bones are mostly bilateral, while the absence of a digit such as a thumb **(ectrodactyly)** is usually unilateral. Polydactyly can be inherited as a dominant trait but may also be induced by teratogens.

Abnormal fusion is usually restricted to the fingers or toes **(syndactyly)**. Normally, mesenchyme between prospective digits in the handplates and footplates breaks down. Not infrequently (1 in 2000 births), this fails to occur, and the result is fusion of one or more fingers and toes (Fig. 9.13B). In some cases, actual fusion of the bones occurs.

Cleft hand and foot (lobster-claw deformity) consists of an abnormal cleft between the 2nd and 4th metacarpal bones and soft tissues.

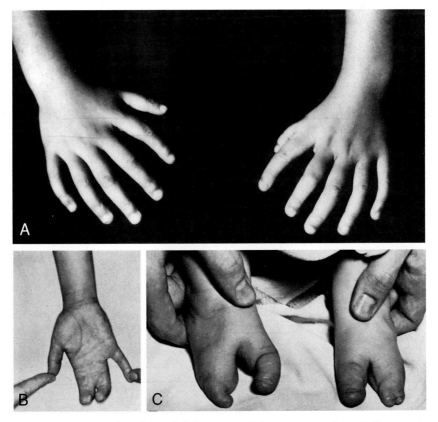

Figure 9.13. Examples of digital defects. **A.** Polydactyly, extra digits. **B.** Syndactyly, fused digits. **C.** Cleft foot, lobster-claw deformity.

The 3rd metacarpal and phalangeal bones are almost always absent, and the thumb and index finger as well as the 4th and 5th fingers may be fused (Fig. 9.13C). The two parts of the hand are somewhat opposed to each other and act like a lobster claw.

Clubfoot is usually present in combination with syndactyly. The sole of the foot is turned inward, and the foot is adducted and plantar flexed. It is observed mainly in males and in some cases is hereditary. Abnormal positioning of the legs in utero may also cause the abnormality.

Congenital absence or deficiency of the radius is usually a genetic abnormality observed with malformations in other structures, such as **craniosynostosis-radial aplasia syndrome.** Associated digital defects, which may include absent thumbs and a short curved ulna, are usually present.

Amniotic bands may cause ring constrictions of the limbs or digits and amputations (Fig. 9.14). The origin of bands is not clear, but they may represent adhesions between the amnion and affected structures in the fetus. Other investigators believe that bands originate from tears in the amnion that detach and surround part of the fetus.

Congenital hip dislocation consists of underdevelopment of the acetabulum and head of the femur. The condition is rather common and occurs mostly in females. Although dislocation usually occurs after birth, the abnormality of the bones develops prenatally. Since many babies with the abnormality are breech deliveries, it has been thought that breech posture may interfere with development of the hip joint. The abnormality is frequently associated with laxity of the joint capsule.

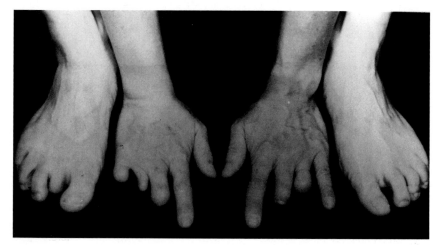

Figure 9.14. Patient showing digit amputations resulting from amniotic bands.

Vertebral Column

During the 4th week of development, cells of the sclerotomes shift their position to surround both the spinal cord and notochord (Fig. 9.1). This positional change is effected by differential growth of the surrounding structures and not by active migration of sclerotome cells. This mesenchymal column retains traces of its segmental origin as the sclerotomic blocks are separated by less dense areas containing **intersegmental arteries** (Fig. 9.15A).

During further development, the caudal portion of each sclerotome segment proliferates extensively and condenses (Fig. 9.15B). This proliferation is so extensive that it proceeds into the subjacent intersegmental tissue and binds the caudal half of one sclerotome to the cephalic half of the subjacent sclerotome (see *arrows* in Fig. 9.15, *A* and *B*). Hence, by incorporation of the intersegmental tissue into the **precartilaginous vertebral body** (Fig. 9.15B), the body of the vertebra becomes intersegmental in origin.

Mesenchymal cells located between cephalic and caudal parts of the original sclerotome segment do not proliferate but fill the space between two precartilaginous vertebral bodies. In this way, they contribute to formation of the **intervertebral disc** (Fig. 9.15B). Although the notochord regresses entirely in the region of the vertebral bodies, it persists and enlarges in the region of the intervertebral disc. Here it contributes to the **nucleus pulposus,** which is later surrounded by circular fibers of the **annulus fibrosus.** Combined, these two structures form the **intervertebral disc** (Fig. 9.15C).

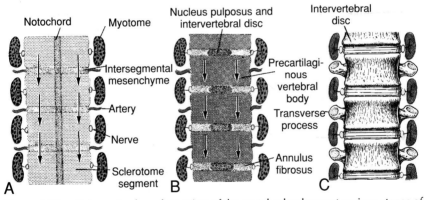

Figure 9.15. Scheme to show formation of the vertebral column at various stages of development. **A.** At the 4th week of development, sclerotomic segments are separated by less dense intersegmental tissue. Note the position of the myotomes, intersegmental arteries, and segmental nerves. **B.** Condensation and proliferation of the caudal half of one sclerotome proceed into the intersegmental mesenchyme and cranial half of the subjacent sclerotome. Note the appearance of the intervertebral discs. Note the position of the *arrows* in **A** and **B.** **C.** Precartilaginous vertebral bodies are formed by the upper and lower halves of two successive sclerotomes and the intersegmental tissue. Myotomes bridge the intervertebral discs and, therefore, can move the vertebral column.

Rearrangement of sclerotomes into definitive vertebrae causes the myotomes to overbridge the intervertebral discs, and this alteration gives them the capacity to move the spine (Fig. 9.15C). For the same reason, intersegmental arteries, at first located between the sclerotomes, now pass midway over the vertebral bodies. Spinal nerves, however, come to lie near the intervertebral discs and leave the vertebral column through the intervertebral foramina.

CLINICAL CORRELATES

The process of formation and subsequent rearrangement of segmental sclerotomes into definitive vertebrae is complicated, and it is not uncommon to have two successive vertebrae fuse asymmetrically or have half a vertebra missing, a cause of **scoliosis (lateral curving of the spine).** Also, the number of vertebrae is frequently increased or decreased. A rather typical example of these abnormalities is found in patients with **Klippel-Feil anomaly.** These patients have a reduced number of cervical vertebrae, and often, other vertebrae are fused or abnormal in shape. The condition is usually associated with other abnormalities.

One of the most serious vertebral defects is the result of imperfect fusion or nonunion of the vertebral arches. Such an abnormality, known as **cleft vertebra (spina bifida),** may involve only the bony vertebral arches, leaving the spinal cord intact. In these cases, the bony defect is covered by skin, and no neurological deficits occur **(spina bifida occulta).** A more severe abnormality is **spina bifida cystica** in which the neural tube fails to close, vertebral arches fail to form, and neural tissue is exposed. Neurological deficits occur and are dependent on the level and extent of the lesion. This defect occurs in 1 in 1000 births and, in many cases, may be prevented by providing mothers with folic acid prior to conception. Spina bifida can be detected prenatally by ultrasound (Fig. 9.16), and in cases where neural tissue is exposed, amniocentesis would detect elevated levels of α-fetoprotein (AFP) in the amniotic fluid. (For the various types of spina bifida, see Figs. 20.14 and 20.15.)

In addition to abnormalities specifically affecting the skull, vertebral column, or limbs, a number of diseases affect almost all the bones of the skeleton. One of the best-known systemic abnormalities of the skeletal system is **achondroplasia.** This condition is caused by a disturbance of endochondral ossification in the epiphysial plates of long bones, resulting in **dwarfism.** The extremities are short, the head has a normal size or is slightly enlarged, and the center of the face is somewhat underdeveloped (Fig. 9.17). Mental development is normal and occasionally high. The condition is inherited as a mendelian dominant trait and occurs in about 1 in 10,000 births.

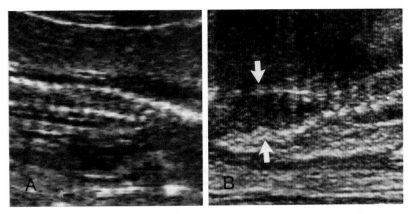

Figure 9.16. Ultrasound scans of the vertebral columns in a normal infant **(A)** and one with spina bifida **(B)** aged 4 months. The cleft vertebrae are readily apparent *(arrows)*.

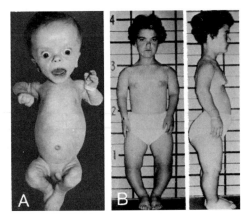

Figure 9.17 **A.** Three-month-old infant with achondroplasia. Note the large head, short extremities, and protruding abdomen. **B.** Achondroplasia in a 15-year-old girl. Note dwarfism of the short limb type, the limbs being disproportionately shorter than the trunk. The limbs are bowed, there is an increase in lumbar lordosis, and the face is small relative to the head.

Acromegaly is caused by congenital hyperpituitarism and excessive production of growth hormone. The abnormality is characterized by disproportional enlargement of the face, hands, and feet. Sometimes, it causes more symmetrical excessive growth and gigantism.

Ribs and Sternum

Ribs form from costal processes of thoracic vertebrae and thus are derived from the sclerotome portion of paraxial mesoderm. The sternum develops independently in somatic mesoderm in the ventral body wall. Two sternal bands are formed on either side of the midline, and these later fuse to form cartilaginous models of the manubrium, sternebrae, and xiphoid process.

SUMMARY

The skeletal system develops from mesenchyme, which is derived from the mesodermal germ layer and from neural crest. Some bones, such as the flat bones of the skull, undergo **membranous ossification;** i.e., mesenchyme cells are directly transformed into osteoblasts (Fig. 9.2). In most bones, such as the long bones of the limbs, mesenchyme condenses and forms hyaline cartilage models of bones (Fig. 9.10). Ossification centers appear in these cartilage models, and the bone gradually ossifies by **endochondral ossification.**

The **vertebral column** and **ribs** develop from the **sclerotome** compartments of the **somites.** A definitive vertebra is formed by condensation of the caudal half of one sclerotome and fusion with the cranial half of the subjacent sclerotome (Fig. 9.15).

The **skull** consists of the **neurocranium** and **viscerocranium** (face). The neurocranium includes a **membranous portion,** which forms the cranial vault, and a cartilaginous portion **(chondrocranium),** which forms the base of the skull. Neural crest cells form the face, most of the cranial vault, and the prechordal part of the chondrocranium (the part that lies rostral to the notochord). Paraxial mesoderm forms the remainder of the skull.

Many abnormalities of the skeletal system occur, including vertebral (spina bifida), skull (cranioschisis and craniosynostosis), and facial (cleft palate) defects. Major malformations of the limbs are rare, but defects of the radius and digits are often associated with other abnormalities **(syndromes).**

PROBLEMS TO SOLVE

1. Why are cranial sutures important? Are they involved in any abnormalities?

2. If you observe congenital absence of the radius or digital defects such as absent thumb or polydactyly, would you consider examining the infant for other malformations? Why?

3. Explain the origin of scoliosis as a vertebral anomaly.

SUGGESTED READINGS

Cohen MM Jr: Syndrome delineation and its implications for the study of pathogenetic mechanisms. *In* Persaud TVN (ed): *Advances in the Study of Birth Defects,* vol 5: *Genetic Disorders.* New York, Alan R Liss, 1982.
Couly GF, Coltey PM, LeDouarin: The triple origin of skull in higher vertebrates: a study in quail-chick chimeras. *Development* 117:409–429, 1993.
Dolle P, Izpisua-Belmonte J-C, Falkenstein H, Rennucci A, Duboule D. Coordinate expression of the murine *Hox-5* complex homeobox-containing genes during limb pattern formation. *Nature (Lond)* 342:767, 1989.
Edgerton MT, Jane JA, Berry FA: Craniofacial osteotomies and reconstruction in infants and children. *J Plast Recontr Surg* 54:13, 1974.

Eichele G, Thaller C: Characterization of concentration gradients of a morphologically active retinoid in the chick limb bud. *J Cell Biol* 105:1917, 1987.

Filly RA: Sonographic anatomy of the normal fetus. *In* Harrison MR, Golbus MS, Filly RA (eds): *The Unborn Patient. Prenatal Diagnosis and Treatment.* 2nd ed. Philadelphia, WB Saunders, 1991.

Filly RA, Golbus MS: Ultrasonography of the normal and pathologic fetal skeleton. *Radiol Clin North Am* 20:311, 1982.

Gans C, Northcutt RG: Neural crest and the origin of vertebrates: a new head. *Science* 220:268–274, 1983.

Gasser RF: Evidence that sclerotomal cells do not migrate medially during normal embryonic development of the rat. *Am J Anat* 154:509, 1979.

Gorlin RJ: *Syndromes of the Head and Neck.* 2nd ed. New York, McGraw-Hill, 1976.

Johnston MC, Listgarten MA: Observations on the migration, interaction, and early differentiation of orofacial tissues. *In* Slavkin HC, Baretta LA (eds): *Developmental Aspects of Oral Biology.* New York, Academic Press, 1972.

Lenz W: Thalidomide and congenital abnormalities. *Lancet* 1:1219, 1962.

Madan M, Ong DE, Summerbell D, Chytil F. The role of retinoid-binding proteins in the generation of pattern in the developing limb and the nervous system. *Dev Suppl* 107:109, 1989.

Noden DM: Interactions and fates of avian craniofacial mesenchyme. *Development* 103:121–140, 1988.

Northcutt RG, Gans C: The genesis of neural crest and epidermal placodes: a reinterpretation of vertebrate origins. *Q Rev Biol* 58:1–28, 1983.

Smith DW: *Recognizable Patterns of Human Malformation: Genetic, Embryologic and Clinical Aspects.* Philadelphia, WB Saunders, 1976.

Tickle C, Summerbell D, Wolpert L. Positional signalling and specification of digits in chick limb morphogenesis. *Nature (Lond)* 254:199, 1975.

chapter 10

Muscular System

The muscular system develops from the mesodermal germ layer (except for the muscles of the iris, which form from optic cup ectoderm (see Chapter 18)) and consists of **skeletal, smooth,** and **cardiac muscle.** Skeletal muscle is derived from **paraxial mesoderm,** which forms somites from the occipital to the sacral regions and somitomeres in the head. Smooth muscle differentiates from **splanchnic mesoderm** surrounding the gut and its derivatives, and cardiac muscle is derived from **splanchnic mesoderm** surrounding the heart tube.

Striated Skeletal Musculature

Somites and **somitomeres** form the musculature of the axial skeleton, body wall, limbs, and head. From the occipital region caudally, somites form and differentiate into the sclerotome and dermomyotome (Fig. 10.1A). Cells of the myotome in the body wall and limb regions dissociate, move to their definitive locations, and become elongated and spindle shaped. These cells, known as **myoblasts,** fuse together and form long, multinucleated muscle fibers. Myofibrils soon appear in the cytoplasm, and by the end of the 3rd month, cross-striations typical for skeletal muscle appear. A similar process occurs in the seven somitomeres located in the head region rostral to the occipital somites. Somitomeres remain loosely organized structures, however, never segregating into sclerotome and dermomyotome segments.

Patterns for muscle formation are controlled by connective tissue into which myoblasts migrate. In the head region, these connective tissues are derived from neural crest cells; in cervical and occipital regions, they come from somitic mesoderm; and in the body wall and limbs, they originate from somatic mesoderm (Fig. 10.1B).

By the end of the 5th week, each myotome is divided into a small dorsal portion, the **epimere,** and a larger ventral part, the **hypomere,** which is formed by migration of myotome cells (Figs. 10.1B and 10.2A). Nerves innervating segmental muscles are also divided into a **dorsal primary ramus** for the epimere and a **ventral primary ramus** for the hypomere (Fig. 10.2B).

Myoblasts of the epimeres form the extensor muscles of the vertebral column, while those of the hypomeres give rise to the lateral and ventral flexor musculature (Fig. 10.2B). Myoblasts from cervical hypomeres form the **scalene, geniohyoid,** and **prevertebral muscles.** Those from thoracic segments split into three layers, which in the thorax are represented by the **external intercostal,**

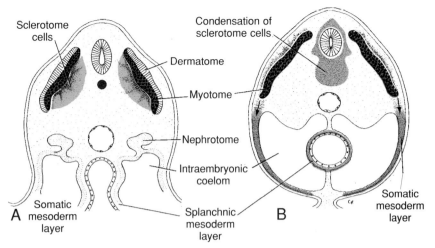

Figure 10.1. A. Diagrammatic transverse section through a 4-week embryo, showing cells of the myotome in close contact with the dermatome. **B.** Similar section as in **A,** showing migration of the myotome cells in a ventral direction until they reach the intraembryonic coelom.

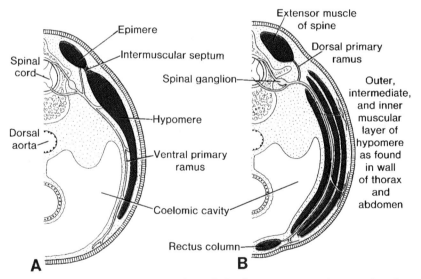

Figure 10.2. A. Transverse section through the thoracic region of a 5-week embryo. The dorsal portion of the body wall musculature (epimere) and the ventral portion (hypomere) are innervated by a dorsal primary ramus and a ventral primary ramus, respectively. **B.** Similar section as in **A** at a later stage of development. The hypomere has formed three separate muscle layers and a ventral longitudinal muscle.

internal intercostal, and **innermost intercostal** or **transverse thoracic muscle** (Fig. 10.2*B*). In the abdominal wall, these three muscle layers consist of the **external oblique,** the **internal oblique,** and the **transverse abdominal muscles.** Due to the presence of the ribs, muscles in the wall of the thorax maintain their segmental character, whereas muscles in the various segments of the abdominal wall fuse to form large sheets of muscle tissue. Myoblasts from the hypoblast of lumbar segments form the **quadratus lumborum muscle,** while those from sacral and coccygeal regions form the **pelvic diaphragm** and **striated muscles of the anus.**

In addition to the three ventrolateral muscle layers, a ventral longitudinal column arises at the ventral tip of the hypomeres (Fig. 10.2*B*). This column is represented by the **rectus abdominis muscle** in the abdominal region and by the **infrahyoid musculature** in the cervical region. In the thorax, the longitudinal muscle normally disappears but is occasionally represented by the **sternalis muscle.**

HEAD MUSCULATURE

All voluntary muscles of the head region are derived from paraxial mesoderm (somitomeres and somites), including musculature of the tongue, eye (except that of the iris, which is derived from optic cup ectoderm), and that associated with the pharyngeal (visceral) arches (Table 10.1). Patterns of muscle formation in the head are directed by connective tissue elements derived from neural crest cells.

LIMB MUSCULATURE

The first indication of limb musculature is observed in the 7th week of development as a condensation of mesenchyme near the base of the limb buds (Fig. 10.3*A*). The mesenchyme is derived from dermomyotome cells of somites that migrate into the limb bud to form the muscles. As in other regions, connective tissue dictates the pattern of muscle formation, and this tissue is derived from somatic mesoderm, which also gives rise to the bones of the limb.

With elongation of the limb buds, the muscular tissue splits into flexor and extensor components (Fig. 10.3*B*). Although muscles of the limbs have a

Table 10.1.
Origins of the Craniofacial Muscles

Mesodermal Origin	Muscles	Innervation
Somitomeres 1, 2	Superior, medial, and ventral recti	Oculomotor (III)
Somitomere 3	Superior oblique	Trochlear (IV)
Somitomere 4	Jaw-closing muscles	Trigeminal (V)
Somitomere 5	Lateral rectus	Abducens (VI)
Somitomere 6	Jaw-opening and other 2nd arch muscles	Facial (VII)
Somitomere 7	Stylopharyngeus	Glossopharyngeal (IX)
Somites 1, 2	Intrinsic laryngeals	Vagus (X)
Somites 2–5[a]	Tongue muscles	Hypoglossal (XII)

[a] Somites 2–5 represent the occipital group (somite 1 degenerates for the most part).

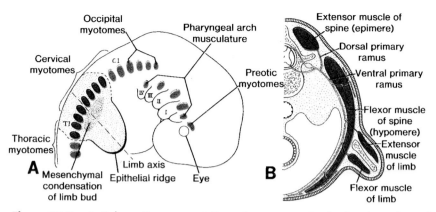

Figure 10.3. A. Schematic representation of myotomes in the head, neck, and thoracic region of a 7-week embryo. Note the localization of the preotic and occipital myotomes and condensation of mesenchyme at the base of the limb bud. **B.** Transverse section through the region of attachment of the limb bud. Note the dorsal (extensor) and ventral (flexor) muscular components of the limb.

segmental character initially, with time they fuse and are then composed of muscle tissue derived from several segments.

The upper limb buds lie opposite the lower five cervical and upper two thoracic segments (Fig. 10.4, *A* and *B*), and the lower limb buds lie opposite the lower four lumbar and upper two sacral segments (Fig. 10.4*C*). As soon as the buds are formed, the appropriate spinal nerves penetrate into the mesenchyme (Fig. 10.5). At first, they enter with isolated dorsal and ventral branches, but soon these branches unite to form large dorsal and ventral nerves. Thus, the **radial nerve,** which supplies the extensor musculature, is formed by a combination of the dorsal segmental branches, whereas the **ulnar** and **median nerves,** which supply the flexor musculature, are formed by combination of the ventral branches. Immediately after the nerves have entered the limb buds, they establish an intimate contact with the differentiating mesodermal condensations, and the early contact between the nerve and muscle cells is a prerequisite for their complete functional differentiation.

Spinal nerves not only play an important role in differentiation and motor innervation of the limb musculature but also provide sensory innervation for the dermatomes. Although the original dermatomal pattern changes with growth of the extremities, an orderly sequence can still be recognized in the adult (Fig. 10.4).

CLINICAL CORRELATES

Partial or complete absence of one or more muscles is a rather common occurrence. One of the best known examples is total or partial absence of the pectoralis major muscle. Similarly, the palmaris longus, the serratus anterior, and the quadratus femoris muscles may be partially or entirely absent.

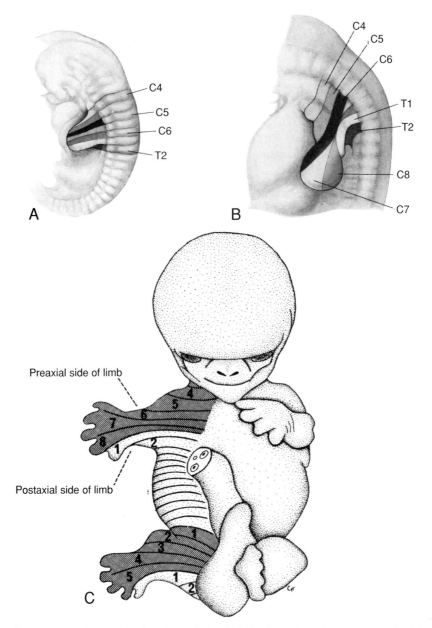

Figure 10.4. Schematic drawings of the limb buds, with their segments of origin indicated. With further development, the segmental pattern disappears; an orderly sequence in the dermatome pattern, however, can still be recognized in the adult. **A.** Upper limb bud at 5 weeks. **B.** Upper limb bud at 6 weeks. **C.** Limb buds at 7 weeks.

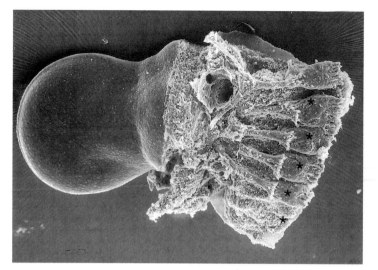

Figure 10.5. Scanning electron micrograph of a mouse upper limb bud, showing spinal nerves entering the limb. *Asterisks,* spinal ganglia.

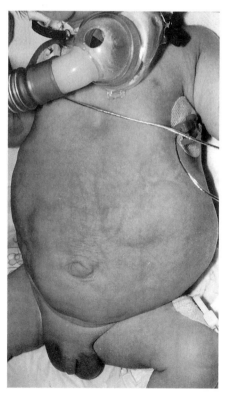

Figure 10.6. Patient with prune belly syndrome, showing a distended abdomen from aplasia of abdominal wall musculature.

Partial or complete absence of abdominal musculature results in prune belly syndrome (Fig. 10.6). Usually, the abdominal wall is so thin that organs are visible and easily palpated. The defect is usually associated with malformations of the urinary tract and bladder.

Cardiac Muscle

Cardiac muscle in the embryo develops from splanchnic mesoderm surrounding the endothelial heart tube. Myoblasts adhere to one another by special attachments that later develop into **intercalated discs.** Myofibrils develop as in skeletal muscle, but myoblasts do not fuse. During later development, a few special bundles of muscle cells with irregularly distributed myofibrils become visible. These bundles are **Purkinje fibers** and form the conducting system of the heart.

SUMMARY

Muscles are of mesodermal origin. Skeletal muscles are derived from paraxial mesoderm, including (a) somites, which give rise to muscles of the axial skeleton, body wall, and limbs, and (b) somitomeres, which give rise to muscles of the head. By the 5th week, each myotome is divided into a small dorsal portion, the **epimere,** innervated by a **dorsal primary ramus,** and a larger ventral portion, the **hypomere,** innervated by a ventral primary ramus. Myoblasts from epimeres form extensor muscles of the vertebral column, while those from hypomeres form muscles of the body wall and limbs. **Connective tissue** derived from somites, somatic mesoderm, and neural crest (head region) provide a template for establishment of muscle patterns. **Most smooth muscles** as well as **cardiac muscle fibers** are derived from **splanchnic mesoderm.**

PROBLEMS TO SOLVE

1. In examining a newborn female, you note that her right nipple is lower than the left and that the right anterior axillary fold is nearly absent. What is your diagnosis?

2. Patterning of muscles is dependent on what type of tissue?

SUGGESTED READINGS

Chevallier A, Kieny M, Mauger A: Limb-somite relationship: origin of the limb musculature. *J Embryol Exp Morphol* 41:245–258, 1977.

Christ B, Jacob HJ, Jacob M: Experimental analysis of the origin of the wing musculature in avian embryos. *Anat Embryol* 150:171–186, 1977.

Christ B, Jacob M, Jacob HJ: On the origin and development of the ventrolateral abdominal muscles in the avian embryo. *Anat Embryol* 166:87–101, 1983.

Levi AC, Borghi F, Garavoglia M: Development of the anal canal muscles. *Dis Colon Rectum* 34:262, 1991.

Noden DM: The embryonic origins of avian cephalic and cervical muscles and associated connective tissues. *Am J Anat* 168:257–276, 1983.

Noden DM: Craniofacial development: new views on old problems. *Anat Rec* 208:1–13, 1984.

Noden DM: Interactions and fates of avian craniofacial mesenchyme. *Development* 103:121–140, 1988.

Body Cavities

Formation of the Intraembryonic Coelom

At the end of the 3rd week, intraembryonic mesoderm on each side of the midline differentiates into a paraxial portion, an intermediate portion, and a lateral plate (Fig. 11.1A). When intercellular clefts appear in the lateral mesoderm, the plates are divided into two layers: the **somatic mesoderm layer** and the **splanchnic mesoderm layer.** The latter is continuous with mesoderm of the wall of the yolk sac (Fig. 11.1B). The space bordered by these layers forms the **intraembryonic coelom (body cavity).**

At first, the right and left sides of the intraembryonic coelom are in open connection with the extraembryonic coelom, but when the body of the embryo folds in cephalocaudal and lateral directions, this connection is lost (Fig. 11.2, A–C). In this manner, a large intraembryonic coelom is formed, extending from the thoracic to the pelvic region.

CLINICAL CORRELATES

Ventral body wall defects may occur in the thorax or abdomen and may involve the heart, abdominal viscera, and urogenital organs. They may be due to a failure of body folding, in which case one or more of the four folds (cephalic, caudal, and two lateral) responsible for closing the ventral body wall at the umbilicus fail to progress to that region. Another cause of these defects is due to incomplete development of body wall structures, including muscle, bone, and skin.

Cleft sternum is a ventral body wall defect that results from lack of fusion of the bilateral bars of mesoderm responsible for formation of this structure. In some cases, the heart may protrude through a sternal defect (either cleft sternum or absence of the lower third of this structure) and lie outside the body **(ectopia cordis)** (Fig. 11.3A). Sometimes, the defect involves both the thorax and abdomen, creating a spectrum of abnormalities known as **Cantrell pentalogy,** which includes cleft sternum, ectopia cordis, omphalocele, diaphragmatic hernia (anterior portion), and congenital heart defects (ventricular septal defect, tetralogy of Fallot). Ectopia cordis defects appear to be due to a failure of progression of cephalic and lateral folds.

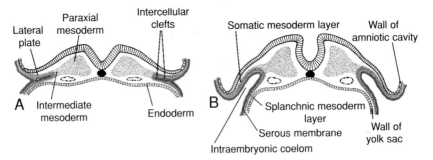

Figure 11.1. **A.** Transverse section through an embryo of approximately 19 days. Intercellular clefts are visible in the lateral plate mesoderm. **B.** Section through an embryo of approximately 20 days. The lateral plate is divided into somatic and splanchnic mesoderm layers that line the intraembryonic coelom. Tissue bordering the intraembryonic coelom differentiates into serous membranes and is indicated by red lines.

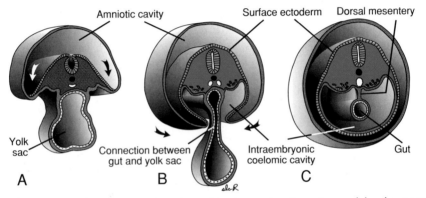

Figure 11.2. Transverse sections through embryos at various stages of development. **A.** The intraembryonic coelom is in open communication with the extraembryonic coelom. **B.** The intraembryonic coelom is about to lose contact with the extraembryonic coelom. **C.** At the end of the 4th week. Splanchnic mesoderm layers are continuous with somatic layers as a double-layered membrane, the dorsal mesentery. Dorsal mesentery extends from the caudal limit of the foregut to the end of the hindgut.

Omphalocele (Fig. 11.3*B*) involves herniation of abdominal viscera through an enlarged umbilical ring. The viscera, which may include liver, small and large intestines, stomach, spleen, or bladder, are covered by amnion. The origin of the defect is a failure of the bowel to return to the body cavity from its physiological herniation during the 6th to 10th weeks. The abnormality occurs in 2.5/10,000 births and is associated with a high rate of mortality (25%) and severe malformations, such as cardiac anomalies (50%) and neural tube defects (40%). Chromosomal abnormalities are present in approximately 50% of liveborn infants with omphalocele.

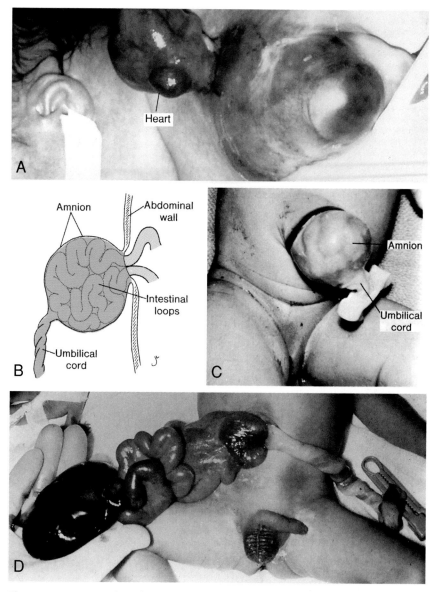

Figure 11.3. Examples of ventral body wall defects. **A.** Infant with ectopia cordis. Mesoderm of the sternum has failed to fuse, and the heart lies outside the body. **B.** Illustration of patient with omphalocele, showing failure of the intestinal loops to return to the body cavity following physiological herniation. The herniated loops are covered by amnion. **C.** Photograph of omphalocele in a newborn. **D.** Photograph of a newborn with gastroschisis. Loops of bowel return to the body cavity but herniate again through the body wall, usually to the right of the umbilicus in the region of the regressing right umbilical vein. Unlike omphalocele, the defect is not covered by amnion.

Gastroschisis (Fig. 11.3C) is a herniation of abdominal contents through the body wall, directly into the amniotic cavity. The defect occurs lateral to the umbilicus, usually on the right, through a region weakened by regression of the right umbilical vein, which normally disappears. Viscera are not covered by peritoneum or amnion, and the bowel may be damaged by exposure to amniotic fluid. Both omphalocele and gastroschisis result in elevated levels of α-fetoprotein in the amniotic fluid that can be detected prenatally.

Gastroschisis occurs in 1/10,000 births but is increasing in frequency, especially among young women, and this increase may be related to cocaine use. Unlike omphalocele, gastroschisis is not associated with chromosome abnormalities or other severe defects, and therefore, the survival rate is excellent. Volvulus (rotation of the bowel) resulting in a compromised blood supply, however, may kill large regions of the intestine and lead to fetal death.

Cells of the somatic mesoderm lining the intraembryonic coelom become mesothelial and form the **parietal layer of the serous membranes** lining the outside of the peritoneal, pleural, and pericardial cavities. In a similar manner, cells of the splanchnic mesoderm layer form the **visceral layer of the serous membranes** covering the abdominal organs, lungs, and heart (Fig. 11.1). Visceral and parietal layers are continuous with each other as the **dorsal mesentery** (Fig. 11.2C), which suspends the gut tube in the peritoneal cavity. Initially, this dorsal mesentery is a thickened band of mesoderm running continuously from the caudal limit of the foregut to the end of the hindgut. **Ventral mesentery** exists only from the caudal foregut to the upper portion of the duodenum and results from thinning of mesoderm of the **septum transversum** (see Chapter 14). These mesenteries represent double layers of peritoneum that provide a pathway for blood vessels, nerves, and lymphatics to the organs.

Diaphragm and Thoracic Cavity

The **septum transversum** is a thick plate of mesodermal tissue occupying the space between the thoracic cavity and the stalk of the yolk sac (Fig. 11.4, *A* and *B*). This septum does not separate the thoracic and abdominal cavities completely but leaves large openings, the **pericardioperitoneal canals,** on each side of the foregut (Fig. 11.4B).

When lung buds begin to grow, they expand in a caudolateral direction within the pericardioperitoneal canals (Fig. 11.4C). As a result of the rapid growth of the lungs, the pericardioperitoneal canals become too small, and the lungs begin to expand into the mesenchyme of the body wall in dorsal, lateral, and ventral

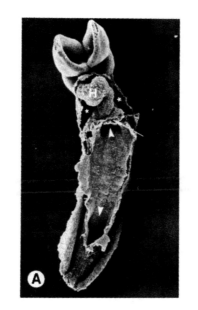

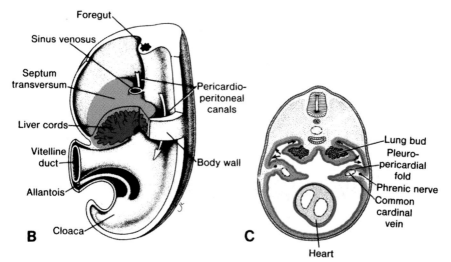

Figure 11.4. **A.** Scanning electron micrograph showing the ventral view of a mouse embryo (equivalent to approximately the 4th week in human development). The gut tube is closing, the anterior and posterior intestinal portals are visible *(arrowheads)*, and the heart *(H)* lies in the primitive pleuropericardial cavity *(asterisks)*, which is partially separated from the abdominal cavity by the septum transversum *(arrow)*. **B.** Model of a portion of an embryo at approximately 5 weeks. Parts of the body wall and septum transversum have been removed to show the pericardioperitoneal canals. Note the size and thickness of the septum transversum and liver cords penetrating the septum. **C.** Drawing to show growth of the lung buds into the pericardioperitoneal canals. Note the pleuropericardial folds. *Arrows* indicate direction of expansion of the lung buds.

directions (Fig. 11.4*C, small arrows*). This expansion in ventral and lateral directions occurs in a plane lateral to the **pleuropericardial folds.** At first, these folds appear as small ridges projecting into the primitive undivided thoracic cavity (Fig. 11.4*C*). With expansion of the lungs, mesoderm of the body wall is split into two components (Fig. 11.5, *A* and *B*): *(a)* the definitive wall of the thorax; and *(b)* the **pleuropericardial membranes,** which are thin layers of mesoderm that contain the common cardinal veins and phrenic nerves. Subsequently, descent of the heart and positional changes of the sinus venosus shift the common cardinal veins toward the midline, and the pleuropericardial membranes are drawn out in mesentery-like fashion (Fig. 11.5*A*). Finally, they fuse with each other and with the root of the lungs, and the thoracic cavity is then divided into the definitive **pericardial cavity** and two **pleural cavities** (Fig. 11.5*B*). In the adult, the pleuropericardial membranes form the **fibrous pericardium.**

Although the pleural cavities are separated from the pericardial cavity, they remain temporarily in open communication with the abdominal cavity, since the diaphragm is incomplete. During further development, the caudal border of the pleural cavities is delineated by crescent-shaped folds, the **pleuroperitoneal folds** (Fig. 11.6*A*). These folds project into the caudal end of the pericardioperitoneal canals. With further development, the folds extend in medial and ventral directions and, by the 7th week, fuse with the mesentery of the esophagus and with the septum transversum (Fig. 11.6*B*). Hence, **the connection between the thoracic and abdominal portions of the coelom is closed by the pleuroperitoneal membranes.** Further expansion of the pleural cavities relative to mesenchyme of the body wall results in addition of a peripheral rim to the pleuroperitoneal

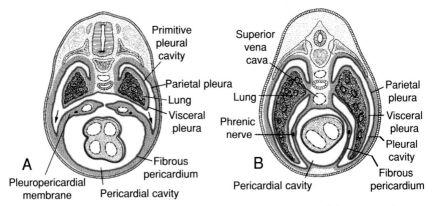

Figure 11.5. **A.** Schematic drawing showing transformation of the pericardioperitoneal canals into the pleural cavities and formation of the pleuropericardial membranes. Note the pleuropericardial folds containing the common cardinal vein and phrenic nerve. Mesenchyme of the body wall splits into the pleuropericardial membranes and the definitive body wall. *Arrows* indicate direction of expansion of the primitive pleural cavity. **B.** Drawing through the thorax after fusion of the pleuropericardial folds with each other and with the root of the lungs. Note the position of the phrenic nerve, which is now in the fibrous pericardium. The right common cardinal vein has developed into the superior vena cava.

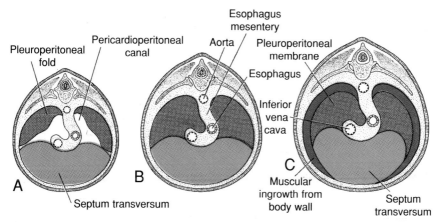

Figure 11.6. Schematic drawings illustrating development of the diaphragm. **A.** Pleuroperitoneal folds appear at the beginning of the 5th week. **B.** Pleuroperitoneal folds fuse with the septum transversum and mesentery of the esophagus in the 7th week, thus separating the thoracic cavity from the abdominal cavity. **C.** Transverse section at the 4th month of development. An additional rim derived from the body wall forms the most peripheral part of the diaphragm.

membranes (Fig. 11.6C). Once this rim is established, myoblasts originating in the body wall penetrate the membranes to form the muscular part of the diaphragm.

Thus, the diaphragm is derived from the following structures: *(a)* the septum transversum, which forms the tendinous part of the diaphragm; *(b)* the two pleuroperitoneal membranes; *(c)* muscular components from the lateral and dorsal body walls; and *(d)* the mesentery of the esophagus, in which the **crura of the diaphragm** develop (Fig. 11.6C).

POSITION AND INNERVATION OF DIAPHRAGM

Initially, the septum transversum lies opposite cervical somites, and nerve components of the **3rd, 4th, and 5th cervical segments** of the spinal cord grow into the septum. At first, the nerves, known as **phrenic nerves,** pass into the septum through the pleuropericardial folds (Fig. 11.4B). This explains why, with further expansion of the lungs and descent of the septum, the phrenic nerves are located in the fibrous pericardium (Fig. 11.5, A and B) on their way to innervate the diaphragm.

Although the septum transversum lies opposite cervical segments during the 4th week, by the 6th week the developing diaphragm is located at the level of thoracic somites. The **descent of the diaphragm** is apparently caused by rapid growth of the dorsal part of the embryo (vertebral column), compared with that of the ventral part. By the beginning of the 3rd month, some of the dorsal bands of the diaphragm originate at the level of the 1st lumbar vertebra.

The phrenic nerves supply the diaphragm with its motor and sensory innervation. Since the most peripheral part of the diaphragm is derived from mesenchyme of the thoracic wall, it is generally accepted that some of the lower intercostal (thoracic) nerves contribute sensory fibers to the peripheral part of the diaphragm.

CLINICAL CORRELATES

A **diaphragmatic hernia** is one of the more common malformations in the newborn (1/2000) and is most frequently caused by failure of one or both of the pleuroperitoneal membranes to close the pericardioperitoneal canals. The peritoneal and pleural cavities are then continuous with one another along the posterior body wall. Such a defect, known as a **congenital diaphragmatic hernia,** allows abdominal viscera to enter the pleural cavity. In 85–90% of the cases, the hernia is on the left side, and intestinal loops, stomach, spleen, and part of the liver may enter the thoracic cavity (Fig. 11.7). Because of the presence of abdominal viscera in the chest, the heart is pushed anteriorly, while the lungs are compressed and often hypoplastic. A large defect is associated with a high rate (75%) of mortality due to pulmonary hypoplasia and dysfunction.

Occasionally, a small part of the muscular fibers of the diaphragm fail to develop, and a hernia may then remain undiscovered until the child is several years old. Such a defect is frequently seen in the anterior portion of the diaphragm and is known as a **parasternal hernia.** A small peritoneal sac containing intestinal loops may then enter the chest between the sternal and costal portions of the diaphragm (Fig. 11.7A).

Another type of diaphragmatic hernia, **esophageal hernia,** is thought to be due to a congenital shortness of the esophagus. The cardia and upper part of the stomach are retained in the thorax, and the stomach is then constricted at the level of the diaphragm.

SUMMARY

At the end of the 3rd week, intercellular clefts appear in the mesoderm on each side of the midline. When these spaces fuse, the **intraembryonic coelom (body cavity),** bordered by **somatic mesoderm** and **a splanchnic mesoderm** layer, is formed (Figs. 11.1 and 11.2). With cephalocaudal and transverse folding of the embryo, the intraembryonic coelom extends from the thoracic to the pelvic region. Somatic mesoderm will form the **parietal layer** of the **serous membranes** lining the outside **of the peritoneal, pleural, and pericardial cavities.** The **splanchnic layer** will form the **visceral layer of the serous membranes** covering the lungs, heart, and abdominal organs. These layers are continuous at the root of these organs in their cavities (as if a finger were stuck into a balloon, with the layer surrounding the finger being the splanchnic or visceral layer and the rest of the balloon representing the somatic or parietal layer surrounding the body cavity). In the abdomen, the serous membranes are called **peritoneum.**

The diaphragm divides the coelom into **thoracic cavity** and **peritoneal cavity.** It develops from four components: *(a)* **septum transversum;** *(b)*

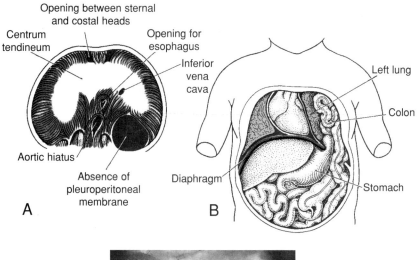

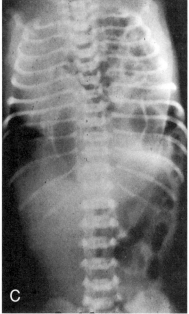

Figure 11.7. Congenital diaphragmatic hernia. **A.** Abdominal surface of the diaphragm, showing a large defect of the pleuroperitoneal membrane. **B.** Hernia of the intestinal loops and part of the stomach into the left pleural cavity. The heart and mediastinum are frequently pushed to the right, while the left lung is compressed. **C.** Radiograph of a newborn with a large defect in the left side of the diaphragm. Abdominal viscera have entered the thorax through the defect.

pleuroperitoneal membranes; (c) dorsal mesentery of the esophagus; and (d) muscular components of the body wall (Fig. 11.6). Congenital diaphragmatic hernias involving a defect of the pleuroperitoneal membrane on the left side occur frequently.

The **thoracic cavity** is divided into the **pericardial cavity** and two **pleural cavities** for the lungs by the **pleuropericardial membranes** (Fig. 11.5).

Double layers of peritoneum form **mesenteries** that suspend the gut tube and provide a pathway for vessels, nerves, and lymphatics to the organs. Initially, the gut tube, from the caudal end of the foregut to the end of the hindgut, is suspended from the dorsal body wall by **dorsal mesentery** (Fig. 11.2C). **Ventral mesentery** derived from the septum transversum exists only in the region of the terminal part of the esophagus, the stomach, and upper portion of the duodenum (see Chapter 14).

PROBLEMS TO SOLVE

1. At birth, an infant is never able to breathe and soon expires. An autopsy reveals a large diaphragmatic defect on the left side, with the stomach and intestines occupying the left side of the thorax. Both lungs are severely hypoplastic. What is the embryological basis for this defect? — *diaphragmatic hernia*

2. A child is born with a large defect in the region of the umbilicus. Most of the large and small bowel are protruding through the defect and are covered by amnion. What is the embryological basis for this abnormality, and should you be concerned that other malformations may be present?

SUGGESTED READINGS

Cunniff C, Jones KL, Jones MC: Patterns of malformations in children with congenital diaphragmatic defects. *J Pediatr* 116:258, 1990.
Puri P, Gormak F: Lethal nonpulmonary anomalies associated with congenital diaphragmatic hernia: implications for early intrauterine surgery. *J Pediatr Surg* 35:29, 1984.
Skandalakis JE, Gray SW: *Embryology for Surgeons. The Embryological Basis for the Treatment of Congenital Anomalies.* 2nd ed. Baltimore, Williams & Wilkins, 1994.

---

chapter 12

Cardiovascular System

CARDIAC DEVELOPMENT

The vascular system of the human embryo appears in the middle of the 3rd week, when the embryo is no longer able to satisfy its nutritional requirements by diffusion alone. At this stage, cells in the splanchnic mesoderm layer of the late presomite embryo are induced by underlying endoderm to form **angioblasts.** These cells proliferate and form isolated endothelial cell clusters known as angiocysts (Fig. 12.1).

At first, the clusters are located on the lateral sides of the embryo, but they rapidly spread in a cephalic direction (Fig. 12.1). With time, they unite and form a **horseshoe-shaped** plexus of small blood vessels. The anterior central portion of this plexus is known as the **cardiogenic area,** and the intraembryonic coelomic cavity located over this region later develops into the **pericardial cavity** (Fig. 12.1*D*).

In addition to the horseshoe-shaped plexus, other clusters of angiogenic cells appear bilaterally, parallel and close to the midline of the embryonic shield. These clusters also acquire a lumen and form a pair of longitudinal vessels, the **dorsal aortae.** At a later stage, these vessels gain connections, via the aortic arches, with the horseshoe-shaped plexus that will form the heart tube.

Formation and Position of the Heart Tube

Initially, the central portion of the cardiogenic area is located anterior to the prechordal plate and the neural plate (Fig. 12.2*A*). With closure of the neural tube and formation of the brain vesicles, however, the central nervous system grows so rapidly in a cephalic direction that it extends over the central cardiogenic area and the future pericardial cavity (Fig. 12.2). As a result of growth of the brain and cephalic folding of the embryo, the prechordal plate (future **buccopharyngeal membrane**) is pulled forward, while the heart and pericardial cavity become located first in the cervical region and finally in the thorax (Fig. 12.2).

As the embryo folds cephalocaudally, it also folds laterally (Fig. 12.3). As a result, the caudal regions of the two endothelial tubes merge with each other, except at their caudalmost ends. Simultaneously, the crescent part of the horseshoe-shaped area expands to form the future outflow tract and ventricular regions. Thus, the heart becomes a continuous expanded tube, receiving venous

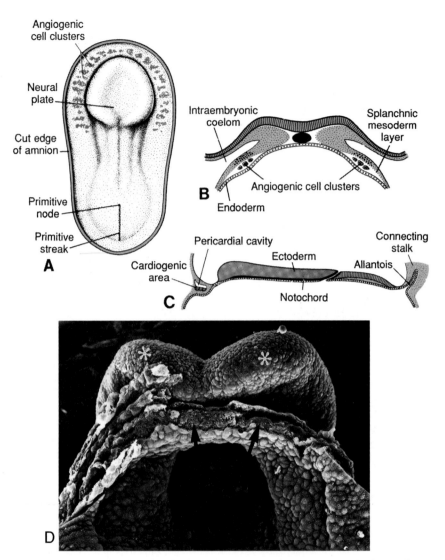

Figure 12.1. **A.** Dorsal view of a late presomite embryo (approximately 18 days) after removal of the amnion. Angiogenic cell clusters formed in the splanchnic mesoderm in front of the neural plate and on each side of the embryo are visible through the overlying ectoderm and somatic mesoderm layers. **B.** Transverse section through a similar-staged embryo to show the position of the angiogenic cell clusters in the splanchnic mesoderm layer. **C.** Cephalocaudal section through a similar-staged embryo, showing the position of the pericardial cavity and cardiogenic area. **D.** Scanning electron micrograph of a mouse embryo equivalent to 19 days in the human, showing coalescence of the angiogenic cells into a horseshoe-shaped heart tube *(arrows)* lying in the primitive pericardial cavity under the cranial neural folds *(asterisks).*

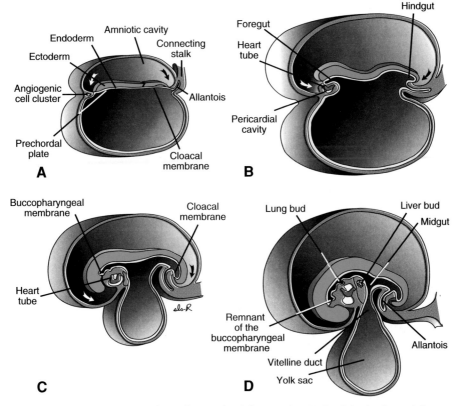

Figure 12.2. Drawings to show the result of the rapid growth of the brain vesicles on the position of the pericardial cavity and the developing heart tube. Initially, the cardiogenic area and the pericardial cavity are located in front of the prechordal plate. **A.** 18 days. **B.** 20 days. **C.** 21 days. **D.** 26 days.

drainage from its caudal pole and beginning to pump blood out the 1st aortic arch into the dorsal aorta (Figs. 12.4 and 12.5).

The developing heart tube bulges more and more into the pericardial cavity. Initially, however, the tube remains attached to the dorsal side of the pericardial cavity by a fold of mesodermal tissue, the **dorsal mesocardium** (Figs. 12.3 and 12.5). A ventral mesocardium is never formed. With further development, the dorsal mesocardium disappears, creating the **transverse pericardial sinus** that connects both sides of the pericardial cavity. The heart is now suspended in the cavity by blood vessels at its cranial and caudal poles (Fig. 12.5).

While these events are occurring, mesoderm adjacent to the endocardial tubes gradually thickens and forms the **myocardium** (Figs. 12.3 and 12.5). In turn, the myocardium secretes a thick layer of extracellular matrix, rich in hyaluronic acid, that separates it from the endothelium. In addition, mesothelial cells from the region of the sinus venosus migrate over the heart to form the **epicardium.** Thus, the heart tube consists of three layers: *(a)* the **endocardium,** forming the internal

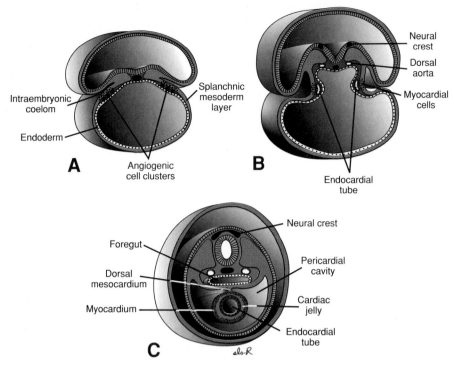

Figure 12.3. Schematic transverse sections through embryos at different stages of development, showing formation of a single heart tube from paired primordia. **A.** Early presomite embryo (17 days). **B.** Late presomite embryo (18 days). **C.** Eight-somite stage (22 days). Fusion occurs only in the caudal region of the horseshoe-shaped tube (see Fig. 12.4). The outflow tract and most of the ventricular region form by expansion and growth of the crescent portion of the horseshoe.

endothelial lining of the heart; *(b)* the **myocardium,** forming the muscular wall; and *(c)* the **epicardium** or **visceral pericardium,** covering the outside of the tube.

FORMATION OF THE CARDIAC LOOP

The heart tube continues to elongate and bend on day 23. The cephalic portion of the tube bends in ventral and caudal directions and to the right (Fig. 12.6, *B* and *C*), while the atrial (caudal) portion shifts in a dorsocranial direction and to the left (Figs. 12.6 and 12.7*A*). This bending, which may be due to cell shape changes, creates the **cardiac loop** and is completed by day 28.

While the cardiac loop is being formed, local expansions become visible throughout the length of the tube. The **atrial portion,** initially a paired structure located outside the pericardial cavity, forms a common atrium and becomes incorporated into the pericardial cavity (Fig. 12.7*A*). The **atrioventricular junction** remains narrow and forms the **atrioventricular canal,** which connects the common atrium and the early embryonic ventricle (Fig. 12.8). The **bulbus**

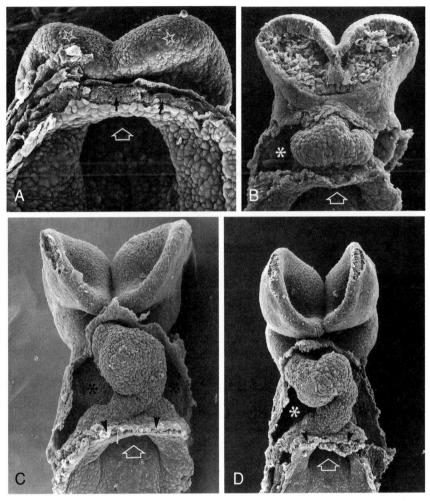

Figure 12.4. Formation of the heart tube on days 19, 20, 21, and 22 as depicted in scanning electron micrographs of mouse embryos at equivalent stages of human development. **A.** The heart tube *(arrows)* is horseshoe shaped in the pericardial cavity beneath the neural folds *(stars)*. **B.** The crescent portion of the horseshoe expands to form the ventricular and outflow tract regions, while lateral folding brings the caudal (venous) poles of the horseshoe together (see Fig. 12.3). **C.** Fusion of the caudal regions is initiated. **D.** Fusion of the caudal regions is complete, leaving the caudal poles embedded in the septum transversum *(arrowheads)*. Cardiac looping has also been initiated. *Asterisk,* pericardial cavity; and *large arrow,* anterior intestinal portal.

cordis is narrow except for its proximal third. This portion will form the **trabeculated part of the right ventricle** (Figs. 12.7*B* and 12.8). The midportion, known as the **conus cordis**, will form the outflow tracts of both ventricles. The distal part of the bulbus, the **truncus arteriosus,** will form the roots and proximal portion of the aorta and pulmonary artery (Fig. 12.8). The junction between the

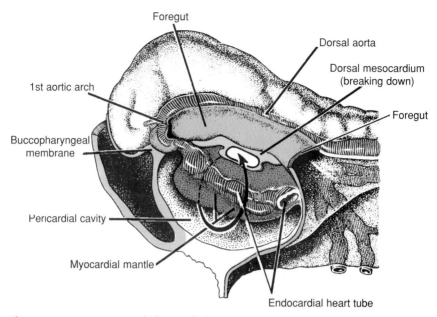

Figure 12.5. Drawing of the cephalic end of an early somite embryo. The developing endocardial heart tube and its investing layer bulge into the pericardial cavity. Note that the dorsal mesocardium is breaking down.

ventricle and the bulbus cordis, externally indicated by the **bulboventricular sulcus** (Fig. 12.6*C*), remains narrow and is called the **primary interventricular foramen** (Fig. 12.8).

At the end of loop formation, the smooth-walled heart tube begins to form primitive trabeculae in two sharply defined areas just proximal and distal to the **primary interventricular foramen** (Fig. 12.8). The atrial portion and the other portions of the bulbus temporarily remain smooth walled. The primitive ventricle, which is now trabeculated, is called the **primitive left ventricle.** Likewise, the trabeculated proximal one-third of the bulbus cordis may be referred to as the **primitive right ventricle** (Fig. 12.8).

The conotruncal portion of the heart tube, initially located on the right side of the pericardial cavity, shifts gradually to a more medial position. This change in position is the result of formation of two transverse dilatations of the atrium, bulging on each side of the bulbus cordis (Figs. 12.7*B* and 12.8).

DEVELOPMENT OF THE SINUS VENOSUS

In the middle of the 4th week, the **sinus venosus** receives venous blood from the **right** and **left sinus horns** (Fig. 12.9*A*). Each horn receives blood from three important veins: *(a)* the **vitelline** or **omphalomesenteric vein,** *(b)* the **umbilical vein,** and *(c)* the **common cardinal vein** (see also Fig. 12.40). At first, communication between the sinus and the atrium is wide. Soon, however, the entrance of the sinus shifts to the right (Fig. 12.9*B*). This shift is primarily caused

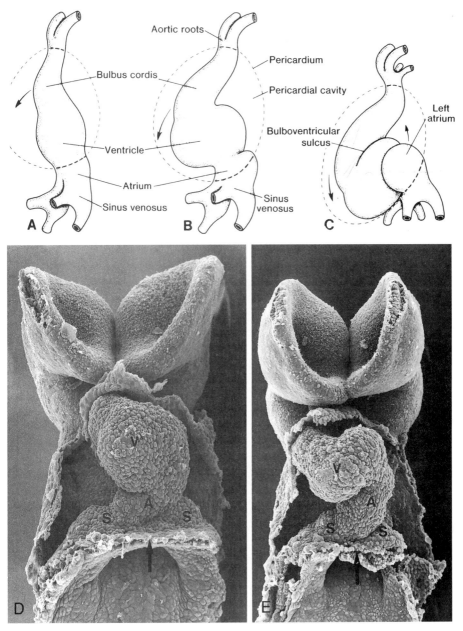

Figure 12.6. Formation of the cardiac loop. **A.** Eight somites. **B.** Eleven somites. **C.** Sixteen somites. *Broken line* indicates the pericardium. **D** and **E.** Scanning electron micrographs of mouse embryos, showing frontal views of the process illustrated in the diagrams. Initially, the cardiac tube is short and relatively straight **(D),** but as it lengthens, it bends (loops), bringing the atrial region cranial and dorsal to the ventricular region **(E).** *A,* primitive atrium; *arrow,* septum transversum; *S,* sinus venosus; and *V,* ventricle.

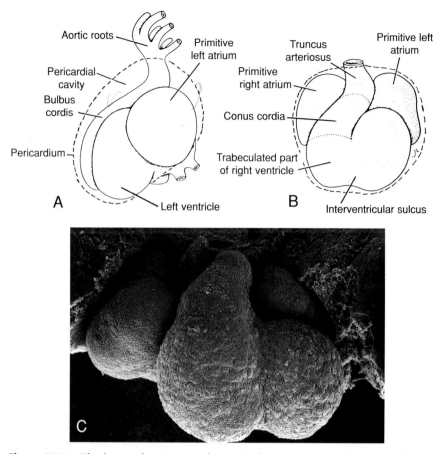

Figure 12.7. The heart of a 5-mm embryo (28 days). **A.** Viewed from the left. **B.** Frontal view. Note that the bulbus cordis is divided into the truncus arteriosus, conus cordis, and trabeculated part of the right ventricle. *Broken line,* pericardium. **C.** Scanning electron micrograph of the heart of a similar-staged mouse embryo, showing a view similar to **B.**

by left-to-right shunts of blood, which occur in the venous system during the 4th and 5th weeks of development.

With obliteration of the right umbilical vein and the left vitelline vein during the 5th week, the left sinus horn rapidly loses its importance (Fig. 12.9*B*). When the left common cardinal vein is obliterated at 10 weeks, all that remains of the left sinus horn is the **oblique vein of the left atrium** and the **coronary sinus** (Fig. 12.10).

As a result of left-to-right shunts of blood, the right sinus horn and veins enlarge greatly. The right horn, which now forms the only communication between the original sinus venosus and the atrium, is incorporated into the right atrium to form the smooth-walled part of the right atrium (Figs. 12.11 and 12.14).

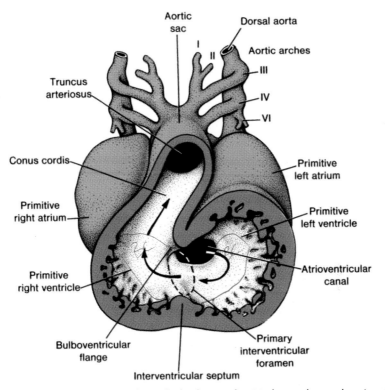

Figure 12.8. Frontal section through the heart of a 30-day embryo, showing the primary interventricular foramen and entrance of the atrium into the primitive left ventricle. Note the bulboventricular flange. *Arrows* indicate direction of blood flow.

Its entrance, the **sinuatrial orifice,** is flanked on each side by a valvular fold, the **right** and **left venous valves** (Fig. 12.11*A*). Dorsocranially, the valves fuse, thereby forming a ridge known as the **septum spurium** (Fig. 12.11*A*). Initially, the valves are large, but when the right sinus horn is incorporated into the wall of the atrium, the left venous valve and the septum spurium fuse with the developing atrial septum (Fig. 12.11*C*). The superior portion of the right venous valve disappears entirely. The inferior portion develops into two parts: *(a)* the **valve of the inferior vena cava,** and *(b)* the **valve of the coronary sinus** (Fig. 12.11*C*). The **crista terminalis** forms the dividing line between the original trabeculated part of the right atrium and the smooth-walled part **(sinus venarum),** which originates from the right sinus horn (Fig. 12.11*C*).

Formation of the Cardiac Septa

The major septa of the heart are formed between the 27th and 37th days of development, when the embryo grows in length from 5 mm to approximately 16–17 mm.

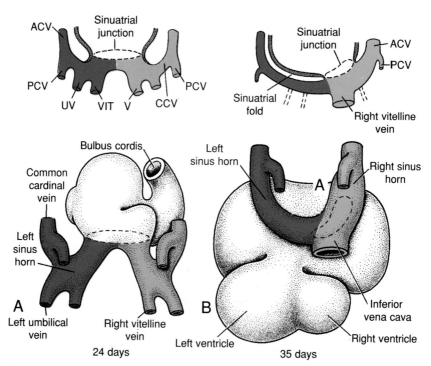

Figure 12.9. Dorsal view of two stages in the development of the sinus venosus at approximately 24 days (**A**) and 35 days (**B**). *Broken line* indicates the entrance of the sinus venosus into the atrial cavity. Each drawing is accompanied by a scheme to show, in transverse section, the great veins and their relationship to the atrial cavity. *ACV,* anterior cardinal vein; *PCV,* posterior cardinal vein; *UV,* umbilical vein; *VIT V,* vitelline vein; and *CCV,* common cardinal vein. (See also Figs. 12.10 and 12.40.)

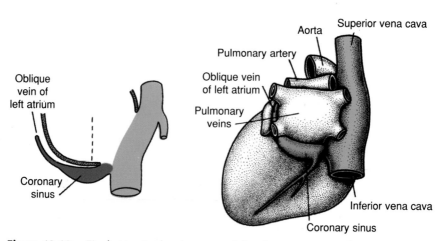

Figure 12.10. Final stage in development of the sinus venosus and great veins.

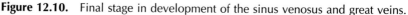

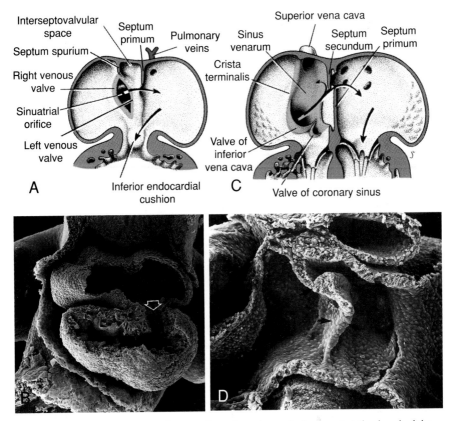

Figure 12.11. Ventral view of coronal sections through the heart at the level of the atrioventricular canal, to show development of the venous valves. **A.** 5 weeks. **B.** Scanning electron micrograph of a similar-staged mouse heart, showing initial formation of the septum primum (septum spurium is not visible). Note the atrioventricular canal *(arrow)*. **C.** Fetal stage. The sinus venarum (indicated in *blue*) is smooth walled and derived from the right sinus horn. *Arrows* indicate blood flow. **D.** High magnification of the interatrial septum *(arrow)* of a mouse embryo at a stage similar to **C.** The foramen ovale is not visible.

One method by which a septum may be formed involves two actively growing masses of tissue that approach each other until they fuse, thereby dividing the lumen into two separate canals (Fig. 12.12, *A* and *B*). Such a septum may also be formed by active growth of a single tissue mass that continues expanding until it reaches the opposite side of the lumen (Fig. 12.12*C*). Formation of such tissue masses is dependent on synthesis and deposition of extracellular matrices and cell proliferation. The masses, known as **endocardial cushions,** develop in the **atrioventricular** and **conotruncal** regions. In these locations, they assist in formation of the **atrial and ventricular (membranous portion) septa,** the **atrioventricular canals,** and the **aortic and pulmonary channels.**

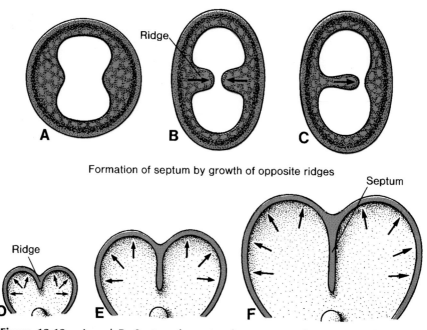

Formation of septum by growth of opposite ridges

Figure 12.12. **A** and **B.** Septum formation by two actively growing ridges that approach each other until they fuse. **C.** Septum formed by a single, actively growing cell mass. **D–F.** Septum formation by fusion of two expanding portions of the wall of the heart. Such a septum never completely separates two cavities.

The other manner in which a septum is formed does not involve endocardial cushions. If, for example, a narrow strip of tissue in the wall of the atrium or ventricle should fail to grow, while areas on each side of it expand rapidly, then a narrow ridge would be formed between the two expanding portions (Fig. 12.12, *D* and *E*). When growth of the expanding portions continues on either side of the narrow portion, the two walls approach each other and eventually fuse, thus forming a septum (Fig. 12.12*F*). Such a septum will never completely divide the original lumen but will leave a narrow communicating canal between the two expanded sections. It is usually closed secondarily by tissue contributed by neighboring proliferating tissues. Such a septum is formed to partially divide the atria and ventricles.

CLINICAL CORRELATES

Because of their key location, abnormalities in <u>endocardial cushion</u> formation <u>play a role in the origin of many cardiac malformations</u>, including **atrial** and **ventricular septal defects** and defects involving the **great vessels** (i.e., **transposition of the great vessels** and **tetralogy of Fallot**). Since cells populating the conotruncal cushions include

neural crest cells and since crest cells also contribute extensively to development of the head and neck, cardiac abnormalities are often associated with craniofacial defects (see Chapter 16).

Septum Formation in the Common Atrium

At the end of the 4th week, a sickle-shaped crest grows from the roof of the common atrium into the lumen. This crest represents the first portion of the **septum primum** (Figs. 12.11*A* and 12.13, *A* and *B*). The two limbs of this septum extend in the direction of the endocardial cushions in the atrioventricular canal. The opening between the lower rim of the septum primum and the endocardial cushions is the **ostium primum** (Fig. 12.13, *A* and *B*). With further

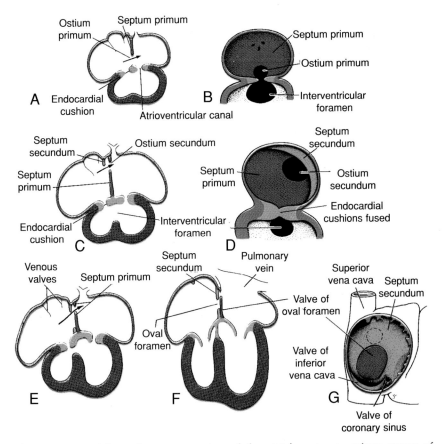

Figure 12.13. Schematic representation of the atrial septa at various stages of development. **A.** 30 days (6 mm). **B.** Same stage as in **A** but viewed from the right. **C.** 33 days (9 mm). **D.** Same stage as in **C** but viewed from the right. **E.** 37 days (14 mm). **F.** Newborn. **G.** View of the atrial septum from the right; same stage as in **F.**

development, extensions of the superior and inferior endocardial cushions grow along the edge of the septum primum, thereby closing the ostium primum (Fig. 12.13, *C* and *D*). Before closure is completed, however, **cell death** produces perforations in the upper portion of the septum primum. When these perforations coalesce, the **ostium secundum** is formed, thus ensuring a free blood flow from the right to the left primitive atrium (Fig. 12.13, *B* and *D*).

When the lumen of the right atrium expands as a result of incorporation of the sinus horn, a new crescent-shaped fold appears. This new fold, the **septum secundum** (Fig. 12.13, *C* and *D*), never forms a complete partition in the atrial cavity (Fig. 12.13*G*). Its anterior limb extends downward to the septum in the atrioventricular canal. When the left venous valve and the septum spurium fuse with the right side of the septum secundum, the free concave edge of the septum secundum begins to overlap the ostium secundum (Fig. 12.11, *A* and *B*). The opening left by the septum secundum is called the **oval foramen (foramen ovale).** When the upper part of the septum primum gradually disappears, the remaining part becomes the **valve of the oval foramen.** The passage between the two atrial cavities consists of an obliquely elongated cleft (Fig. 12.13, *E–G*), and blood from the right atrium flows to the left side through this cleft (see *arrows* in Figs. 12.11*B* and 12.13*E*).

After birth, when lung circulation begins and pressure in the left atrium increases, the valve of the oval foramen is pressed against the septum secundum, thus obliterating the oval foramen and separating the right and left atria. In about 20% of cases, fusion of the septum primum and septum secundum is incomplete, and a narrow oblique cleft remains between the two atria. This condition is known as **probe patency** of the oval foramen; it does not allow intracardiac shunting of blood.

FURTHER DIFFERENTIATION OF THE ATRIA

While the primitive right atrium enlarges by incorporation of the right sinus horn, the primitive left atrium is likewise expanding greatly. Initially, a single embryonic **pulmonary vein** develops as an outgrowth of the posterior left atrial wall, just to the left of the septum primum (Fig. 12.14*A*). This vein gains

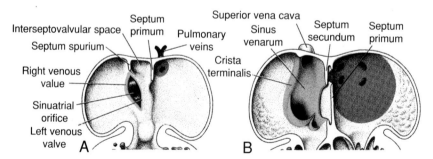

Figure 12.14. Coronal sections through the heart, to show development of the smooth-walled portions of the right and left atrium. Both the wall of the right sinus horn *(blue)* and the pulmonary veins *(red)* are incorporated into the heart to form the smooth-walled parts of the atria.

connection with veins of the developing lung buds. During further development, the pulmonary vein and its branches become incorporated into the left atrium, thus forming the large **smooth-walled** part of the adult atrium. Although initially one vein enters the left atrium, ultimately four pulmonary veins enter (Fig. 12.14*B*) as the branches are incorporated into the expanding atrial wall.

In the fully developed heart, the original embryonic left atrium is represented by little more than the **trabeculated atrial appendage,** while the smooth-walled part originates from the pulmonary veins (Fig. 12.14). On the right side, the original embryonic right atrium becomes the trabeculated **right atrial appendage** containing the pectinate muscles, while the smooth-walled **sinus venarum** originates from the right horn of the sinus venosus.

Septum Formation in the Atrioventricular Canal

At the end of the 4th week, two mesenchymal cushions, the **atrioventricular endocardial cushions,** appear at the superior and inferior borders of the atrioventricular canal (Figs. 12.15 and 12.16). Initially, the atrioventricular canal gives access only to the primitive left ventricle and is separated from the bulbus cordis by the **bulbo(cono)ventricular flange** (Fig. 12.8). Near the end of the 5th week, however, the posterior extremity of the flange terminates almost midway along the base of the superior endocardial cushion and is much less prominent than before (Fig. 12.16). Since the atrioventricular canal enlarges to the right, blood passing through the atrioventricular orifice now has direct access to the primitive left as well as the primitive right ventricle.

In addition to the superior and inferior endocardial cushions, two other cushions, the **lateral atrioventricular cushions,** appear on the right and left borders of the canal (Figs. 12.15 and 12.16). The superior and inferior cushions, in the meantime, project further into the lumen and fuse with each other, resulting in a complete division of the canal into right and left atrioventricular orifices by the end of the 5th week (Fig. 12.15).

ATRIOVENTRICULAR VALVES

After the atrioventricular endocardial cushions fuse, each atrioventricular orifice is surrounded by localized proliferations of mesenchymal tissue (Fig. 12.17*A*). When tissue located on the ventricular surface of these proliferations becomes hollowed out and thinned by the bloodstream, valves are formed that remain attached to the ventricular wall by muscular cords (Fig. 12.17*B*). Finally, muscular tissue in the cords degenerates and is replaced by dense connective tissue. The valves then consist of connective tissue covered by endocardium and are connected to thickened trabeculae in the wall of the ventricle, the **papillary muscles,** by means of **chordae tendineae** (Fig. 12.17*C*). In this manner, two valve leaflets are formed in the left atrioventricular canal, the **bicuspid** or **mitral valve,** and three on the right side, the **tricuspid valve.**

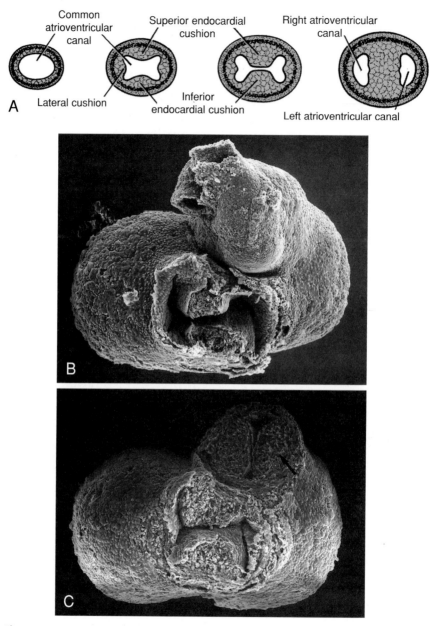

Figure 12.15. Formation of the septum in the atrioventricular canal. **A.** From left to right, days 23, 26, 31, and 35, respectively. The initial circular opening becomes widened in a transverse direction. **B** and **C.** Scanning electron micrographs of hearts from mouse embryos, showing growth and fusion of the superior and inferior endocardial cushions in the atrioventricular canal. In **C,** cushions of the outflow tract *(arrow)* are also fusing.

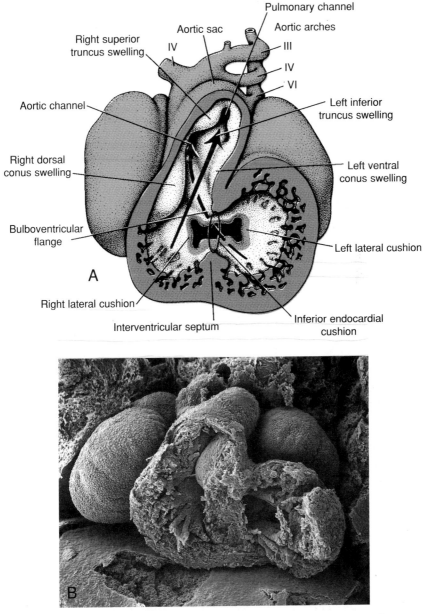

Figure 12.16. **A.** Frontal section through the heart of a day 35 embryo. At this stage of development, blood from the atrial cavity enters the primitive left ventricle as well as the primitive right ventricle. Note development of the cushions in the atrioventricular canal. Cushions in the truncus and conus are also visible. The *ring* indicates the primitive interventricular foramen. *Arrows* indicate blood flow. **B.** Scanning electron micrograph of a mouse embryo at a slightly later stage, showing fusion of the atrioventricular cushions and contact between those in the outflow tract.

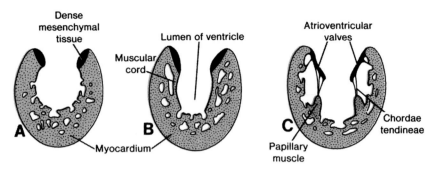

Figure 12.17. Formation of the atrioventricular valves and chordae tendineae. Note how the valves are hollowed out from the ventricular side but remain attached to the ventricular wall by the chordae tendineae.

CLINICAL CORRELATES

Atrial septal defects (ASDs) are common congenital heart abnormalities occurring with an incidence of 6.4/10,000 births and with a 2:1 prevalence in female versus male infants. One of the most significant defects is the **ostium secundum defect**. This anomaly is characterized by a large opening between the left and right atria and is caused either by excessive cell death and resorption of the septum primum (Fig. 12.18, *B* and *C*) or by inadequate development of the septum secundum (Fig. 12.18, *D* and *E*). Depending on the size of the opening, considerable intracardiac shunting may occur from left to right.

The most serious abnormality in this group is complete absence of the atrial septum (Fig. 12.18*F*). This condition, known as common atrium or **cor triloculare biventriculare,** is always associated with serious defects elsewhere in the heart.

Occasionally, the oval foramen closes during prenatal life. This abnormality, known as **premature closure of the oval foramen,** leads to massive hypertrophy of the right atrium and ventricle and underdevelopment of the left side of the heart. Death usually occurs shortly after birth.

Endocardial cushions of the atrioventricular canal not only divide this canal into a right and left orifice but also participate in formation of the membranous portion of the interventricular septum and in closure of the ostium primum. This region has the appearance of a cross, with the atrial and ventricular septa forming the post and the atrioventricular cushions the crossbar. The integrity of this cross is an important sign in ultrasound scans of the heart (Fig. 12.28*C*). Whenever the cushions fail to fuse, the result is a **persistent atrioventricular canal,** combined with a defect in the cardiac septum (Fig. 12.19*A*). This septal defect has an atrial and a ventricular component, separated by abnormal valve leaflets in the single atrioventricular orifice (Fig. 12.19*C*).

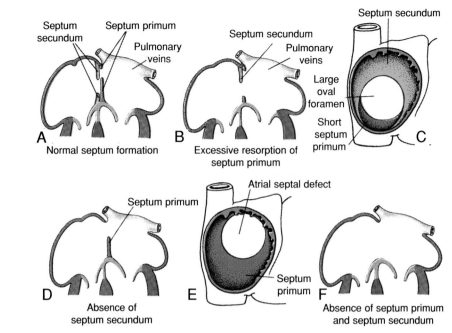

Figure 12.18. **A.** Normal atrial septum formation. **B** and **C.** Ostium secundum defect caused by excessive resorption of the septum primum. **D** and **E.** Similar defect caused by failure of development of the septum secundum. **F.** Common atrium or cor triloculare biventriculare resulting from complete failure of the septum primum and septum secundum to form.

Occasionally, endocardial cushions in the atrioventricular canal fuse partially. The defect in the atrial septum is then similar to that in the above-described abnormality, but the interventricular septum is closed (Fig. 12.19, *D* and *E*). This defect, known as the **ostium primum defect,** is usually combined with a cleft in the anterior leaflet of the tricuspid valve (Fig. 12.19*C*).

    Tricuspid atresia involves obliteration of the right atrioventricular orifice (Fig. 12.20*B*) and is characterized by the absence or fusion of the tricuspid valves. The defect is always associated with *(a)* patency of the oval foramen, *(b)* ventricular septal defect, *(c)* underdevelopment of the right ventricle, and *(d)* hypertrophy of the left ventricle.

Septum Formation in the Truncus Arteriosus and Conus Cordis

    During the 5th week, pairs of opposing ridges appear in the truncus. These ridges, the **truncus swellings** or **cushions,** are located on the right superior wall

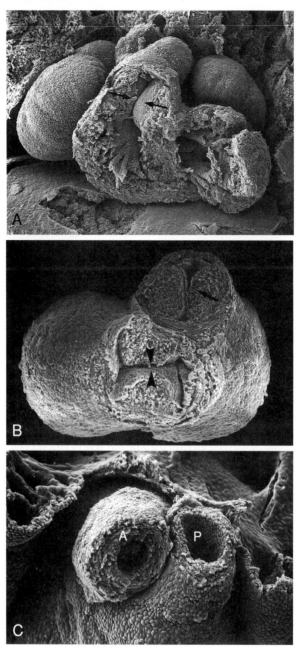

Figure 12.21. Scanning electron micrographs of hearts from mouse embryos, showing formation of the conotruncal ridges (cushions) that form a septum in the outflow tract to divide this region into aortic and pulmonary channels. **A.** Frontal section showing cushion contact in the outflow tract (*arrows* show cushions). **B.** Cross section through the atrioventricular canal (*arrowheads*) and outflow tract (*arrow*). Cushions in both regions have made initial contact. **C.** Cross section through the aortic (*A*) and pulmonary (*P*) vessels, showing their spiral course caused by spiraling of the conotruncal ridges (see Fig. 12.22). Note the thickness of the aorta.

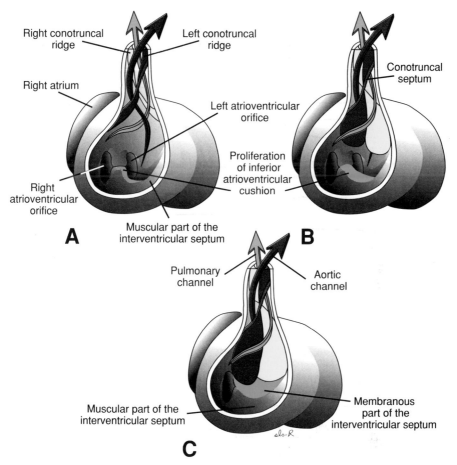

Right conotruncal ridge

Left conotruncal ridge

Right atrium

Conotruncal septum

Left atrioventricular orifice

Proliferation of inferior atrioventricular cushion

Right atrioventricular orifice

Muscular part of the interventricular septum

A

B

Pulmonary channel

Aortic channel

Muscular part of the interventricular septum

Membranous part of the interventricular septum

C

Figure 12.22. Schematic drawings showing development of the conotruncal ridges (cushions) and closure of the interventricular foramen. Proliferations of the right and left conus cushions, combined with proliferation of the inferior endocardial cushion, close the interventricular foramen and form the membranous portion of the interventricular septum. **A.** 6 weeks (12 mm). **B.** Beginning of the 7th week (14.5 mm). **C.** End of the 7th week (20 mm).

interventricular foramen becomes the **membranous part of the interventricular septum.**

SEMILUNAR VALVES

When partitioning of the truncus has almost been completed, primordia of the semilunar valves become visible as small tubercles. These tubercles are found on the main truncus swellings, and one of each pair is assigned to the pulmonary and aortic channels, respectively (Fig. 12.25). Opposite the fused truncus swellings, a third tubercle appears in both channels. Gradually, the tubercles are hollowed out at their upper surface, thus forming the **semilunar valves** (Fig. 12.26).

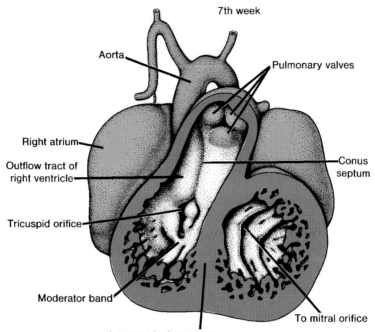

Figure 12.23. Frontal section through the heart of a 7-week embryo. Note the conus septum and position of the pulmonary valves.

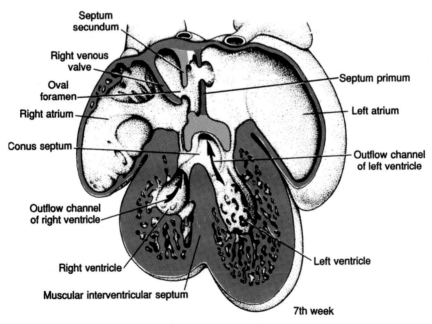

Figure 12.24. Frontal section through the heart of an embryo at the end of the 7th week. The conus septum is complete, and blood from the left ventricle enters the aorta. Note the septum in the atrial region.

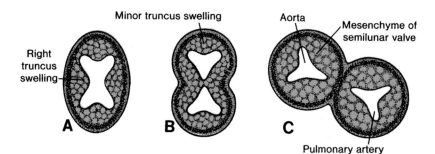

Figure 12.25. Transverse sections through the truncus arteriosus at the level of the semilunar valves at 5, 6, and 7 weeks of development (**A, B,** and **C,** respectively).

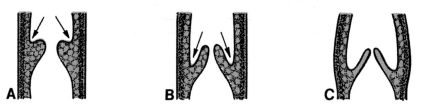

Figure 12.26. Longitudinal sections through the semilunar valves at the 6th (**A**), 7th (**B**), and 9th (**C**) weeks of development.

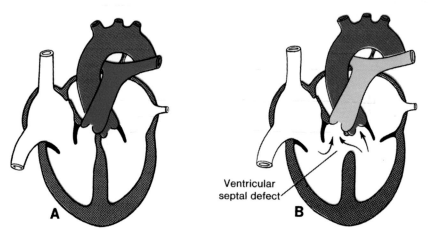

Figure 12.27. **A.** Drawing of a normal heart. **B.** Drawing of an isolated defect in the membranous portion of the interventricular septum. Note blood from the left ventricle flows to the right through the interventricular foramen.

CLINICAL CORRELATES

Ventricular septal defects (VSD) involving the membranous portion of the septum (Fig. 12.27) are the most common congenital cardiac malformation, occurring as an isolated condition in 12/10,000 births.

Although it may be found as an isolated lesion, the defect is also often associated with abnormalities in partitioning of the conotruncal region. Depending on the size of the opening, blood carried by the pulmonary artery may be 1.2–1.7 times more abundant than that carried by the aorta. Occasionally, the defect is not restricted to the membranous part but also involves the muscular part of the septum.

Tetralogy of Fallot is the most frequently occurring abnormality of the **conotruncal** region (Fig. 12.28). The defect is due to an unequal division of the conus, resulting from anterior displacement of the conotruncal septum. Displacement of the septum produces four cardiovascular alterations: (a) a narrow right ventricular outflow region, i.e., a **pulmonary infundibular stenosis;** (b) a large defect of the interventricular septum; (c) an overriding aorta that arises directly above the septal defect; and (d) hypertrophy of the right ventricular wall that is due to resulting higher pressure on the right side. The defect occurs at a rate of 9.6/10,000 births and is compatible with life.

Persistent truncus arteriosus results when the conotruncal ridges fail to fuse and to descend toward the ventricles (Fig. 12.29). In such a case, which occurs in 0.8/10,000 births, the pulmonary artery arises some distance above the origin of the undivided truncus. Since the ridges also participate in formation of the interventricular septum, the persistent truncus is always accompanied by a defective interventricular septum. The undivided truncus thus overrides both ventricles and receives blood from both sides.

Transposition of the great vessels occurs when the conotruncal septum fails to follow its normal spiral course and descends straight downward (Fig. 12.30A). As a consequence, the aorta originates from the right ventricle, and the pulmonary artery originates from the left ventricle. This condition occurs in 4.8/10,000 births and sometimes is associated with a defect in the membranous part of the interventricular septum. It is usually accompanied by an open ductus arteriosus. Since neural crest cells contribute to the formation of the truncal cushions, insults to these cells contribute to cardiac defects involving the outflow tract.

Valvular stenosis of the pulmonary artery or aorta occurs when the semilunar valves are fused for a variable distance. The incidence of the abnormality is similar for both regions, being approximately 3–4/10,000 births. In the case of a **valvular stenosis of the pulmonary artery,** the trunk of the pulmonary artery is narrow or even atretic (Fig. 12.30B). The patent oval foramen then forms the only outlet for blood from the right side of the heart. The ductus arteriosus is always patent and represents the only access route to the pulmonary circulation.

In the case of **aortic valvular stenosis** (Fig. 12.31A), fusion of the thickened valves may be so complete that only a pinhole opening remains. The size of the aorta itself, however, is usually normal.

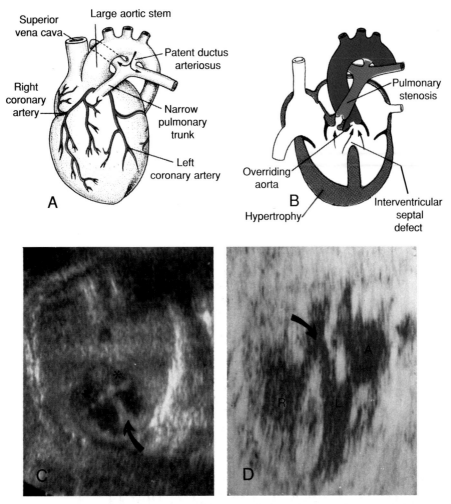

Figure 12.28. Tetralogy of Fallot. **A.** Surface view. **B.** Schematic drawing to show the four components of the defect: *(a)* pulmonary stenosis; *(b)* overriding aorta; *(c)* interventricular septal defect; and *(d)* hypertrophy of the right ventricle. **C.** Ultrasound scan showing a normal heart with atria *(asterisks)*, ventricles *(V)*, and interventricular septum *(arrow)*. **D.** Scan of a heart showing the characteristic features of the tetralogy, including hypertrophy of the right ventricle *(R)* and overriding aorta *(arrow)*. *A*, atrium; and *L*, left ventricle.

When fusion of the semilunar aortic valves is complete—a condition known as **aortic valvular atresia** (Fig. 12.31*B*)—the aorta, left ventricle, and left atrium are markedly underdeveloped. The abnormality is usually accompanied by an open ductus arteriosus, which delivers blood into the aorta.

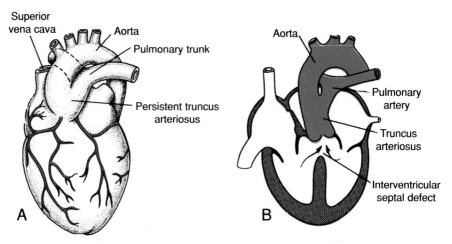

Figure 12.29. Persistent truncus arteriosus. The pulmonary artery originates from a common truncus. The septum in the truncus and conus has failed to form. This abnormality is always accompanied by an interventricular septal defect.

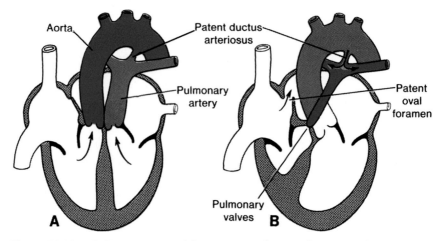

Figure 12.30. **A.** Transposition of the great vessels. **B.** Pulmonary valvular atresia with a normal aortic root. The only access route to the lungs is by way of a patent ductus arteriosus.

Dextrocardia is caused by formation of the cardiac loop to the left rather than the right. In this condition, the heart is located in the right side of the thorax, and the abnormality is usually associated with a total or partial **situs inversus** (transposition of the viscera).

Ectopia cordis is a rare anomaly in which the heart is located on the surface of the chest. This malformation is caused by failure of the embryo to close the ventral body wall (see Chapter 5).

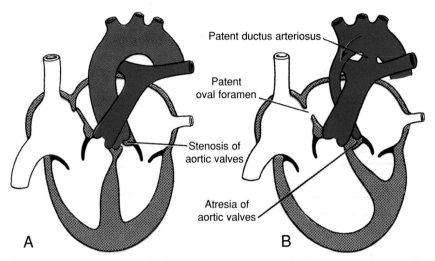

Figure 12.31. **A.** Aortic valvular stenosis. **B.** Aortic valvular atresia. *Arrow* in the arch of the aorta indicates direction of blood flow. The coronary arteries are supplied by this retroflux. Note the small left ventricle and the large right ventricle.

It is estimated that 8% of cardiac malformations are due to genetic factors, 2% are due to environmental agents, and the vast majority are due to a complex interplay between genetic and environmental influences (**multifactorial** causes). Classic examples of environmental cardiovascular teratogens include **rubella virus** and **thalidomide,** but others exist, including **isotretinoin (vitamin A), alcohol,** and many other compounds. Maternal diseases such as insulin-dependent **diabetes** and **hypertension** have also been linked to cardiac defects. Chromosomal abnormalities are associated with heart malformations, with 6–10% of newborns with cardiac defects having an unbalanced chromosomal abnormality. Furthermore, 33% of all children with chromosomal abnormalities will have a congenital heart defect, with an incidence of nearly 100% in children with trisomy 18. Finally, cardiac malformations are associated with a number of genetic syndromes, including **DiGeorge, Goldenhar,** and **Down** syndromes (see Chapter 16).

Formation of the Conducting System of the Heart

Initially, the **pacemaker** for the heart lies in the caudal part of the left cardiac tube. Later, the sinus venosus assumes this function, and as the sinus is incorporated into the right atrium, pacemaker tissue lies near the opening of the superior vena cava. Thus, the **sinuatrial node** is formed.

The **atrioventricular node and bundle (bundle of His)** are derived from two sources: *(a)* cells in the left wall of the sinus venosus, and *(b)* cells from the atrioventricular canal. Once the sinus venosus is incorporated into the right atrium, these cells are located in their final position at the base of the interatrial septum.

VASCULAR DEVELOPMENT

Arterial System

AORTIC ARCHES

When pharyngeal arches are formed during the 4th and 5th weeks of development, each arch receives its own cranial nerve and its own artery (see Chapter 16). These arteries are known as **aortic arches** and arise from the **aortic sac,** the most distal part of the truncus arteriosus (Figs. 12.8 and 12.32). The aortic arches are embedded in mesenchyme of the pharyngeal arches and terminate in the right and left dorsal aortae (in the region of the arches the dorsal aortae remain paired, but caudal to this region they fuse to form a single vessel). The pharyngeal arches and their vessels appear in a cranial to caudal sequence, such that they are not all present simultaneously. The aortic sac contributes a branch to each new arch as it forms, thus giving rise to a total of five pairs of arteries. (The 5th arch either never forms or forms incompletely and then regresses. Consequently, the five arches are numbered I, II, III, IV, and VI (Fig. 12.33).) During further development, this arterial pattern becomes modified, and some vessels regress completely.

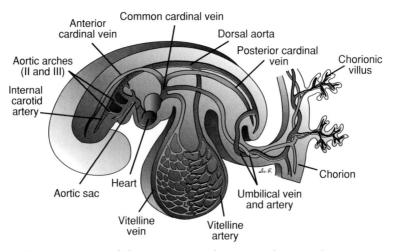

Figure 12.32. Drawing of the main intraembryonic and extraembryonic arteries *(red)* and veins *(blue)* in a 4-mm embryo (end of the 4th week). Only the vessels on the left side of the embryo are represented.

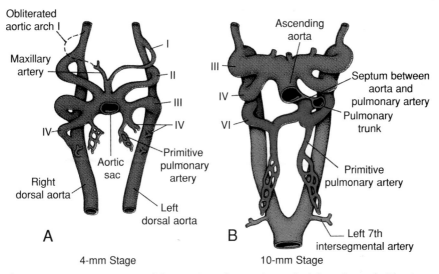

Obliterated
aortic arch I

Maxillary
artery

III

IV

Right
dorsal aorta

Aortic
sac

I

II

III

IV

Primitive
pulmonary
artery

Left
dorsal aorta

A

4-mm Stage

Ascending
aorta

III

IV

VI

Septum between
aorta and
pulmonary artery

Pulmonary
trunk

Primitive
pulmonary artery

Left 7th
intersegmental artery

B

10-mm Stage

Figure 12.33. **A.** Drawing of the aortic arches at the end of the 4th week. The 1st arch is obliterated before the 6th is formed. **B.** Aortic arch system at the beginning of the 6th week. Note the aorticopulmonary septum and the large pulmonary arteries.

Division of the truncus arteriosus by the aorticopulmonary septum divides the outflow channel of the heart into the **ventral aorta** and the **pulmonary artery.** The aortic sac then forms right and left horns, which subsequently give rise to the **brachiocephalic artery** and the proximal segment of the **aortic arch,** respectively (Fig. 12.34, *B* and *C*).

By day 27, most of the **1st aortic arch** has disappeared (Fig. 12.33). A small portion persists, however, to form the **maxillary artery.** Similarly, the **2nd aortic arch** soon disappears. The remaining portions of this arch are the **hyoid and stapedial arteries.** The 3rd arch is large; the 4th and 6th arches are in the process of formation. Even though the 6th arch is not completed, the **primitive pulmonary artery** is already present as a major branch (Fig. 12.33A).

In a 29-day embryo, the 1st and 2nd aortic arches have disappeared (Fig. 12.33B). The 3rd, 4th, and 6th arches are large. The truncoaortic sac has been divided so that the 6th arches are now continuous with the pulmonary trunk.

Since with further development the aortic arch system loses its original symmetrical form, the basic vascular pattern is schematically shown in Figure 12.34A, while the definitive pattern is given in Figure 12.34, *B* and *C.* This representation may be of help in understanding the transformation from the original into the adult arterial system.

The following changes occur:

① The **3rd aortic arch** forms the **common carotid artery** and the first part of the **internal carotid artery.** The remainder of the internal carotid is formed by the cranial portion of the dorsal aorta. The **external carotid artery** is a sprout of the 3rd aortic arch.

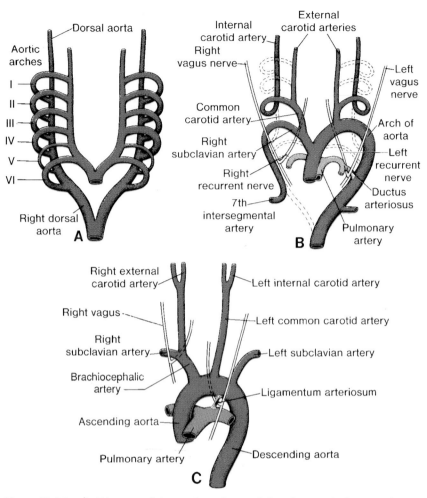

Figure 12.34. **A.** Diagram of the aortic arches and dorsal aortas before transformation into the definitive vascular pattern. **B.** Diagram of the aortic arches and dorsal aortas after the transformation. Obliterated components are indicated by *broken lines.* Note the patent ductus arteriosus and position of the 7th intersegmental artery on the left. **C.** The great arteries in the adult. Compare the distance between the place of origin of the left common carotid artery and the left subclavian in **B** and **C**. After disappearance of the distal part of the 6th aortic arch (the 5th arches never form completely), the right recurrent laryngeal nerve hooks around the right subclavian artery. On the left, the nerve remains in place and hooks around the ligamentum arteriosum.

  ② The **4th aortic arch** persists on both sides, but its ultimate fate is different on the right and left sides. On the left, it forms part of the arch of the aorta, between the left common carotid and the left subclavian arteries. On the right, it forms the most proximal segment of the right subclavian artery, the distal part of which is formed by a portion of the right dorsal aorta and the 7th intersegmental artery (Fig. 12.34*B*).

---

③ The **5th aortic arch** either never forms or forms incompletely and then regresses.

④ The **6th aortic arch,** also known as the **pulmonary arch,** gives off an important branch that grows toward the developing lung bud (Fig. 12.33*B*). On the right side, the proximal part becomes the proximal segment of the right pulmonary artery. The distal portion of this arch loses its connection with the dorsal aorta and disappears. On the left, the distal part persists during intrauterine life as the **ductus arteriosus.**

OTHER CHANGES IN THE ARCH SYSTEM

Simultaneously, with alterations in the aortic arch system, a number of other changes occur. *(a)* The dorsal aorta located between the entrance of the 3rd and 4th arches, known as the **carotid duct,** is obliterated (Fig. 12.35). *(b)* The right dorsal aorta disappears between the origin of the 7th intersegmental artery and the junction with the left dorsal aorta (Fig. 12.35). *(c)* Cephalic folding, growth of the forebrain, and elongation of the neck cause the heart to descend into the thoracic cavity. Hence, the carotid and brachiocephalic arteries elongate considerably (Fig. 12.34*C*). As a further result of this caudal shift, the left subclavian artery, distally fixed in the arm bud, shifts its point of origin from the aorta at the level of the 7th intersegmental artery (Fig. 12.34*B*) to an increasingly higher point, until it comes close to the origin of the left common carotid artery (Fig. 12.34*C*). *(d)* As a result

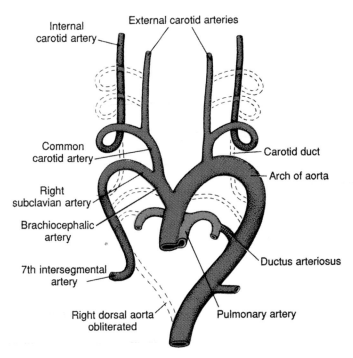

Figure 12.35. Drawing demonstrating the changes from the original aortic arch system.

of the caudal shift of the heart and the disappearance of various portions of the aortic arches, the course of the **recurrent laryngeal nerves** becomes different on the right and left sides. Initially, these nerves, branches of the vagus, supply the 6th pharyngeal arches. When the heart descends, they hook around the 6th aortic arches and then ascend again to the larynx, thus accounting for their recurrent course. On the right, when the distal part of the 6th aortic arch and the 5th aortic arch disappear, the recurrent laryngeal nerve moves up and hooks around the right subclavian artery. On the left, the nerve does not move up, since the distal part of the 6th aortic arch persists as the **ductus arteriosus,** which later forms the **ligamentum arteriosum.**

VITELLINE AND UMBILICAL ARTERIES

The **vitelline arteries,** initially a number of paired vessels supplying the yolk sac (Fig. 12.32), gradually fuse and form the arteries located in the dorsal mesentery of the gut. In the adult, they are represented by the **celiac, superior mesenteric,** and **inferior mesenteric arteries.** These vessels supply derivatives of the **foregut, midgut,** and **hindgut,** respectively.

The **umbilical arteries,** initially paired ventral branches of the dorsal aorta, course to the placenta in close association with the allantois (Fig. 12.32). During the 4th week, however, each artery acquires a secondary connection with the dorsal branch of the aorta, the **common iliac artery,** and loses its original origin. After birth, the proximal portions of the umbilical arteries persist as the **internal iliac** and **superior vesical arteries,** while the distal parts are obliterated to form the **medial umbilical ligaments.**

CLINICAL CORRELATES

Under normal conditions, the **ductus arteriosus** is functionally closed through contraction of its muscular wall shortly after birth to form the **ligamentum arteriosum.** Anatomical closure by means of intima proliferation, however, takes 1–3 months. A **patent ductus arteriosus** is one of the most frequently occurring abnormalities of the great vessels (8/10,000 births), especially in premature infants, and may occur either as an isolated abnormality or in combination with other heart defects (Figs. 12.28A and 12.30). In particular, defects that cause large differences between aortic and pulmonary pressures may cause increased blood flow through the ductus, thus preventing its normal closure.

Coarctation of the aorta (Fig. 12.36, A and B) occurs in 3.2/10,000 births and is a condition in which the aortic lumen below the origin of the left subclavian artery is significantly narrowed. Since the constriction may be located above or below the entrance of the ductus arteriosus, two types may be distinguished: **preductal** and **postductal.** The cause of aortic narrowing is primarily an abnormality in the media of the aorta, followed by intima proliferations. In the preductal type,

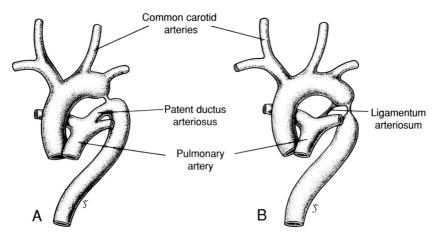

Figure 12.36. Coarctation of the aorta. **A.** Preductal type. **B.** Postductal type. The caudal part of the body is supplied by large, hypertrophied intercostal and internal thoracic arteries.

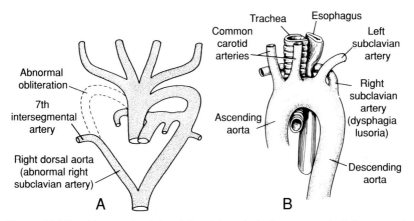

Figure 12.37. Abnormal origin of the right subclavian artery. **A.** Scheme to show obliteration of the right 4th aortic arch and the proximal portion of the right dorsal aorta with persistence of the distal portion of the right dorsal aorta. **B.** The abnormal right subclavian artery crosses the midline behind the esophagus and may compress this structure.

the ductus arteriosus persists, whereas in the postductal type, which is more common, this channel is usually obliterated. In the latter case, collateral circulation between the proximal and distal parts of the aorta is established by way of large intercostal and internal thoracic arteries. In this manner, the lower part of the body is supplied with blood.

Abnormal origin of the right subclavian artery (Fig. 12.37, *A* and *B*) occurs when the artery is formed by the distal portion of the right dorsal aorta and the 7th intersegmental artery. The right 4th aortic arch and the proximal part of the right dorsal aorta are obliterated. With shortening of the aorta between the left common carotid and left subclavian arteries, the origin of the abnormal right subclavian artery is finally located just below that of the left subclavian artery. Since its stem is derived from the right dorsal aorta, it must cross the midline behind the esophagus to reach the right arm. This location does not usually cause problems with swallowing or breathing, however, since neither the esophagus nor the trachea is severely compressed.

With a **double aortic arch,** the right dorsal aorta persists between the origin of the 7th intersegmental artery and its junction with the left dorsal aorta (Fig. 12.38). A **vascular ring** is formed that surrounds the trachea and esophagus and frequently compresses these structures, causing difficulties in breathing and swallowing.

A **right aortic arch** exists when the left 4th arch and left dorsal aorta are completely obliterated and replaced by the corresponding vessels on the right side. Occasionally, when the ligamentum arteriosum is situated on the left side and passes behind the esophagus, it may cause complaints with swallowing.

An **interrupted aortic arch** is caused by obliteration of the 4th aortic arch on the left side (Fig. 12.39, A and B). It is frequently combined with an abnormal origin of the right subclavian artery. The ductus arteriosus remains open, and the descending aorta and subclavian arteries are supplied with blood of low oxygen content. The aortic trunk supplies the two common carotid arteries.

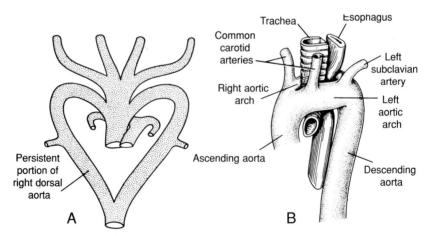

Figure 12.38. Double aortic arch. **A.** Scheme showing persistence of the distal portion of the right dorsal aorta. **B.** The double aortic arch forms a vascular ring around the trachea and esophagus.

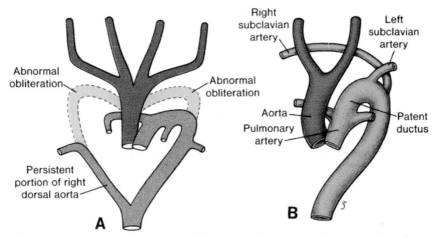

Figure 12.39. **A.** Scheme showing obliteration of the 4th aortic arch on the right as well as on the left and persistence of the distal portion of the right dorsal aorta. **B.** Case of interrupted aortic arch. The aorta supplies the head; the pulmonary artery, by way of the ductus arteriosus, supplies the remaining parts of the body.

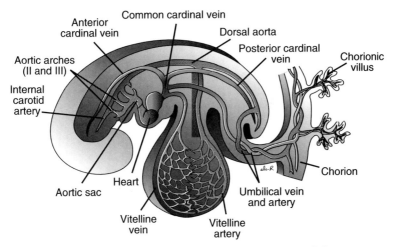

Figure 12.40. Schematic drawing of the main components of the venous and arterial systems in a 4-mm embryo (end of the 4th week).

Venous System

In the 5th week, three pairs of major veins can be distinguished: *(a)* the **vitelline or omphalomesenteric veins,** carrying blood from the yolk sac to the sinus venosus; *(b)* the **umbilical veins,** originating in the chorionic villi and carrying oxygenated blood to the embryo; and *(c)* the **cardinal veins,** draining the body of the embryo proper (Fig. 12.40).

VITELLINE VEINS

Before entering the sinus venosus, the vitelline veins form a plexus around the duodenum and pass through the septum transversum. The liver cords growing into the septum interrupt the course of the veins, and an extensive vascular network is formed, known as the **hepatic sinusoids** (Fig. 12.41).

With reduction of the left sinus horn, blood from the left side of the liver is rechanneled toward the right, resulting in an enlargement of the right vitelline vein (right hepatocardiac channel). Ultimately, the right hepatocardiac channel forms the **hepatocardiac portion of the inferior vena cava.** The proximal part of the left vitelline vein disappears (Fig. 12.42, *A* and *B*). The anastomotic network around the duodenum develops into a single vessel, the **portal vein** (Fig. 12.42*B*). The **superior mesenteric vein,** which drains the primary intestinal loop, is derived from the right vitelline vein. The distal portion of the left vitelline vein also disappears (Fig. 12.42, *A* and *B*).

UMBILICAL VEINS

Initially, the umbilical veins pass on each side of the liver, but some become connected to the hepatic sinusoids (Fig. 12.41, *A* and *B*). The proximal part of both umbilical veins and the remainder of the right umbilical vein then disappear, so that the left vein is the only one to carry blood from the placenta to the liver (Fig. 12.42). With the increase of the placental circulation, a direct communication is formed between the left umbilical vein and the right hepatocardiac channel, the ductus venosus (Fig. 12.42, *A* and *B*). This vessel bypasses the sinusoidal plexus of the liver. After birth, the left umbilical vein and ductus venosus are obliterated and form the **ligamentum teres hepatis** and **ligamentum venosum,** respectively (see "Circulatory Changes at Birth").

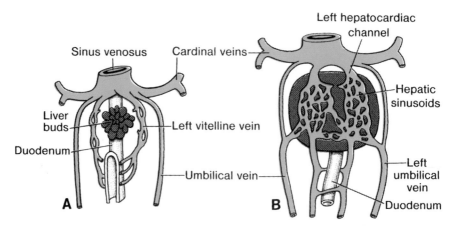

Figure 12.41. Schematic drawings to show development of the vitelline and umbilical veins during the 4th **(A)** and 5th weeks **(B)**. Note the plexus around the duodenum, formation of the hepatic sinusoids, and initiation of left-to-right shunts between the vitelline veins.

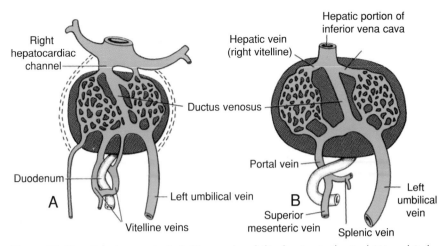

Figure 12.42. Development of vitelline and umbilical veins in the 2nd **(A)** and 3rd **(B)** months. Note formation of the ductus venosus, portal vein, and hepatic portion of the inferior vena cava. The splenic and superior mesenteric veins enter the portal vein.

CARDINAL VEINS

Initially, the cardinal veins form the main venous drainage system of the embryo. This system consists of the **anterior cardinal veins,** which drain the cephalic part of the embryo, and the **posterior cardinal veins,** which drain the remaining part of the body of the embryo. The anterior and posterior veins join before entering the sinus horn and form the short **common cardinal veins.** During the 4th week, the cardinal veins form a symmetrical system (Fig. 12.43*A*).

During the 5th to the 7th week, a number of additional veins are formed: *(a)* the **subcardinal veins,** which mainly drain the kidneys; *(b)* the **sacrocardinal veins,** which drain the lower extremities; and *(c)* the **supracardinal veins,** which drain the body wall by way of the intercostal veins, thereby taking over the functions of the posterior cardinal veins (Fig. 12.43).

Formation of the vena cava system is characterized by the appearance of anastomoses between left and right in such a manner that the blood from the left is channeled to the right side.

The **anastomosis between the anterior cardinal veins** develops into the **left brachiocephalic vein** (Fig. 12.43, *A* and *B*). Most of the blood from the left side of the head and the left upper extremity is then channeled to the right. The terminal portion of the left posterior cardinal vein entering into the left brachiocephalic vein is retained as a small vessel, the **left superior intercostal vein** (Fig. 12.43*B*). This vessel receives blood from the 2nd and 3rd intercostal spaces. The **superior vena cava** is formed by the right common cardinal vein and the proximal portion of the right anterior cardinal vein.

The **anastomosis between the subcardinal veins** forms the **left renal vein.** When this communication has been established, the left subcardinal vein

---

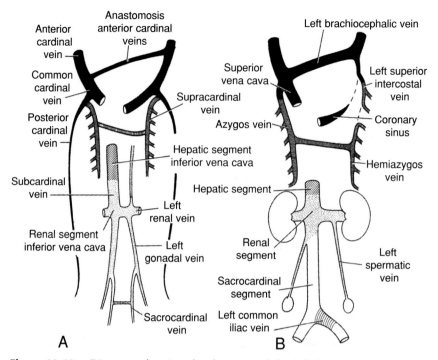

Figure 12.43. Diagrams showing development of the inferior vena cava, azygos vein, and superior vena cava. **A.** 7th week. Note the anastomosis formed between the subcardinals, supracardinals, sacrocardinals, and anterior cardinals. **B.** The venous system at birth. Note the three components of the inferior vena cava.

disappears, and only its distal portion remains as the **left gonadal vein.** Hence, the right subcardinal vein becomes the main drainage channel and develops into the **renal segment of the inferior vena cava** (Fig. 12.43B).

The **anastomosis between the sacrocardinal veins** forms the **left common iliac vein** (Fig. 12.43B). The right sacrocardinal vein becomes the sacrocardinal segment of the inferior vena cava. When the renal segment of the inferior vena cava connects with the hepatic segment, which is derived from the right vitelline vein, the inferior vena cava is complete. It consists then of a hepatic segment, a renal segment, and a sacrocardinal segment.

With obliteration of the major portion of the posterior cardinal veins, the supracardinal veins gain in importance. The 4th to 11th right intercostal veins empty into the right supracardinal vein, which, together with a portion of the posterior cardinal vein, forms the **azygos vein** (Fig. 12.43). On the left, the 4th to 7th intercostal veins enter into the left supracardinal vein, and the left supracardinal vein empties into the azygos vein and is then known as the **hemiazygos vein** (Fig. 12.43B).

CLINICAL CORRELATES

The complicated development of the venae cavae accounts for the fact that deviations from the normal pattern occur frequently.

A **double inferior vena cava** occurs when the left sacrocardinal vein fails to lose its connection with the left subcardinal (Fig. 12.44A). The left common iliac vein may or may not be present, but the left gonadal vein remains as in normal conditions.

Absence of the inferior vena cava arises when the right subcardinal vein fails to make its connection with the liver and shunts its blood directly into the right supracardinal vein (Figs. 12.43 and 12.44B). Hence, the bloodstream from the caudal part of the body reaches the heart by way of the azygos vein and superior vena cava. The hepatic vein enters into the right atrium at the site of the inferior vena cava. Usually, this abnormality is associated with other heart malformations.

Left superior vena cava is an abnormality caused by persistence of the left anterior cardinal vein and obliteration of the common cardinal and proximal part of the anterior cardinal veins on the right (Fig. 12.45A). In such a case, blood from the right is channeled toward the left by way of the brachiocephalic vein. The left superior vena cava drains into the right atrium by way of the left sinus horn, i.e., the coronary sinus.

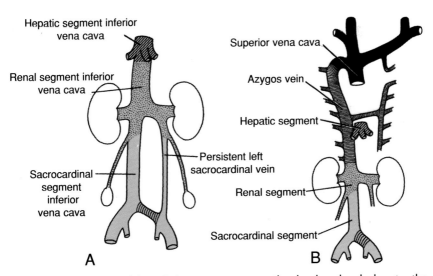

Figure 12.44. A. Double inferior vena cava at the lumbar level due to the persistence of the left sacrocardinal vein. **B.** Absent inferior vena cava. The lower half of the body is drained by the azygos vein, which enters the superior vena cava. The hepatic vein enters the heart at the site of the inferior vena cava.

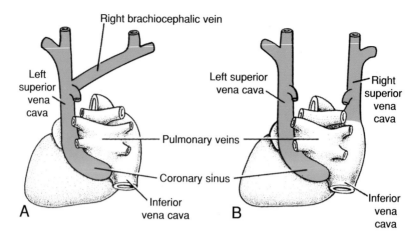

Figure 12.45. **A.** Left superior vena cava draining into the right atrium by way of the coronary sinus (dorsal view). **B.** Double superior vena cava. The communicating (brachiocephalic) vein between the two anterior cardinals has failed to develop (dorsal view).

A **double superior vena cava** is characterized by the persistence of the left anterior cardinal vein and failure of the left brachiocephalic vein to form (Fig. 12.45B). The persistent left anterior cardinal vein, which is called the **left superior vena cava,** drains into the right atrium by way of the coronary sinus.

Circulatory Changes at Birth

FETAL CIRCULATION

Before birth, blood from the placenta—about 80% saturated with oxygen—returns to the fetus by way of the umbilical vein. On approaching the liver, the main portion of this blood flows through the ductus venosus directly into the inferior vena cava, thereby short-circuiting the liver. A smaller portion enters the liver sinusoids and mixes with blood from the portal circulation (Fig. 12.46). A **sphincter mechanism** in the **ductus venosus,** close to the entrance of the umbilical vein, regulates flow of umbilical blood through the liver sinusoids. It is thought that this sphincter closes when, because of a uterine contraction, the venous return is too high, thus preventing a sudden overloading of the heart.

After a short course in the inferior vena cava, where placental blood mixes with deoxygenated blood returning from the lower limbs, it enters the right atrium. Here it is guided toward the oval foramen by the valve of the inferior vena cava, and the major portion of the bloodstream passes directly into the left atrium. A small portion, however, is prevented from doing so by the lower edge

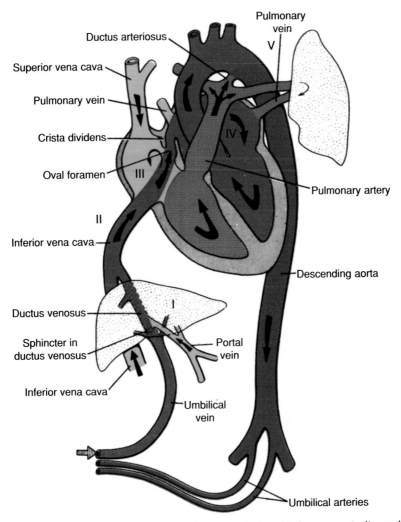

Figure 12.46. Diagram of the human circulation before birth. *Arrows* indicate the direction of blood flow. Note where oxygenated blood mixes with deoxygenated blood: in the liver *(I),* in the inferior vena cava *(II),* in the right atrium *(III),* in the left atrium *(IV),* and at the entrance of the ductus arteriosus into the descending aorta *(V).*

of the septum secundum, the **crista dividens,** and remains in the right atrium. Here it mixes with desaturated blood returning from the head and arms by way of the superior vena cava.

From the left atrium, where it mixes with a small amount of desaturated blood returning from the lungs, blood enters the left ventricle and ascending aorta. Since the coronary and carotid arteries are the first branches of the ascending aorta, the heart musculature and the brain are supplied with well-oxygenated blood. Desaturated blood from the superior vena cava flows by way of the right ventricle into the pulmonary trunk. Since resistance in the pulmonary vessels during fetal life is high, the main portion of this blood passes directly through the **ductus arteriosus** into the descending aorta, where it mixes with blood from the proximal aorta. After coursing through the descending aorta, blood flows toward the placenta by way of the two umbilical arteries. The oxygen saturation in the umbilical arteries is approximately 58%.

During its course from the placenta to the organs of the fetus, blood in the umbilical vein has its high oxygen content gradually decreased by mixing with desaturated blood. Theoretically, mixing may occur in the following places (Fig. 12.46, *I–V*): in the liver *(I)*, by mixture with a small amount of blood returning from the portal system; in the inferior vena cava *(II)*, which carries deoxygenated blood returning from the lower extremities, pelvis, and kidneys; in the right atrium *(III)*, by mixture with blood returning from the head and limbs; in the left atrium *(IV)*, by mixture with blood returning from the lungs; and at the entrance of the ductus arteriosus into the descending aorta *(V)*.

CHANGES AT BIRTH

Changes occurring in the vascular system at birth are caused by cessation of placental blood flow and the beginning of respiration. Since, at the same time, the ductus arteriosus closes by muscular contraction of its wall, the amount of blood flowing through the lung vessels increases rapidly. This, in turn, results in a rise in pressure in the left atrium. Simultaneously, pressure in the right atrium decreases as a result of interruption of placental blood flow. The septum primum is then apposed to the septum secundum, and functionally, the oval foramen closes.

In summary, the following changes occur in the vascular system after birth (Fig. 12.47):

① **Closure of the umbilical arteries** is accomplished by contraction of the smooth musculature in their walls and is probably caused by thermal and mechanical stimuli and a change in oxygen tension. Functionally, the arteries are closed a few minutes after birth. The actual obliteration of the lumen by fibrous proliferation, however, may take 2–3 months. Distal parts of the umbilical arteries form the **medial umbilical ligaments,** while the proximal portions remain open as the **superior vesical arteries** (Fig. 12.47).

② **Closure of the umbilical vein and ductus venosus** occurs shortly after that of the umbilical arteries. Hence, blood from the placenta may enter the newborn for some time after birth. After obliteration, the umbilical vein forms the **ligamentum teres hepatis** in the lower margin of the falciform ligament. The ductus venosus, which courses from the ligamentum teres to the inferior vena cava, is also obliterated and forms the **ligamentum venosum.**

③ **Closure of the ductus arteriosus** by contraction of its muscular wall occurs almost immediately after birth and is mediated by **bradykinin,** a substance released from the lungs during initial inflation. Angiocardio-

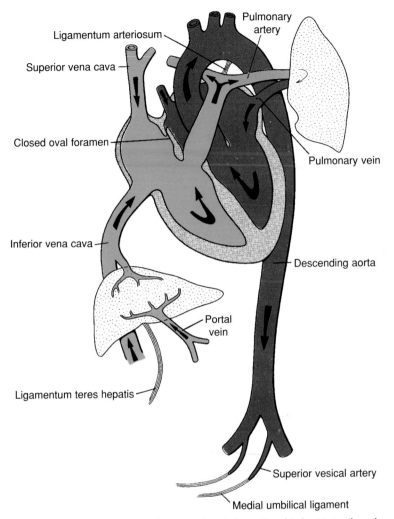

Figure 12.47. Diagram of the human circulation after birth. Note the changes occurring as a result of the beginning of respiration and interruption of placental blood flow.

graphy and cardiac catheterization have, however, revealed that during the first days after birth a left-to-right shunt is not unusual. Complete anatomical obliteration by proliferation of the intima is thought to take 1–3 months. In the adult, the obliterated ductus arteriosus forms the **ligamentum arteriosum.**

④ **Closure of the oval foramen** is caused by an increased pressure in the left atrium, combined with a decrease in pressure on the right side. With the first breath the septum primum is pressed against the septum secundum. During the first days of life, however, this closure is reversible. Crying of the baby creates a shunt from right to left, thus accounting for cyanotic periods in the newborn. Constant apposition gradually leads to fusion of the two septa in about 1 year. In 20% of all individuals, however, perfect anatomical closure may never be obtained (probe patent foramen ovale).

Lymphatic System

The **lymphatic system** begins its development later than the cardiovascular system and does not appear until the 5th week of gestation. The origin of lymphatic vessels is not clear, but they may form from mesenchyme in situ or may arise as sac-like outgrowths from the endothelium of veins. As a result, six primary lymph sacs are formed: two **jugular,** at the junction of the subclavian and anterior cardinal veins; two **iliac,** at the junction of the iliac and posterior cardinal veins; one **retroperitoneal,** near the root of the mesentery; and the **cisterna chyli,** dorsal to the retroperitoneal sac. Numerous channels connect the sacs with each other and also drain lymph from the limbs, body wall, and head and neck. Two main channels, the right and left thoracic ducts, join the jugular sacs with the cisterna chyli, and soon an anastomosis forms between these ducts. The **thoracic duct** then develops from the distal portion of the right thoracic duct, the anastomosis, and the cranial portion of the right thoracic duct. The **right lymphatic duct** is derived from the cranial portion of the right thoracic duct. Both ducts maintain their original connections with the venous system and empty into the junction of the internal jugular and subclavian veins. Due to numerous anastomoses, many variations exist in the final form of the thoracic duct.

SUMMARY: CARDIAC DEVELOPMENT

The entire cardiovascular system—heart, blood vessels, and blood cells—originate from the mesodermal germ layer. Although initially paired, by the 22nd day of development the two tubes (Figs. 12.4 and 12.5) form a single, slightly bent heart tube (Fig. 12.6) consisting of an inner endocardial tube and a surrounding myocardial mantle. During the 4th to 7th weeks, the heart becomes divided into a typical four-chambered structure.

Septum formation in the heart is, in part, due to development of **endocardial cushion** tissue in the atrioventricular canal **(atrioventricular cushions)** and in the conotruncal region **(conotruncal swellings).** Because of the key location of cushion tissue, many cardiac malformations are related to abnormal cushion morphogenesis.

Septum Formation in the Atrium. The septum primum, a sickle-shaped crest descending from the roof of the atrium, begins to divide the atrium in two but leaves a lumen, the ostium primum, for communication between the two sides (Fig. 12.13). Later, when the ostium primum is obliterated due to fusion of the septum primum with the endocardial cushions, the **ostium secundum** is formed by cell death that creates an opening in the septum primum. Finally, a septum secundum is formed, but an interatrial opening, the **oval foramen,** is maintained. Only **at birth,** when pressure in the left atrium increases, are the two septa pressed against each other, and the communication between the two is closed. Abnormalities in the atrial septum may vary from total absence (Fig. 12.18) to a small opening known as **probe patency** of the oval foramen.

Septum Formation in the Atrioventricular Canal. Four **endocardial cushions** surround the atrioventricular canal. Fusion of the opposing superior and inferior cushions divides the orifice into right and left atrioventricular canals. Cushion tissue then becomes fibrous and forms the mitral (bicuspid) valve on the left and the tricuspid valve on the right (Fig. 12.16). Persistence of the common atrioventricular canal (Fig. 12.19) and abnormal division of the canal (Fig. 12.20B) are well-known defects.

Septum Formation in the Ventricles. The interventricular septum consists of a thick **muscular** part and a thin **membranous** portion (Fig. 12.24) formed by *(a)* an inferior endocardial atrioventricular cushion, *(b)* the right conus swelling, and *(c)* the left conus swelling (Fig. 12.22). In many cases, these three components fail to fuse, resulting in an open interventricular foramen. Although this abnormality may be isolated, it is frequently combined with other compensatory defects (Figs. 12.27 and 12.28).

Septum Formation in the Bulbus. The bulbus is divided into *(a)* the truncus (aorta and pulmonary trunk), *(b)* the conus (outflow tract of the aorta and pulmonary trunk), and *(c)* the trabeculated portion of the right ventricle. The truncus region is divided by the spiral-shaped **aorticopulmonary septum** into the two main arteries (Fig. 12.21). The conus swellings divide the outflow tracts of the aortic and pulmonary channels and, with tissue from the inferior endocardial cushion, close the interventricular foramen (Fig. 12.23). Many vascular abnormalities, such as **transposition of the great vessels** and **pulmonary valvular atresia,** result from abnormal division of the conotruncal region and may involve neural crest cells that contribute to formation of the truncal swellings.

SUMMARY: VASCULAR DEVELOPMENT

Arterial System. Although each of the five pharyngeal arches has its own artery (Figs. 12.34 and 16.4), many changes occur (Figs. 12.34C and 12.35A). Three important derivatives of the original system are *(a)* the arch of the aorta (left 4th aortic arch); *(b)* the pulmonary artery (6th aortic arch), which during fetal life is connected to the aorta through the ductus arteriosus; and *(c)* the right subclavian artery formed by the right 4th aortic arch, distal portion of the right dorsal aorta, and the 7th intersegmental artery (Fig. 12.34B). The most common vascular aortic arch abnormalities include *(a)* open ductus arteriosus and coarctation of the aorta (Fig. 12.36) and *(b)* persistent right aortic arch and abnormal right subclavian artery (Figs. 12.37 and 12.38), both causing respiratory and swallowing complaints.

The **vitelline arteries** initially supply the yolk sac but later form the **celiac, superior mesenteric,** and **inferior mesenteric arteries,** which supply the **foregut, midgut,** and **hindgut** regions, respectively.

The **umbilical arteries** are paired and arise from the common iliac arteries. After birth, the distal portions of these arteries are obliterated to form the **medial umbilical ligaments,** whereas the proximal portions persist as the **internal iliac** and **vesicular arteries.**

Venous System. Three systems can be recognized: *(a)* the **vitelline system,** which develops into the **portal system;** *(b)* the cardinal system, which forms the **caval system;** and *(c)* the **umbilical system,** which disappears after birth. The complicated caval system is characterized by many abnormalities, such as double inferior and superior vena cava and left superior vena cava (Fig. 12.45).

Changes at Birth. During prenatal life, the placental circulation provides the fetus with its oxygen, but after birth, the lungs assume the function of gas exchange. In the circulatory system, the following changes take place at birth and in the first postnatal months: *(a)* the ductus arteriosus closes; *(b)* the oval foramen closes; *(c)* the umbilical vein and ductus venosus close and remain as the **ligamentum teres hepatis** and **ligamentum venosum;** and *(d)* the umbilical arteries close and form the **medial umbilical ligaments.**

Lymphatic System. The lymphatic system develops later than the cardio-vascular system, originating as five sacs: two jugular, two iliac, one retroperitoneal, and the cisterna chyli. Numerous channels form to connect the sacs and provide drainage from other structures. Ultimately, the **thoracic duct** forms from anastomosis of the right and left thoracic ducts, the distal part of the right thoracic duct, and the cranial part of the left thoracic duct. The **right lymphatic duct** develops from the cranial part of the right thoracic duct.

PROBLEMS TO SOLVE

1. A prenatal ultrasound on a 35-year-old woman in her 12th week of gestation reveals an abnormal image of the fetal heart. Instead of a four-chambered view provided by the typical "cross," a portion just below the crosspiece was missing. What structures comprise the cross, and what defect does this infant probably have?

2. A child is born with severe craniofacial defects and transposition of the great vessels. What cell population might play a role in both abnormalities, and what type of insult might have produced this effect?

3. What type of tissue is critical for dividing the heart into four chambers and the outflow tract into pulmonary and aortic channels?

4. A patient complains about having difficulty swallowing. What vascular abnormality or abnormalities might produce this complaint? What is its embryological origin?

SUGGESTED READINGS

Adkins RB, Maples MD, Graham BS, Whitt TT, Davies J: Dysphagia associated with aortic arch anomaly in adults. *Am Surg* 52:238, 1986.
Aikawa E, Kawano J: Formation of coronary arteries sprouting from the primitive aortic sinus wall of the chick embryo. *Experientia* 38:816, 1982.

Barry A: The aortic arch derivatives in the human adult. *Anat Rec* 111:221, 1951.

Bruyer HJ, Kargas SA, Levy JM: The causes and underlying developmental mechanisms of congenital cardiovascular malformation: a critical review. *Am J Med Genet* 3:411, 1987.

Clark EB: Cardiac embryology: its relevance to congenital heart disease. *Am J Dis Child* 140:41, 1986.

Coceani F, Olly PM: The control of cardiovascular shunts in the fetal and neonatal period. *Am J Physiol Pharmacol* 66:1129, 1988.

Coffin D, Poole TJ: Embryonic vascular development: immunohistochemical identification of the origin and subsequent morphogenesis of the major vessel primordia of quail embryos. *Development* 102:735, 1988.

Deanfield JE: Transposition of the great arteries: to switch or not to switch? *Curr Opin Pediatr* 1:85, 1989.

Hirakow R: Development of the cardiac blood vessels in staged human embryos. *Acta Anat* 115:220, 1983.

Ho E, Shimada Y: Formation of the epicardium studied with the scanning electron microscope. *Dev Biol* 66:579,1978.

Kirby ML, Gale TF, Stewart DE: Neural crest cells contribute to normal aorticopulmonary septation. *Science* 220:1059–1061, 1983.

Kirklin JW, Colvin EV, McConnell ME, et al: Complete transposition of the great arteries: treatment in the current era. *Pediatr Clin North Am* 37:171, 1990.

Manasek FJ, Burnside MB, Waterman RE: Myocardial cell shape change as a mechanism of embryonic heart looping. *Dev Biol* 29:349, 1972.

McClure FW, Butler FG: The development of the vena cava inferior in man. *Am J Anat* 35:331, 1925.

Noden DM: Origins and assembly of avian embryonic blood vessels. *Ann N Y Acad Sci* 588:236, 1990.

Schmidt KG, Silverman WH: Evaluation of the fetal heart by ultrasound. *In* Callen PW (ed): *Ultrasonography in Obstetrics and Gynecology.* Philadelphia, WB Saunders, 1988.

Skandalakis JE, Gray SW: *Embryology for Surgeons. The Embryological Basis for the Treatment of Congenital Anomalies.* 2nd ed. Baltimore, Williams & Wilkins, 1994.

Van Mierop LHS, Alley RD, Kausei MW, Stranahan A: The anatomy and embryology of endocardial cushion defect. *J Thorac Cardiovasc Surg* 43:71, 1962.

chapter 13

Respiratory System

When the embryo is approximately 4 weeks old, the **respiratory diverticulum (lung bud)** appears as an outgrowth from the ventral wall of the foregut (Fig. 13.1*A*). Hence, **epithelium** of the internal lining of the larynx, trachea, and bronchi, as well as that of the lungs, is entirely of **endodermal origin.** The **cartilaginous** and **muscular** components of the trachea and lungs, however, are derived from **splanchnic mesoderm** surrounding the foregut.

Initially, the lung bud is in open communication with the foregut (Fig. 13.1*B*). When the diverticulum expands in a caudal direction, however, it becomes separated from the foregut by development of two longitudinal ridges, the **esophagotracheal ridges** (Fig. 13.2*A*). Subsequently, when these ridges fuse to form a septum **(esophagotracheal septum),** the foregut is divided into a dorsal portion, the **esophagus,** and a ventral portion, the **trachea** and **lung buds** (Fig. 13.2, *B* and *C*). The respiratory primordium, however, maintains its communication with the pharynx through the **laryngeal orifice** (Fig. 13.2*D*).

CLINICAL CORRELATES

Abnormalities in partitioning of the esophagus and trachea by the esophagotracheal septum results in esophageal atresia (EA) with or without **tracheoesophageal fistulas (TEFs).** These defects occur in approximately 1 in 3000 births, and 90% result in the upper portion of the esophagus ending in a blind pouch and the lower segment forming a fistula with the trachea (Fig. 13.3*A*). Isolated esophageal atresia (Fig. 13.3*B*) and H-type TEF without esophageal atresia (Fig. 13.3*C*) account for 4% each of these defects. Other variations (Fig. 13.3, *D* and *E*) account for approximately 1% each of these defects. These abnormalities are associated with other birth defects, including cardiac abnormalities, which occur in 33% of these cases. In this regard, TEFs are a component of the VACTERL association (**v**ertebral anomalies, **a**nal atresia, **c**ardiac defects, **t**racheoesophageal fistula/**e**sophageal atresia, **r**enal anomalies, and **l**imb defects), a collection of defects of unknown etiology but occurring more frequently than predicted by chance alone (see Chapter 8).

A complication of some TEFs is polyhydramnios, since amniotic fluid may not pass to the stomach and intestines (depending on the

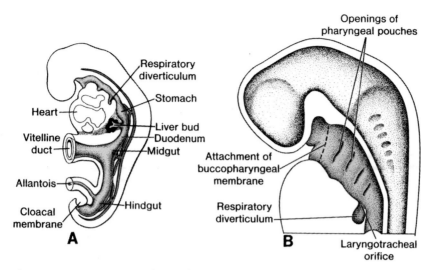

Figure 13.1. **A.** Drawing of an embryo of approximately 25 days gestation to show the relationship of the respiratory diverticulum to the heart, stomach, and liver. **B.** Sagittal section through the cephalic end of a 5-week embryo, showing the openings of the pharyngeal pouches and the laryngotracheal orifice.

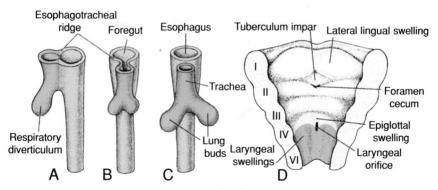

Figure 13.2. **A–C.** Successive stages in development of the respiratory diverticulum. Note the esophagotracheal ridges and formation of the septum, splitting the foregut into esophagus and trachea with lung buds. **D.** The ventral portion of the pharynx seen from above. Note the laryngeal orifice and surrounding swelling.

type of TEF). Also, gastric contents and/or amniotic fluid may enter the trachea through a fistula, causing pneumonitis and pneumonia.

Larynx

The internal lining of the larynx is of endodermal origin, but the cartilages and muscles originate from mesenchyme of the **4th** and **6th pharyngeal arches** (see

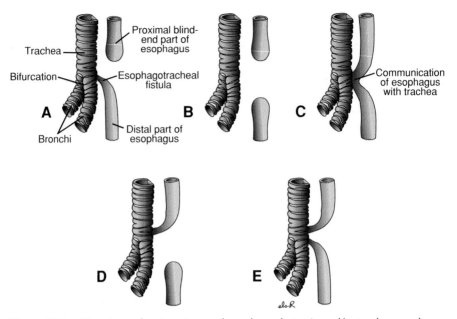

Figure 13.3. Drawings of various types of esophageal atresia and/or tracheoesophageal fistula. **A.** The most frequent abnormality (90% of cases) occurs with the upper esophagus ending in a blind pouch and the lower segment forming a fistula with the trachea. **B.** Isolated esophageal atresia (4% of cases). **C.** H-type tracheoesophageal fistula (4% of cases). **D** and **E.** Other variations (1% each of cases).

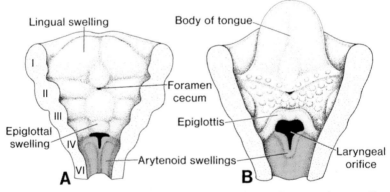

Figure 13.4. Drawings showing the laryngeal orifice and surrounding swellings at successive stages of development. **A.** 6 weeks. **B.** 12 weeks.

Fig. 16.9). As a result of rapid proliferation of this mesenchyme, the laryngeal orifice changes in appearance from a sagittal slit to a T-shaped opening (Fig. 13.4A). When, subsequently, mesenchyme of the two arches is transformed into the **thyroid, cricoid,** and **arytenoid cartilages,** the characteristic adult shape of the laryngeal orifice can be recognized (Fig. 13.4B).

At about the time that the cartilages are formed, the laryngeal epithelium also proliferates rapidly, resulting in a temporary occlusion of the lumen. When, subsequently, vacuolization and recanalization occur, a pair of lateral recesses, the **laryngeal ventricles,** are formed. These recesses are bounded by folds of tissue that do not disappear but do differentiate into the **false** and **true vocal cords.**

Since musculature of the larynx is derived from mesenchyme of the 4th and 6th pharyngeal arches, all laryngeal muscles are innervated by branches of the 10th cranial nerve, the **vagus nerve.** The **superior laryngeal nerve innervates derivatives of the 4th pharyngeal arch,** and **the recurrent laryngeal nerve innervates derivatives of the 6th pharyngeal arch.** (For further details on the laryngeal cartilages, see Chapter 16.)

Trachea, Bronchi, and Lungs

During its separation from the foregut, the **lung bud** forms the trachea and two lateral outpocketings, the **bronchial buds** (Fig. 13.2, *B* and *C*). At the beginning of the 5th week, each of these buds enlarges to form right and left main bronchi. The right then forms three secondary bronchi, and the left, two (Fig. 13.5*A*), thus foreshadowing the presence of three lobes on the right side and two on the left (Fig. 13.5, *B* and *C*).

With subsequent growth in caudal and lateral directions, the lung buds penetrate into the coelomic cavity (Fig. 13.6). This space is rather narrow and is known as the **pericardioperitoneal canal.** It is found on either side of the foregut (Figs. 11.4 and 13.5) and is gradually filled by the expanding lung buds. Ultimately, the pericardioperitoneal canals are separated from the peritoneal and pericardial cavities by the pleuroperitoneal and pleuropericardial folds, respectively, and the remaining spaces are the **primitive pleural cavities** (see Fig. 11.5). The mesoderm, which covers the outside of the lung, develops into the **visceral pleura.** The somatic mesoderm layer, covering the body wall from the inside, becomes the **parietal pleura** (Fig. 13.6*A*). The space between the parietal and visceral pleura is the **pleural cavity** (Fig. 13.7).

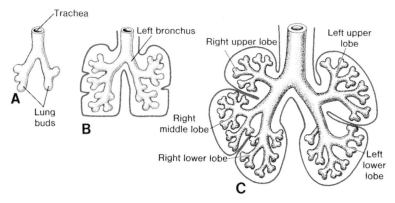

Figure 13.5. Successive stages in development of the trachea and lungs. **A.** 5 weeks. **B.** 6 weeks. **C.** 8 weeks.

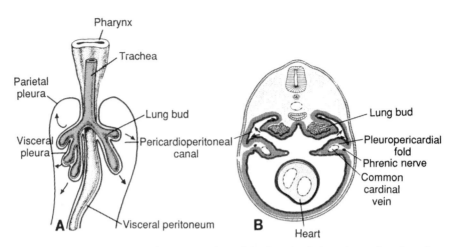

Figure 13.6. Drawings to show expansion of the lung buds into the pericardioperitoneal canals. At this stage of development, the canals are in communication with the peritoneal and pericardial cavities. **A.** Lung buds seen from a ventral view. **B.** Transverse section through the lung buds. Note the pleuropericardial folds that will divide the thoracic portion of the coelomic cavity into the pleural and pericardial cavities.

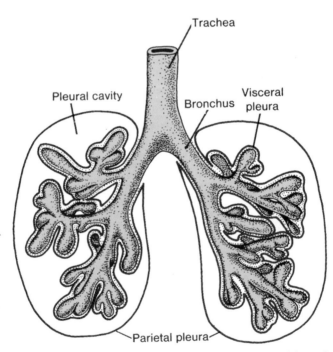

Figure 13.7. Once the pericardioperitoneal canals are separated from the pericardial and peritoneal cavities, respectively, the lungs expand in the pleural cavities. Note the visceral and parietal pleura and definitive pleural cavity. The visceral pleura extends between the lobes of the lungs.

During further development, secondary bronchi divide repeatedly in a dichotomous fashion, forming 10 **tertiary (segmental)** bronchi in the right lung and 8 in the left, thereby creating the **bronchopulmonary segments** of the adult lung. By the end of the 6th month, approximately 17 generations of subdivisions have been formed. Before the bronchial tree has reached its final shape, however, **an additional 6 divisions will be formed during postnatal life.** While all of these new subdivisions are forming and the bronchial tree is developing, the lungs assume a more caudal position, such that by the time of birth the bifurcation of the trachea is located opposite the 4th thoracic vertebra.

MATURATION OF THE LUNGS (SUMMARIZED IN TABLE 13.1)

Up to the 7th prenatal month, the bronchioles divide continuously into more and smaller canals (canalicular phase) (Fig. 13.8A), and the vascular supply increases steadily. Respiration becomes possible when some of the cells of the cuboidal **respiratory bronchioles** change into thin, flat cells (Fig. 13.8B). These cells are intimately associated with numerous blood and lymph capillaries, and the surrounded spaces are now known as **terminal sacs** or **primitive alveoli.** During the 7th month, sufficient capillaries are present to guarantee adequate gas exchange, and the premature infant is able to survive.

During the last 2 months of prenatal life and for several years of postnatal life, the number of terminal sacs increases steadily. In addition, cells lining the sacs, known as **type I alveolar epithelial cells,** become thinner, so that surrounding capillaries protrude into the alveolar sacs (Fig. 13.9). This intimate contact between epithelial and endothelial cells makes up the **blood-air barrier.** Characteristic **mature alveoli** are not present before birth. In addition to endothelial cells and flat alveolar epithelial cells, another cell type develops at the end of the 6th month. These cells, **type II alveolar epithelial cells,** produce **surfactant,** a phospholipid-rich fluid capable of lowering surface tension at the air-alveolar interface.

Table 13.1.
Maturation of the Lungs

Pseudoglandular period	5–16 weeks	Branching has continued to form terminal bronchioles. No respiratory bronchioles or alveoli are present.
Canalicular period	16–26 weeks	Each terminal bronchiole divides into 2 or more respiratory bronchioles, which, in turn, divide into 3–6 alveolar ducts.
Terminal sac period	26 weeks to birth	Terminal sacs (primitive alveoli) form, and capillaries establish close contact.
Alveolar period	8 months to childhood	Mature alveoli with well-developed epithelial endothelial (capillary) contacts.

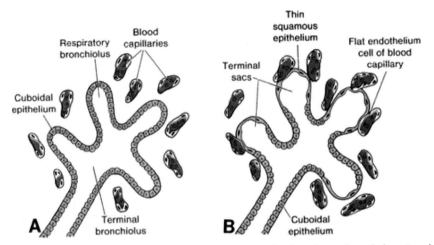

Figure 13.8. Schematic drawings representing the histological and functional development of the lung. **A.** The canalicular period lasts from 16 to 26 weeks. Note the cuboidal cells lining the respiratory bronchioli. **B.** The terminal sac period begins at the end of the 6th and beginning of the 7th prenatal month. Cuboidal cells become very thin and intimately associated with the endothelium of blood and lymph capillaries or form terminal sacs (primitive alveoli).

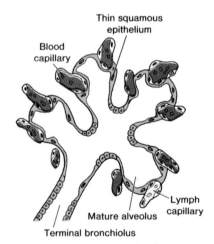

Figure 13.9. Lung tissue in a newborn. Note the thin squamous epithelial cells (also known as alveolar epithelial cells, type I) and surrounding capillaries protruding into mature alveoli.

Before birth, the lungs are filled with fluid that contains a high chloride concentration, little protein, some mucus from the bronchial glands, and surfactant from the alveolar epithelial cells (type II). The amount of surfactant in the fluid increases, particularly during the last 2 weeks before birth.

Fetal **breathing movements** begin before birth and cause aspiration of amniotic fluid. These movements are important for stimulating lung development and conditioning respiratory muscles. When respiration begins at birth, most of the lung fluid is rapidly resorbed by the blood and lymph capillaries, while a small amount is probably expelled via the trachea and bronchi during the delivery process. When the fluid is resorbed from alveolar sacs, surfactant remains deposited as a thin, phospholipid coat on alveolar cell membranes. With air entering alveoli during the first breath, the surfactant coat prevents the development of an air-water (blood) interface with high surface tension. Without the fatty surfactant layer, the alveoli would collapse during expiration (atelectasis).

Respiratory movements after birth cause air to enter the lungs, which subsequently expand and fill the pleural cavity. Although the alveoli increase somewhat in size, growth of the lungs after birth is due primarily to an increase in the **number** of respiratory bronchioles and alveoli. It is estimated that only one-sixth of the adult number of alveoli are present at birth. The remaining alveoli are formed during the first 10 years of postnatal life through the continuous formation of new primitive alveoli.

CLINICAL CORRELATES

Surfactant appears to be particularly important for survival of the **premature infant.** When insufficient amounts of surfactant are present, the air-water (blood) surface membrane tension becomes high, and the risk is great that alveoli will collapse during expiration. As a result, **respiratory distress syndrome** (RDS) develops. This is a common cause of death in the premature infant. In these cases, the partially collapsed alveoli contain a fluid with a high protein content, many hyaline membranes, and lamellar bodies, probably derived from the surfactant layer. The disease is, therefore, also known as **hyaline membrane disease** and accounts for approximately 20% of all infant deaths in the newborn period. Recent development of artificial surfactant and of treatment of premature babies with glucocorticoids to stimulate surfactant production has reduced the mortality produced by RDS and allowed some babies as young as 5½ months of age to survive.

Although many abnormalities of the lung and bronchial tree have been described (e.g., blind-ending trachea with absence of lungs and agenesis of one lung), most of these gross abnormalities are rare. Abnormal divisions of the bronchial tree occur more frequently, sometimes resulting in the presence of supernumerary lobules. These variations of the bronchial tree are of little functional significance but may cause unexpected difficulties in bronchoscopy.

More interesting are **ectopic lung lobes** that arise from the trachea or esophagus. It is believed that these lobes are formed from additional respiratory buds of the foregut that develop independently of the main respiratory system.

Most important clinically are **congenital cysts of the lung,** which are formed by dilation of terminal or larger bronchi. These cysts may be small and multiple, giving the lung a honeycombed appearance on x-ray, or they may be restricted to one or more larger ones. Cystic structures of the lung usually drain poorly and frequently cause chronic infections.

SUMMARY

The **respiratory system** is an outgrowth of the ventral wall of the foregut, and the epithelium of the larynx, trachea, bronchi, and alveoli is of endodermal origin. The cartilaginous and muscular components are of mesodermal origin. In the 4th week of development, the trachea is separated from the foregut by the **esophagotracheal septum,** thus dividing the foregut into the lung bud anteriorly and the esophagus posteriorly. Contact between the two is maintained through the larynx, which is formed by tissue of the 4th and 6th pharyngeal arches (see Fig. 16.9). The lung bud develops into two main bronchi: the right forms three secondary bronchi and three lobes; the left forms two secondary bronchi and two lobes. Faulty partitioning of the foregut by the esophagotracheal septum causes esophageal atresias and tracheoesophageal fistulas (Fig. 13.3).

After a pseudoglandular (5–16 weeks) and canalicular (16–26 weeks) phase, cells of the cuboidal lined bronchioles change into thin, flat cells, **type I alveolar epithelial cells,** intimately associated with blood and lymph capillaries. In the 7th month, gas exchange between the blood and air in the **primitive alveoli** is possible. Before birth, the lungs are filled with fluid with little protein, some mucus, and **surfactant.** This substance is produced by **type II alveolar epithelial cells** and forms a phospholipid coat on the alveolar membranes. At the beginning of respiration, the lung fluid is resorbed, except for the surfactant coat, which prevents the collapse of the alveoli during expiration by reducing the surface tension at the air-blood capillary interface. Absence or insufficient amount of surfactant in the premature baby causes **RDS** due to collapse of the primitive alveoli **(hyaline membrane disease).**

Growth of the lungs after birth is primarily due to an increase in the **number** of respiratory bronchioles and alveoli and not to an increase in the **size** of the alveoli. New alveoli are formed during the first 10 years of postnatal life.

PROBLEMS TO SOLVE

1. A prenatal ultrasound revealed polyhydramnios, and at birth the baby had excessive fluids in its mouth. What type of birth defect might be present, and what is its embryological origin? Would you examine the child carefully for other birth defects? Why?

2. A baby born at 6 months gestation is having trouble breathing. Why?

SUGGESTED READINGS

Boyden EA: The pattern of terminal airspaces in a premature infant of 30–32 weeks that lived nineteen and a quarter hours. *Am J Anat* 126:31, 1969.

Behrman RE (ed): *Nelson Textbook of Pediatrics.* 14th ed. Philadelphia, WB Saunders, 1992.

Endo H, Oka T: An immunohistochemical study of bronchial cells producing surfactant protein A in the developing human fetal lung. *Early Hum Dev* 25:149, 1991.

Kozuma S, Nemoto A, Okai T, Mizuno M: Maturational sequence of fetal breathing movements. *Biol Neonate* 60(suppl 1):36, 1991.

Whitsett JA: Molecular aspects of the pulmonary surfactant system in the newborn. *In* Chernick V, Mellins RB (eds): *Basic Mechanisms of Pediatric Respiratory Disease: Cellular and Integrative.* Philadelphia, BC Decker, 1991.

chapter 14

Digestive System

As a result of cephalocaudal and lateral folding of the embryo, a portion of the endoderm-lined yolk sac cavity is incorporated into the embryo to form the **primitive gut.** Two other portions of the endoderm-lined cavity, the **yolk sac** and the **allantois, remain outside the embryo** (Fig. 14.1, A–D).

In the cephalic and caudal parts of the embryo, the primitive gut forms a blind-ending tube, the **foregut** and **hindgut,** respectively. The middle part, the **midgut,** remains temporally connected to the yolk sac by means of the **vitelline duct** or **yolk stalk** (Fig. 14.1D).

Development of the primitive gut and its derivatives is usually discussed in four sections: *(a)* the **pharyngeal gut** or **pharynx,** which extends from the buccopharyngeal membrane to the tracheobronchial diverticulum (Fig. 14.1D) (since this section is of particular importance for development of the head and neck, it is discussed in Chapter 16); *(b)* the **foregut,** lying caudal to the pharyngeal tube and extending as far caudally as the liver outgrowth; *(c)* the **midgut,** beginning caudal to the liver bud and extending to a point where, in the adult, the junction of the right two-thirds and left one-third of the transverse colon is located; and *(d)* the **hindgut,** extending from the left one-third of the transverse colon to the cloacal membrane (Fig. 14.1). Endoderm forms the epithelial lining of the digestive tract and gives rise to the parenchyma of glands, such as the liver and pancreas. Muscular and peritoneal components of the wall of the gut are derived from splanchnic mesoderm.

Mesenteries

Portions of the gut tube and its derivatives are suspended from the dorsal and ventral body wall by **mesenteries.** A mesentery is a double layer of peritoneum that encloses an organ and connects it to the body wall. Such organs are referred to as **intraperitoneal,** whereas organs that lie against the posterior body wall and are covered by peritoneum on their anterior surface only (e.g., the kidneys) are considered **retroperitoneal.** Peritoneal ligaments are double layers of peritoneum (mesenteries) that pass from one organ to another or from an organ to the body wall. Mesenteries and ligaments provide pathways for vessels, nerves, and lymphatics to and from abdominal viscera (Figs. 14.2 and 14.3).

Initially, the foregut, midgut, and hindgut are in broad contact with the mesenchyme of the posterior abdominal wall (Fig. 14.2). By the 5th week, however, the connecting tissue bridge has become narrow, and the caudal part of

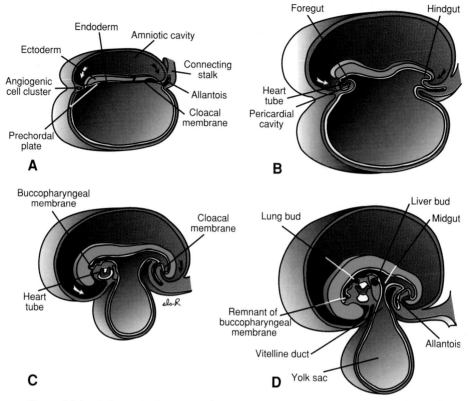

Figure 14.1. Schematic drawings of sagittal sections through embryos at various stages of development to demonstrate the effect of cephalocaudal and lateral flexion on position of the endoderm-lined cavity. Note formation of the foregut, midgut, and hindgut. **A.** Presomite embryo. **B.** 7-somite embryo. **C.** 14-somite embryo. **D.** At the end of the 1st month.

the foregut, the midgut, and a major part of the hindgut are suspended from the abdominal wall by the **dorsal mesentery** (Figs. 14.2*C* and 14.3). Dorsal mesentery extends from the lower end of the esophagus to the cloacal region of the hindgut. In the region of the stomach, it is known as the **dorsal mesogastrium** or **greater omentum;** in the region of the duodenum, it is known as the dorsal **mesoduodenum;** and in the region of the colon, it is known as the **dorsal mesocolon.** Dorsal mesentery of the jejunal and ileal loops is known as the **mesentery proper.**

Ventral mesentery exists only in the region of the terminal part of the esophagus, the stomach, and the upper part of the duodenum (Fig. 14.3) and is derived from the **septum transversum.** Growth of the liver into the mesenchyme of the septum transversum divides the ventral mesentery into *(a)* the **lesser omentum,** extending from the lower portion of the esophagus, the stomach, and the upper portion of the duodenum to the liver, and *(b)* the **falciform ligament,** extending from the liver to the ventral body wall (Fig. 14.3).

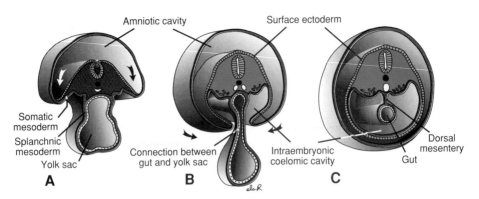

Figure 14.2. Transverse sections through embryos at various stages of development. **A.** The intraembryonic coelom, bordered by splanchnic and somatic layers of lateral plate mesoderm, is in open communication with the extraembryonic cavity. **B.** The intraembryonic coelom is losing its wide connection with the extraembryonic cavity. **C.** At the end of the 4th week, splanchnic mesoderm layers are fused in the midline and form a double-layered membrane (dorsal mesentery) between right and left halves of the body cavity. Ventral mesentery exists only in the region of the septum transversum (not shown).

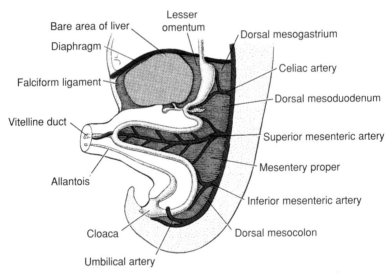

Figure 14.3. Schematic drawing showing the primitive dorsal and ventral mesenteries. Note that the liver is connected to the ventral abdominal wall and to the stomach by the falciform ligament and lesser omentum, respectively. The superior mesenteric artery runs through the mesentery proper and continues toward the yolk sac as the vitelline artery.

Foregut

ESOPHAGUS

When the embryo is approximately 4 weeks old, the **respiratory diverticulum (lung bud)** appears at the ventral wall of the foregut at the border with the pharyngeal gut (Fig. 14.4). This **diverticulum** is gradually separated from the dorsal part of the foregut through a partition, which is known as the **esophagotracheal septum** (Fig. 14.5). In this manner the foregut is divided into a ventral portion, the **respiratory primordium,** and a dorsal portion, the **esophagus** (see Chapter 13).

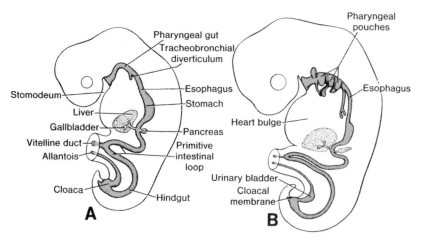

Figure 14.4. Schematic drawings of embryos during the 4th (**A**) and 5th (**B**) weeks of development to show formation of the gastrointestinal tract and the various derivatives originating from the endodermal germ layer.

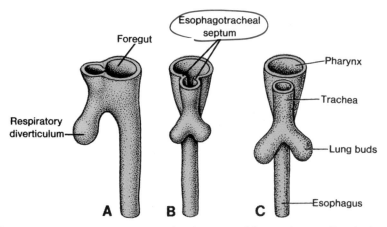

Figure 14.5. Successive stages in development of the respiratory diverticulum and esophagus through partitioning of the foregut. **A.** At the end of the 3rd week (lateral view). **B** and **C.** During the 4th week (ventral view).

Initially, the esophagus is short (Fig. 14.4*A*), but with descent of the heart and lungs, it lengthens rapidly (Fig. 14.4*B*). The muscular coat, which is formed by surrounding mesenchyme, is striated in its upper two-thirds and innervated by the vagus; the muscle coat is smooth in the lower one-third and is innervated by the splanchnic plexus.

CLINICAL CORRELATES

Esophageal atresia (EA) and/or tracheoesophageal fistula (TEF) results either from spontaneous deviation of the **esophagotracheal septum** in a posterior direction or from some mechanical factor pushing the dorsal wall of the foregut anteriorly. In its most common form, the proximal part of the esophagus ends as a blind sac, whereas the distal part is connected to the trachea by a narrow canal at a point just above the bifurcation (Fig. 14.6*A*). Other types of defects in this region occur much less frequently (Fig. 14.6, *B–E*) (see Chapter 13).

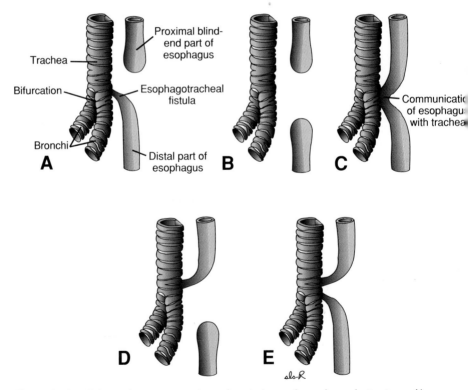

Figure 14.6. Schematic representation of variations of esophageal atresia and/or tracheoesophageal fistula in order of their frequency of appearance: **A,** 90%; **B,** 4%; **C,** 4%; **D,** 1%; and **E,** 1%.

Atresia of the esophagus prevents normal passage of amniotic fluid into the intestinal tract, resulting in accumulation of excess fluid in the amniotic sac (polyhydramnios).

In addition to atresias, the lumen of the esophagus may become narrowed, producing esophageal stenosis. Stenosis usually occurs in the lower one-third and may be caused by incomplete recanalization or vascular abnormalities or accidents that compromise blood flow.

Occasionally, the esophagus fails to lengthen sufficiently, and consequently, the stomach is pulled upward into the esophageal hiatus through the diaphragm. The result is a congenital hiatal hernia.

STOMACH

The stomach appears as a fusiform dilatation of the foregut in the 4th week of development (Fig. 14.7). During the following weeks, its appearance and position change greatly as a result of the different rates of growth in various regions of its wall and the changes in position of surrounding organs. Positional

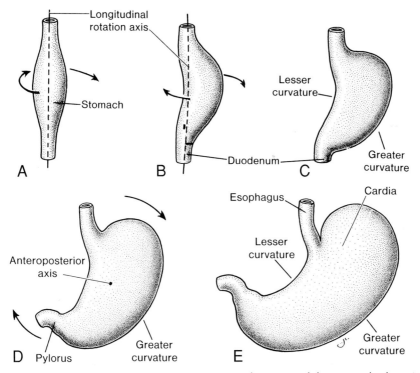

Figure 14.7. A–C. Schematic representations of rotation of the stomach along its longitudinal axis as seen anteriorly. **D** and **E.** Schematic drawings to show rotation of the stomach around the anteroposterior axis. Note the change in position of the pylorus and cardia.

changes of the stomach are most easily explained by assuming that it rotates around a longitudinal and an anteroposterior axis (Fig. 14.7).

Around its longitudinal axis, the stomach rotates 90° clockwise, causing its left side to face anteriorly and its right side to face posteriorly (Fig. 14.7, A–C). Hence, the left vagus nerve, initially innervating the left side of the stomach, now innervates the anterior wall; similarly, the right vagus nerve innervates the posterior wall. During this rotation, the original posterior wall of the stomach grows faster than the anterior portion, and this results in formation of the **greater** and **lesser curvatures** (Fig. 14.7C).

The cephalic and caudal ends of the stomach are originally located in the midline, but during further growth the stomach rotates around an anteroposterior axis, such that the caudal or **pyloric part** moves to the right and upward and the cephalic or **cardiac portion** moves to the left and slightly downward (Fig. 14.7, D and E). The stomach thus assumes its final position, and its axis runs from above left to below right.

Since the stomach is attached to the dorsal body wall by the **dorsal mesogastrium** and to the ventral body wall by the ventral **mesogastrium** (Figs. 14.3 and 14.8A), its rotation and disproportionate growth alter the position of these mesenteries. Thus, rotation about the longitudinal axis pulls the dorsal mesogastrium to the left, creating a space, called the **omental bursa (lesser peritoneal sac),** behind the stomach (Figs. 14.8 and 14.9). This rotation also pulls the ventral mesogastrium to the right. As this process continues in the 5th week of development, the spleen primordium appears as a mesodermal proliferation between the two leaves of the dorsal mesogastrium (Figs. 14.9 and 14.10). With continued rotation of the stomach, the dorsal mesogastrium

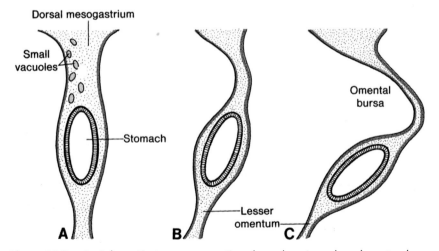

Figure 14.8. **A.** Schematic transverse section through a 4-week embryo to show intercellular clefts appearing in the dorsal mesogastrium. **B** and **C.** The clefts have fused, and the omental bursa is formed as an extension of the right side of the coelomic cavity behind the stomach.

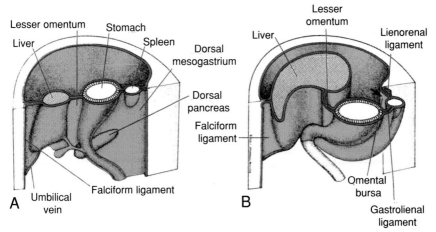

Figure 14.9. **A.** Drawing of the positions of the spleen, stomach, and pancreas at the end of the 5th week. Note the position of the spleen and pancreas in the dorsal mesogastrium. **B.** Position of spleen and stomach at the 11th week. Note formation of the omental bursa or lesser peritoneal sac.

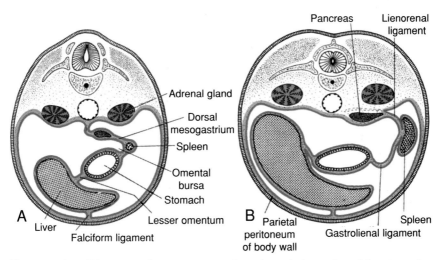

Figure 14.10. Diagrammatic transverse sections through the region of the stomach, liver, and spleen, showing formation of the lesser peritoneal sac, rotation of the stomach, and position of the spleen and tail of the pancreas between the two leaves of the dorsal mesogastrium. With further development, the pancreas assumes a retroperitoneal position.

lengthens, and the portion between the spleen and dorsal midline swings to the left and fuses with the peritoneum of the posterior abdominal wall (Figs. 14.9 and 14.10). The posterior leaf of the dorsal mesogastrium and the peritoneum along this line of fusion degenerate. The spleen, which always maintains an intraperitoneal position, is then connected to the body wall in the region of the left kidney by the **lienorenal ligament** and to the stomach by the **gastrolienal ligament** (Figs. 14.9 and 14.10). Lengthening and fusion of the dorsal mesogastrium to the posterior body wall also determine the final position of the pancreas. Initially, the organ grows into the dorsal mesoduodenum, but eventually its tail extends into the dorsal mesogastrium (Fig. 14.9A). Since this portion of the dorsal mesogastrium fuses with the dorsal body wall, the tail of the pancreas lies against this region (Fig. 14.10). Once the posterior leaf of the dorsal mesogastrium and the peritoneum of the posterior body wall degenerate along the line of fusion, the tail of the pancreas is covered by peritoneum on its anterior surface only and therefore lies in a **retroperitoneal** position. (Organs, such as the pancreas, that are originally covered by peritoneum but later fuse with the posterior body wall to become retroperitoneal are referred to as being **secondarily retroperitoneal**.)

As a result of rotation of the stomach about its anteroposterior axis, the dorsal mesogastrium bulges in a downward direction (Fig. 14.11). It continues to grow in this direction and forms a double-layered sac extending over the transverse colon and small intestinal loops like an apron (Fig. 14.12A). This double-leaved apron is the **greater omentum,** and later its layers fuse to form a single sheet hanging from the greater curvature of the stomach (Fig. 14.12B). The posterior layer of the greater omentum also fuses with the mesentery of the transverse colon (Fig. 14.12B).

The **lesser omentum** and **falciform ligament** form from the ventral mesogastrium, which itself is derived from mesoderm of the septum transversum. When liver cords grow into the septum, it becomes thinned to form (a) the peritoneum of the liver, (b) the **falciform ligament,** extending from the liver to the ventral body wall, and (c) the **lesser omentum,** extending from the stomach

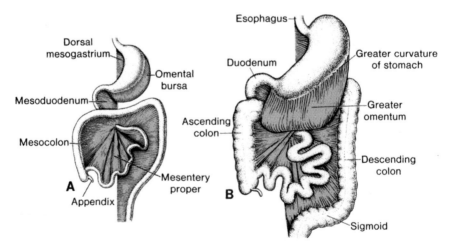

Figure 14.11. **A.** Schematic drawing of derivatives of the dorsal mesentery at the end of the 3rd month. The dorsal mesogastrium bulges out on the left side of the stomach, where it forms part of the border of the omental bursa. **B.** The greater omentum hangs down from the greater curvature of the stomach in front of the transverse colon.

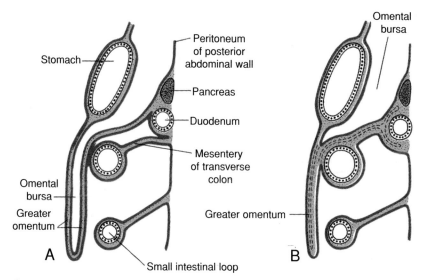

Figure 14.12. **A.** Schematic sagittal section showing the relationship between the greater omentum, stomach, transverse colon, and small intestinal loops at 4 months. The pancreas and duodenum have already acquired a retroperitoneal position. **B.** Similar section as in **A,** in the newborn. The leaves of the greater omentum have fused with each other and with the transverse mesocolon. The transverse mesocolon covers the duodenum, which fuses with the posterior body wall to assume a retroperitoneal position.

and upper duodenum to the liver (Figs. 14.13 and 14.14). The free margin of the falciform ligament contains the umbilical vein (Fig. 14.9A), which, after birth, is obliterated to form the **round ligament of the liver (ligamentum teres hepatis).** The free margin of the lesser omentum connecting the duodenum and liver **(hepatoduodenal ligament)** contains the bile duct, portal vein, and hepatic artery **(portal triad).** This free margin also forms the roof of the **epiploic foramen of Winslow,** which is the opening connecting the omental bursa (lesser sac) with the rest of the peritoneal cavity (greater sac) (Fig. 14.15).

CLINICAL CORRELATES

Pyloric stenosis occurs when the circular and, to a lesser degree, the longitudinal musculature of the stomach in the region of the pylorus is hypertrophied. This is one of the most common abnormalities of the stomach in infants and is believed to develop during fetal life. There is an extreme narrowing of the pyloric lumen, and the passage of food is obstructed, resulting in severe vomiting. A few cases have been described in which the pylorus was atretic.

Other malformations of the stomach, such as duplications and the presence of a prepyloric septum, are rare.

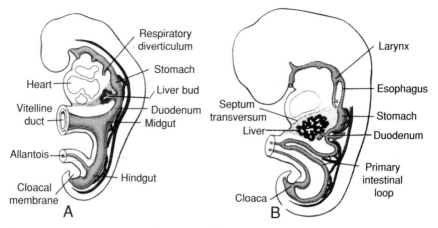

Figure 14.13. **A.** Drawing of a 3-mm embryo (approximately 25 days) to show the primitive gastrointestinal tract and formation of the liver bud. The bud is formed by endoderm lining the foregut. **B.** Drawing of a 5-mm embryo (approximately 32 days). Epithelial liver cords penetrate the mesenchyme of the septum transversum.

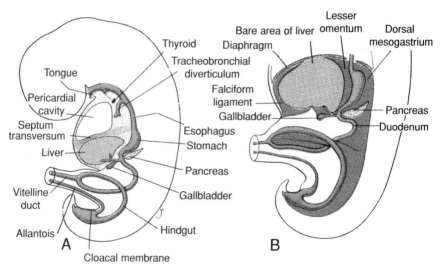

Figure 14.14. **A.** Drawing of a 9-mm embryo (approximately 36 days). The liver expands caudally into the abdominal cavity. Note condensation of mesenchyme in the area between the liver and the pericardial cavity, foreshadowing formation of the diaphragm from part of the septum transversum. **B.** Drawing of a slightly older embryo. Note the falciform ligament extending between the liver and the anterior abdominal wall and the lesser omentum extending between the liver and the foregut (stomach and duodenum). The liver is entirely surrounded by peritoneum, except in its contact area with the diaphragm. This area is known as the bare area of the liver.

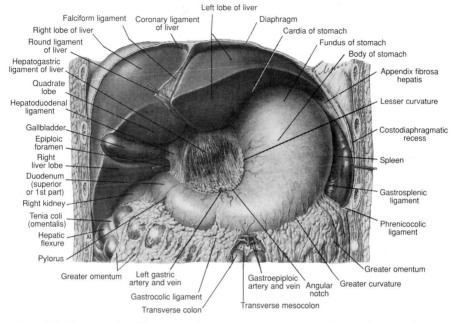

Figure 14.15. Drawing illustrating the lesser omentum extending as the gastrohepatic and duodenal hepatic ligaments. In its free margin are the hepatic artery portal vein and the bile duct (portal triad) lying anterior to the epiploic foramen (of Winslow) that connects the omental bursa with the rest of the peritoneal cavity.

DUODENUM

This portion of the intestinal tract is formed by the terminal part of the foregut and the cephalic part of the midgut. The junction of the two parts is located directly distal to the origin of the liver bud (Figs. 14.13 and 14.14). As the stomach rotates, the duodenum takes on the form of a C-shaped loop and rotates to the right. This rotation, together with rapid growth of the head of the pancreas, causes the duodenum to swing from its initial midline position to the left side of the abdominal cavity (Figs. 14.9A and 14.16). The duodenum and head of the pancreas are pressed against the dorsal body wall, and the right surface of the dorsal mesoduodenum fuses with the adjacent peritoneum. Both layers subsequently disappear, and the duodenum and head of the pancreas become fixed in a **retroperitoneal position.** The entire pancreas thus obtains a retroperitoneal position. The dorsal mesoduodenum disappears entirely except in the region of the pylorus of the stomach, where a small portion of the duodenum **(duodenal cap)** remains intraperitoneal.

During the 2nd month, the lumen of the duodenum is obliterated by proliferation of cells in its walls. However, the lumen is recanalized shortly thereafter (Fig. 14.17, A and B). Since the **foregut** is supplied by the **celiac artery** and the midgut is supplied by the **superior mesenteric artery,** the duodenum is supplied by branches of both arteries (Fig. 14.13).

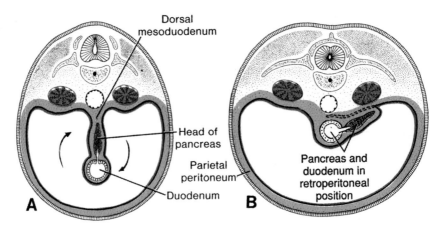

Figure 14.16. Transverse sections through the region of the duodenum at various stages of development. At first, the duodenum and head of the pancreas are located in the median plane (**A**), but later they swing to the right and acquire a retroperitoneal position (**B**).

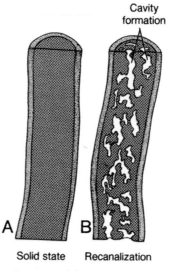

Figure 14.17. Schematic drawings of the upper portion of the duodenum, showing the solid stage (**A**) and cavity formation (**B**) produced by recanalization.

LIVER AND GALLBLADDER

The liver primordium appears in the middle of the 3rd week as an outgrowth of the endodermal epithelium at the distal end of the foregut (Figs. 14.13 and 14.14). This outgrowth, known as the **hepatic diverticulum** or **liver bud,** consists of rapidly proliferating cells that penetrate the **septum transversum,** i.e., the mesodermal plate between the pericardial cavity and the stalk of the yolk sac (Figs. 14.13 and 14.14). While hepatic cells continue to penetrate the septum, the connection between the hepatic diverticulum and the foregut (duodenum) narrows, thus forming the **bile duct.** A small ventral outgrowth is formed by the bile duct, and this outgrowth gives rise to the **gallbladder** and the **cystic duct** (Fig. 14.14). During further development, epithelial liver cords intermingle with the vitelline and umbilical veins, which form hepatic sinusoids. Liver cords differentiate into the **parenchyma** and form the lining of the biliary ducts. **Hematopoietic cells, Kupffer cells,** and **connective tissue cells** are derived from mesoderm of the septum transversum.

When liver cells have invaded the entire septum transversum such that the organ bulges caudally into the abdominal cavity, mesoderm of the septum transversum located between the liver and the foregut and the liver and ventral abdominal wall becomes membranous, thus forming the **lesser omentum** and **falciform ligament,** respectively. Together, they form the peritoneal connection between the foregut and the ventral abdominal wall and are known as the **ventral mesogastrium** (Fig. 14.14).

Mesoderm on the surface of the liver differentiates into visceral peritoneum except on its cranial surface (Fig. 14.14*B*). In this region, the liver remains in contact with the rest of the original septum transversum. This portion of the septum consists of densely packed mesoderm and will form the tendinous portion of the **diaphragm.** The surface of the liver that is in contact with the future diaphragm is never covered by peritoneum and is known as the **bare area of the liver** (Fig. 14.14).

In the 10th week of development, the weight of the liver is approximately 10% of the total body weight. Although this may be attributed partly to the presence of large numbers of sinusoids, another important factor is its **hematopoietic function.** Large nests of proliferating cells, which produce red and white blood cells, are found between hepatic cells and walls of the vessels. Gradually, this activity subsides during the last 2 months of intrauterine life, and only small hematopoietic islands remain at birth. The weight of the liver is then only 5% of the total body weight.

Another important function of the liver begins at approximately the 12th week. At this time, bile is formed by hepatic cells. Meanwhile, since the **gallbladder** and **cystic duct** have developed and the cystic duct has joined the hepatic duct to form the **bile duct** (Fig. 14.14), bile can enter the gastrointestinal tract. As a result, its contents obtain a dark green color. Because of positional changes of the duodenum, the entrance of the bile duct gradually shifts from its initial anterior position to a posterior one, and consequently, the bile duct passes behind the duodenum (Fig. 14.19).

CLINICAL CORRELATES

Variations frequently occur in liver lobulation but are not significant clinically. **Accessory hepatic ducts** and **duplication of the gallbladder**

(Fig. 14.18) are also common and are usually asymptomatic. They become important clinically, however, under pathologic conditions. In some cases, the ducts, which pass through a solid phase in their development, fail to recanalize (Fig. 14.18). This defect is known as **extrahepatic biliary atresia (EHBA)** and occurs with a frequency of 1 in 15,000 live births. Fifteen to 20% of patients with EHBA have patent proximal ducts and a correctable defect, but the remainder usually die without a liver transplant. Another problem with duct formation lies within the liver itself and is known as **intrahepatic biliary duct atresia and hypoplasia.** This abnormality is rare (1 in 100,000 live births) and may be caused by fetal infections. The condition may be lethal but usually runs an extended benign course.

PANCREAS

The pancreas is formed by two buds originating from the endodermal lining of the duodenum (Fig. 14.19). Whereas the dorsal pancreatic bud is located in the dorsal mesentery, the ventral pancreatic bud is located close to the bile duct (Fig. 14.19). When the duodenum rotates to the right and becomes C-shaped, the ventral pancreatic bud migrates dorsally in a manner similar to the shifting of the entrance of the bile duct (Fig. 14.19). Finally, the ventral bud comes to lie immediately below and behind the dorsal bud (Fig. 14.20). Later, the parenchyma and the duct systems of the dorsal and ventral pancreatic buds fuse (Fig. 14.20*B*). The ventral bud forms the **uncinate process** and inferior part of the head of the pancreas. The remaining part of the gland is derived from the dorsal bud. The **main pancreatic duct (of Wirsung)** is formed by the distal part of the dorsal pancreatic duct and the entire ventral pancreatic duct (Fig. 14.20*B*). The proximal part of the dorsal

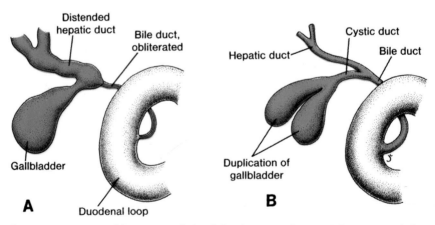

Figure 14.18. **A.** Obliteration of the bile duct, resulting in distention of the gallbladder and hepatic ducts distal to the obliteration. **B.** Duplication of the gallbladder.

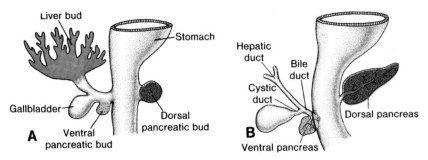

Figure 14.19. Successive stages in development of the pancreas. **A.** 30 days (approximately 5 mm). **B.** 35 days (approximately 7 mm). Initially, the ventral pancreatic bud is located close to the liver bud, but later it migrates posteriorly around the duodenum in the direction of the dorsal pancreatic bud.

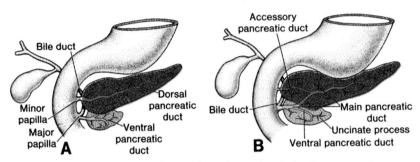

Figure 14.20. **A.** Pancreas during the 6th week of development. The ventral pancreatic bud is in close contact with the dorsal pancreatic bud. **B.** Drawing showing fusion of the pancreatic ducts. The main pancreatic duct enters the duodenum in combination with the bile duct at the major papilla. The accessory pancreatic duct (when present) enters the duodenum at the minor papilla.

pancreatic duct either is obliterated or persists as a small channel, the **accessory pancreatic duct (of Santorini).** The main pancreatic duct, together with the bile duct, enters the duodenum at the site of the **major papilla;** the entrance of the accessory duct (when present) is at the site of the **minor papilla.** In about 10% of all cases the duct system fails to fuse, and the original double system persists.

Pancreatic islets or the **islets of Langerhans** develop from the parenchymatous pancreatic tissue in the 3rd month of fetal life and are scattered throughout the gland. **Insulin secretion** begins at approximately the 5th month. Glucagon- and somatostatin-secreting cells also develop from parenchymal cells. Splanchnic mesoderm surrounding the pancreatic buds forms the connective tissue of the gland.

CLINICAL CORRELATES

The ventral pancreatic bud consists of two components that, under normal conditions, fuse and rotate around the duodenum in such a manner that they come to lie below the dorsal pancreatic bud. Occasionally, however, the right portion of the ventral bud migrates along its normal route, but the left migrates in the opposite direction. In this manner, the duodenum is surrounded by pancreatic tissue, and an **annular pancreas** is formed (Fig. 14.21). The malformation sometimes constricts the duodenum and causes complete obstruction.

Accessory pancreatic tissue may be found anywhere from the distal end of the esophagus to the tip of the primary intestinal loop. Most frequently, it is found in the mucosa of the stomach and in Meckel's diverticulum. Here, it may show all the histological characteristics of the pancreas itself.

Midgut

In the 5-week-old embryo, the midgut is suspended from the dorsal abdominal wall by a short mesentery and communicates with the yolk sac by way of the **vitelline duct** or **yolk stalk** (Figs. 14.1 and 14.14). In the adult, the midgut begins immediately distal to the entrance of the bile duct into the duodenum (Fig. 14.14) and terminates at the junction of the proximal two-thirds of the transverse colon with the distal one-third. Over its entire length, the midgut is supplied by the **superior mesenteric artery** (Fig. 14.22).

Development of the midgut is characterized by rapid elongation of the gut and its mesentery, resulting in formation of the **primary intestinal loop** (Figs. 14.22 and 14.23). At its apex, the loop remains in open connection with the yolk sac by way of the narrow **vitelline duct** (Figs. 14.22). The cephalic limb of the loop develops into the distal part of the duodenum, the jejunum, and part of the ileum. The caudal limb becomes the lower portion of the ileum, the cecum, the appendix, the ascending colon, and the proximal two-thirds of the transverse colon.

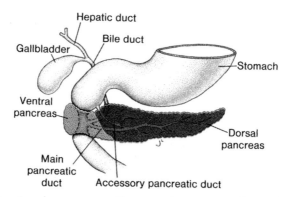

Figure 14.21. Annular pancreas. The ventral pancreas splits and forms a ring around the duodenum, occasionally resulting in duodenal stenosis.

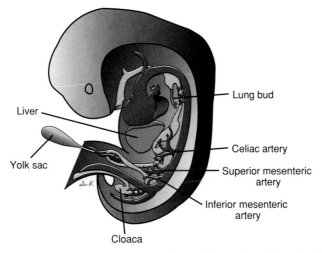

Figure 14.22. Schematic drawing of an embryo during the 6th week of development, showing blood supply to the segments of the gut and formation and rotation of the primary intestinal loop. The superior mesenteric artery forms the axis of this rotation and supplies the midgut. The celiac and inferior mesenteric arteries supply the foregut and hindgut, respectively.

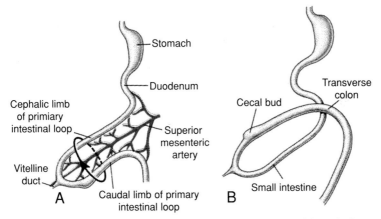

Figure 14.23. **A.** Schematic drawing of the primary intestinal loop before rotation (lateral view). The superior mesenteric artery forms the axis of the loop. *Arrow* indicates the direction of the counterclockwise rotation. **B.** Similar view as in **A,** showing the primary intestinal loop after 180° counterclockwise rotation. Note that the transverse colon passes in front of the duodenum.

PHYSIOLOGICAL HERNIATION

Development of the primary intestinal loop is characterized by rapid elongation, particularly of the cephalic limb. As a result of the rapid growth and expansion of the liver, the abdominal cavity temporarily becomes too small to contain all the intestinal loops, and they enter the extraembryonic coelom in the umbilical cord during the 6th week of development (**physiological umbilical herniation**) (Fig. 14.24)

ROTATION OF THE MIDGUT

Coincident with growth in length, the primary intestinal loop rotates around an axis formed by the **superior mesenteric artery** (Fig. 14.23). When viewed from the front, this rotation is counterclockwise and amounts to approximately 270° when it is completed (Figs. 14.22 and 14.23). Even during rotation, elongation of the small intestinal loop continues, and the jejunum and ileum form a number of coiled loops (Fig. 14.24). The large intestine likewise grows considerably in length but fails to participate in the coiling phenomenon. Rotation occurs during herniation (about 90°) as well as during return of the intestinal loops into the abdominal cavity (remaining 180°) (Fig. 14.25).

RETRACTION OF HERNIATED LOOPS

During the 10th week, herniated intestinal loops begin to return to the abdominal cavity. Although the factors responsible for this return are not

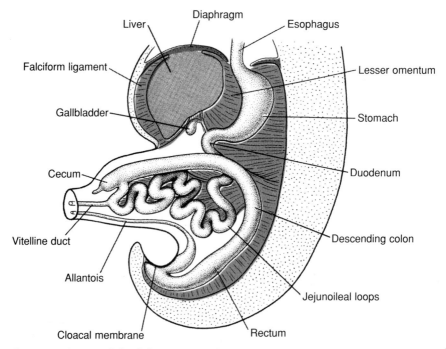

Figure 14.24. Umbilical herniation of the intestinal loops in an embryo of approximately 8 weeks (crown-rump length, 35 mm). Coiling of the small intestinal loops and formation of the cecum occur during the herniation. The first 90° of rotation occurs during herniation, while the remaining 180° occurs during the return of the gut to the abdominal cavity in the 3rd month.

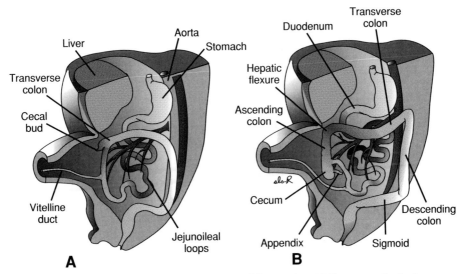

Figure 14.25. **A.** Anterior view of the intestinal loops after 270° counterclockwise rotation. Note the coiling of the small intestinal loops and the position of the cecal bud in the right upper quadrant of the abdomen. **B.** Similar view as in **A,** with the intestinal loops in their final position. Displacement of the cecum and appendix caudally places them in the right lower quadrant of the abdomen.

precisely known, it is thought that regression of the mesonephric kidney, reduced growth of the liver, and actual expansion of the abdominal cavity play important roles.

The proximal portion of the jejunum is the first part to reenter the abdominal cavity and comes to lie on the left side (Fig. 14.25*A*). The later returning loops gradually settle more and more to the right. The **cecal bud,** which appears at about the 6th week as a small conical dilatation of the caudal limb of the primary intestinal loop, is the last part of the gut to reenter the abdominal cavity. Temporarily, it is located in the right upper quadrant directly below the right lobe of the liver (Fig. 14.25*A*). From here it descends into the right iliac fossa, thereby placing the **ascending colon** and **hepatic flexure** on the right side of the abdominal cavity (Fig. 14.25*B*). During this process, the distal end of the cecal bud forms a narrow diverticulum, the **primitive appendix** (Fig. 14.26).

Since the appendix develops during descent of the colon, it is understandable that its final position frequently is posterior to the cecum or colon. These positions of the appendix are referred to as **retrocecal** or **retrocolic,** respectively (Fig. 14.27).

MESENTERIES OF INTESTINAL LOOPS

The mesentery of the primary intestinal loop, the **mesentery proper,** undergoes profound changes with rotation and coiling of the loops. When the caudal limb of the loop moves to the right side of the abdominal cavity, the dorsal mesentery twists around the origin of the **superior mesenteric artery** (Fig.

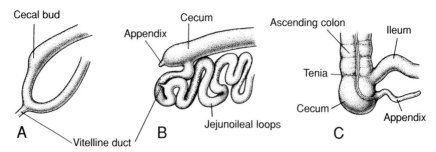

Figure 14.26. Drawings showing successive stages in development of the cecum and appendix. **A.** 7 weeks. **B.** 8 weeks. **C.** In the newborn.

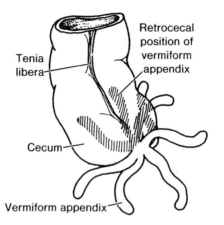

Figure 14.27. Drawing of various positions of the appendix. In about 50% of cases, the appendix is found in a retrocecal or retrocolic position.

14.22). Later, when the ascending and descending portions of the colon obtain their definitive positions, their mesenteries are pressed against the peritoneum of the posterior abdominal wall (Fig. 14.28). After fusion of these layers, the ascending and descending colons are permanently anchored in a retroperitoneal position. The appendix, lower end of the cecum, and sigmoid colon, however, retain their free mesentery (Fig. 14.28*B*).

The fate of the transverse mesocolon is different. It fuses with the posterior wall of the greater omentum (Fig. 14.12) but maintains its mobility. Its line of attachment finally extends from the hepatic flexure of the ascending colon to the splenic flexure of the descending colon (Fig. 14.28*B*).

The mesentery of the jejunoileal loops is at first continuous with that of the ascending colon (Fig. 14.11*A*). When the mesentery of the ascending mesocolon fuses with the posterior abdominal wall, the mesentery of the jejunoileal loops obtains a new line of attachment that extends from the area where the duodenum becomes intraperitoneal to the ileocecal junction (Fig. 14.28*B*).

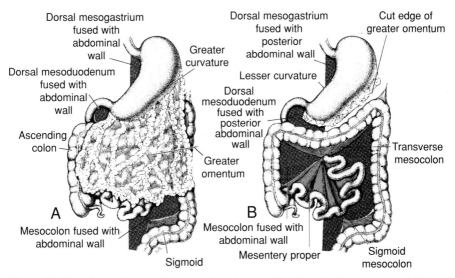

Figure 14.28. Frontal view of the intestinal loops with (**A**) and after removal of (**B**) the greater omentum. *Gray areas* indicate parts of the dorsal mesentery that fuse with the posterior abdominal wall. Note the line of attachment of the mesentery proper.

CLINICAL CORRELATES

Normally, the ascending colon, except for its most caudal part (approximately 1 inch), is fused to the posterior abdominal wall and is covered by peritoneum on its anterior surface and sides. Persistence of a portion of the mesocolon gives rise to what is termed a **mobile cecum.** In its most extreme form, the mesentery of the ascending colon fails to fuse with the posterior body wall, so that the root of the common mesentery is limited to a small area around the origin of the superior mesenteric artery. Such an unusually long mesentery allows for abnormal movements of the gut or even **volvulus** of the cecum and colon. Similarly, retrocolic pockets may occur behind the ascending mesocolon due to incomplete fusion of the mesentery with the posterior body wall. A **retrocolic hernia** represents entrapment of portions of the small intestine behind the mesocolon.

Omphalocele (Fig. 14.29, *A* and *B*) involves herniation of abdominal viscera through an enlarged umbilical ring. The viscera, which may include liver, small and large intestines, stomach, spleen, or gallbladder, are covered by amnion. The origin of the defect is a failure of the bowel to return to the body cavity from its physiological herniation during the 6th to 10th weeks. The abnormality occurs in 2.5 in 10,000 births and is associated with a high rate of mortality (25%) and severe malformations, such as cardiac anomalies (50%) and

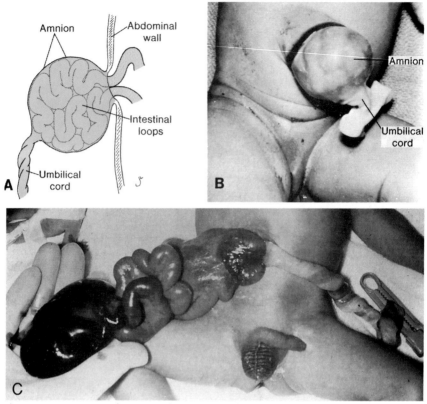

Figure 14.29. **A.** Schematic showing omphalocele, illustrating failure of the intestinal loops to return to the body cavity following physiological herniation. The herniated loops are covered by amnion. **B.** Photograph of omphalocele in a newborn. **C.** Photograph of a newborn with gastroschisis. Loops of bowel return to the body cavity but herniate again through the body wall, usually to the right of the umbilicus in the region of the regressing right umbilical vein. Unlike omphalocele, the defect is not covered by amnion.

neural tube defects (40%). Chromosomal abnormalities are present in approximately 50% of liveborn infants with omphalocele.

Gastroschisis (Fig. 14.29C) is a herniation of abdominal contents through the body wall directly into the amniotic cavity. The defect occurs lateral to the umbilicus, usually on the right, through a region weakened by regression of the right umbilical vein, which normally disappears. Viscera are not covered by peritoneum or amnion, and the bowel may be damaged by exposure to amniotic fluid. Gastroschisis occurs in 1 in 10,000 births but is increasing in frequency, especially among young women, and this increase may be related to cocaine use.

Unlike omphalocele, gastroschisis is not associated with chromosome abnormalities or other severe defects, and therefore, the survival rate is excellent. Volvulus (rotation of the bowel) resulting in a compromised blood supply may, however, kill large regions of the intestine and lead to fetal death.

In 2–4% of people, a small portion of the vitelline duct persists, forming an outpocketing of the ileum, known as **Meckel's** or **ileal diverticulum** (Fig. 14.30A). In the adult, this diverticulum is located approximately 40–60 cm from the ileocecal valve on the antimesenteric border of the ileum and does not usually cause any symptoms. When it contains heterotopic pancreatic tissue or gastric mucosa, however, ulceration, bleeding, or even perforation may occur.

Sometimes, the vitelline duct remains patent over its entire length, thus forming a direct communication between the umbilicus and the intestinal tract. This abnormality is known as an **umbilical or vitelline fistula** (Fig. 14.30C). A fecal discharge may then be found at the umbilicus. In another variation, both ends of the vitelline duct are transformed into fibrous cords, while the middle portion forms a large cyst known as an **enterocystoma** or **vitelline cyst** (Fig. 14 30B). Since the fibrous cords traverse the peritoneal cavity, intestinal loops may twist around such fibrous strands and become obstructed, thereby causing strangulation or volvulus.

Abnormal rotation of the intestinal loop may result in twisting of the intestine **(volvulus)** and a compromise of the blood supply. Normally, the primary intestinal loop rotates 270° counterclockwise. Occasionally, however, rotation amounts to 90° only. When this occurs, the colon and cecum are the first portions of the gut to return from the umbilical cord, and they settle on the left side of the **abdomin-**

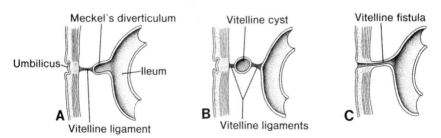

Figure 14.30. Drawings of the remnants of the vitelline duct. **A.** Meckel's or ileal diverticulum combined with fibrous cord (vitelline ligament). **B.** Vitelline cyst attached to the umbilicus and wall of the ileum by vitelline ligaments. **C.** Vitelline fistula connecting the lumen of the ileum with the umbilicus.

al cavity (Fig. 14.31*A*). The later returning loops then become located more and more to the right, resulting in **left-sided colon.**

Reversed rotation of the intestinal loop occurs when the primary loop rotates 90° in a clockwise direction. In such an abnormality, the transverse colon passes behind the duodenum (Fig. 14.31*B*) and lies behind the superior mesenteric artery.

Duplications of intestinal loops and cysts may occur anywhere along the length of the gut tube. They are most frequently located in the region of the ileum, where they may vary from a long segment to a small diverticulum. Symptoms usually occur early in life, and 33% are associated with other defects, such as intestinal atresias, imperforate anus, gastroschisis, and omphalocele. Their origin is unknown, although they may result from abnormal proliferations of gut parenchyma.

Atresia and stenosis may occur anywhere along the intestine. Most occur in the duodenum, fewest occur in the colon, and equal numbers occur in the jejunum and ileum (1/1500 births). Atresias in the upper duodenum are probably due to a lack of recanalization (Fig. 14.17). From the distal portion of the duodenum caudally, however, stenosis and atresias are most likely caused by vascular "accidents." These accidents may be caused by malrotation, volvulus, gastroschisis, omphalocele, and other factors. As a result, blood supply to a region of the bowel is compromised, and a segment dies, resulting in narrowing or complete loss of that region. In 50% of cases a region of the bowel is lost, whereas in 20% a fibrous cord remains (Fig. 14.32, *A* and *B*). In another 20% there is narrowing, with a thin diaphragm separating the larger and smaller pieces of bowel (Fig. 14.32*C*). Stenoses and multiple atresias account for the remaining 10% of these defects, with a

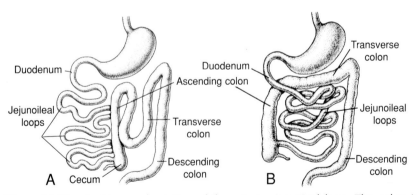

Figure 14.31. A. Abnormal rotation of the primary intestinal loop. The colon is located on the left side of the abdomen, and the small intestinal loops are located on the right side of the abdomen. Note that the ileum enters the cecum from the right. **B.** The primary intestinal loop is rotated 90° in a clockwise direction (reversed rotation). The transverse colon passes behind the duodenum.

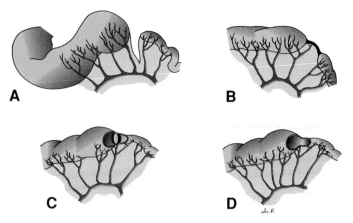

A

B

C

D

Figure 14.32. Schematic drawings of the most commonly occurring bowel atresias and stenoses. **A,** the most common, occurs in 50% of cases, **B** and **C** occur in 20% of cases each, and **D** occurs in 5% of cases. Most are caused by vascular accidents, except for those in the upper duodenum that may also be caused by a lack of recanalization. Atresias **(A–C)** occur in 95% of all cases, and stenoses **(D),** in only 5%.

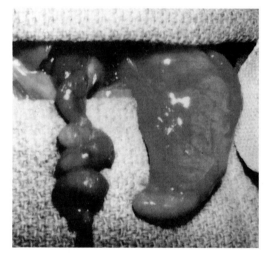

Figure 14.33. Infant with apple peel atresia, which occurs in the jejunum and accounts for 10% of all bowel atresias. The affected portion of the bowel is coiled around a remnant of mesentery.

frequency of 5% each (Fig. 14.32*D*). **Apple peel atresia** is a unique type of defect accounting for 10% of atresias. The atresia is located in the proximal jejunum, and the intestine is short, with the portion distal to the lesion coiled around a mesenteric remnant (Fig. 14.33). Babies with this defect have low birth weight and other abnormalities.

Hindgut

The hindgut gives rise to the distal third of the transverse colon, the descending colon, the sigmoid, the rectum, and the upper part of the anal canal. The endoderm of the hindgut also forms the internal lining of the bladder and urethra (see Chapter 15).

The terminal portion of the hindgut enters into the cloaca, an endoderm-lined cavity in direct contact with surface ectoderm. The contact area involving endoderm and ectoderm forms the **cloacal membrane** (Fig. 14.34).

During further development, a transverse ridge, the **urorectal septum,** arises in the angle between the allantois and hindgut (Fig. 14.34). This septum grows caudally, thereby dividing the cloaca into an anterior portion, the **primitive urogenital sinus,** and a posterior part, the **anorectal canal** (Fig. 14.34C). When the embryo is 7 weeks old, the urorectal septum reaches the cloacal membrane, and in this region the **perineal body** is formed. The cloacal membrane is then divided into the posterior **anal membrane** and the anterior **urogenital membrane** (for discussion of further development of the urogenital sinus, see Chapter 15).

In the meantime, the anal membrane is surrounded by mesenchymal swellings, and in the 8th week it is located at the bottom of an ectodermal depression known as the **anal pit** or **proctodeum** (Fig. 14.35). In the 9th week, the anal membrane ruptures, and an open pathway is formed between the rectum and the outside. The upper part of the anal canal is thus endodermal in origin and is supplied by the artery of the hindgut, the **inferior mesenteric artery.** The lower third of the anal canal, however, is of ectodermal origin and is supplied by the systemic **rectal arteries,** branches of the **internal pudendal artery.** The junction

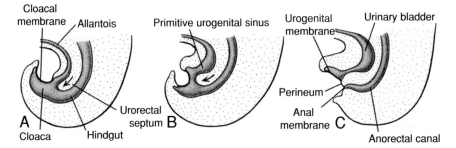

Figure 14.34. Drawings of the cloacal region in embryos at successive stages of development. *Arrow* indicates the route of descent of the urorectal septum. Note the anorectal canal and perineum.

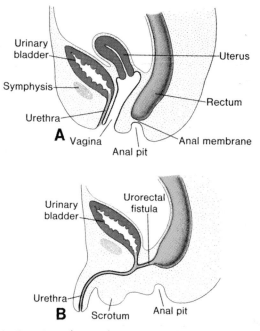

Figure 14.35. A. Drawing of imperforate anus. The anal membrane persists as a diaphragm between the upper and lower portions of the anal canal. **B.** Drawing of urorectal fistula combined with rectal atresia due to a high defect in formation of the urorectal septum.

between the endodermal and ectodermal parts is formed by the **pectinate line,** which is located just below the anal columns. At this line, the epithelium changes from columnar to stratified squamous epithelium.

CLINICAL CORRELATES

Rectoanal atresias occur in 1 in 5000 live births when there is incomplete formation of the hindgut, resulting in **imperforate anus** (Fig. 14.35) with or without a fistula connecting the rectum with the perineum or parts of the urogenital system. Deviation of the **urorectal septum** probably causes many of these anomalies. The defects may be classified as high (usually with fistulas connecting the rectum and urinary or genital tract) (Fig. 14.35B), intermediate (without fistulas in males, with fistulas to the lower vagina or vestibule in females), and low (no fistulas, but the rectum is not continuous with the anal canal). Low lesions are twice as common as high ones, with the intermediate variety being the least frequently occurring. Approximately 50% of children with rectoanal atresias will have other birth defects.

Congenital megacolon may be due to atresia or agenesis of the distal colon or anorectal areas or, more likely, to an absence of parasympathetic ganglia in the bowel wall (**aganglionic megacolon** or **Hirschsprung's disease**). These ganglia are derived from neural crest cells that migrate from the neural folds to the wall of the bowel. In most cases the rectum is involved, and in 80% the defect extends to the midpoint of the sigmoid. In only 10–20% are the transverse and right-side colonic segments involved, and in 3% the entire colon is affected.

SUMMARY

The epithelium of the digestive system and the parenchyma of its derivatives are of endodermal origin; the stromal, muscular, and peritoneal components are of mesodermal origin. The system extends from the buccopharyngeal membrane to the cloacal membrane (Fig. 14.1) and is divided into the pharyngeal gut, foregut, midgut, and hindgut. The pharyngeal gut gives rise to the pharynx and related glands and is discussed in Chapter 16.

The foregut gives rise to the esophagus, the trachea and lung buds, the stomach, and the duodenum proximal to the entrance of the bile duct. In addition, the liver, pancreas, and biliary apparatus develop as outgrowths of the endodermal epithelium of the upper part of the duodenum (Fig. 14.14). Since the upper part of the foregut is divided by a septum (the esophagotracheal septum) into the esophagus posteriorly and the trachea and lung buds anteriorly, deviation of the septum may result in abnormal openings between the trachea and esophagus. The epithelial liver cords and biliary system growing out into the septum transversum (Fig. 14.14) differentiate into parenchyma. Hematopoietic cells (present in the liver in greater numbers before birth), the Kupffer cells, and connective tissue cells are of mesodermal origin. The pancreas develops from a ventral bud and a dorsal bud that later fuse to form the definitive pancreas (Figs. 14.19 and 14.20). Sometimes, the two parts surround the duodenum (annular pancreas), causing constriction of the gut (Fig. 14.21).

The midgut forms the primary intestinal loop (Fig. 14.22), gives rise to the duodenum distal to the entrance of the bile duct, and continues to the junction of the proximal two-thirds of the transverse colon with the distal one-third. At its apex, the primary loop remains temporarily in open connection with the yolk sac through the vitelline duct. During the 6th week, the loop grows so rapidly that it protrudes into the umbilical cord (physiological herniation) (Fig. 14.24). During the 10th week, it returns into the abdominal cavity. While these processes are occurring, the midgut loop rotates 270° counterclockwise (Fig. 14.23). Remnants of the vitelline duct, failure of the midgut to return to the abdominal cavity, malrotation, stenosis, and duplications of parts of the gut are common abnormalities.

The **hindgut** gives rise to the region from the distal one-third of the transverse colon to the upper part of the anal canal (the distal part of the anal canal originates from the ectodermal anal pit). The caudal part of the hindgut is divided by the urorectal septum into the rectum and anal canal posteriorly and the urinary bladder and urethra anteriorly (Fig. 14.34). Deviation of the urorectal septum may result in rectal atresia and abnormal openings between the rectum and the urethra, bladder, or vagina.

PROBLEMS TO SOLVE

1. Prenatal ultrasound showed polyhydramnios at 36 weeks, and at birth the infant had excessive fluids in its mouth and difficulty breathing. What birth defect might cause these conditions?

2. Prenatal ultrasound at 20 weeks revealed a midline mass that appeared to contain intestines and was membrane bound. What diagnosis would you make, and what would be the prognosis for this infant?

3. At birth, a female infant has no anal opening and meconium in her vagina. What type of birth defect does she have, and what was its embryological origin?

SUGGESTED READINGS

Brassett C, Ellis H: Transposition of the viscera. *Clin Anat* 4:139, 1991.
Galloway J: A handle on handedness. *Nature (Lond)* 346:223, 1990.
Severn CB: A morphological study of the development of the human liver. I. Development of the hepatic diverticulum. *Am J Anat* 131:133, 1971.
Severn CB: A morphological study of the development of the human liver. II. Establishment of liver parenchyma, extrahepatic ducts, and associated venous channels. *Am J Anat* 133:85, 1972.
Stephens FD: Embryology of the cloaca and anorectal malformations. *Birth Defects* 24:177, 1988.
Stevenson RE, Hall JG, Goodman RM (eds): *Human Malformations and Related Anomalies.* New York, Oxford University Press, 1993.
Torfs C, Curry C, Roeper P: Gastroschisis. *J Pediatr* 116:1, 1990.
Vellguth S, van Gaudecker B, Muller-Hermelink H-K: The development of the human spleen. *Cell Tissue Res* 242:579, 1985.
Yokoh Y: Differentiation of the dorsal mesentery in man. *Acta Anat* 76:56, 1970.

chapter 15

Urogenital System

Functionally, the urogenital system can be divided into two entirely different components: the **urinary system** and the **genital system**. Embryologically and anatomically, however, they are intimately interwoven. Both develop from a common mesodermal ridge (**intermediate mesoderm**) along the posterior wall of the abdominal cavity, and initially, the excretory ducts of both systems enter a common cavity, the cloaca.

With further development, overlapping of the two systems is particularly evident in the male. The primitive excretory duct first functions as a urinary duct but later is transformed into the main genital duct. Moreover, in the adult, the urinary and the genital organs discharge urine and semen through a common duct, the penile urethra.

Urinary System

FORMATION OF EXCRETORY UNITS

In the beginning of the 4th week, the intermediate mesoderm in the cervical region loses its contact with the somites and forms segmentally arranged cell clusters known as **nephrotomes** (Figs. 15.1 and 15.2). These primitive excretory units form only rudimentary excretory tubules (Figs. 15.1*B* and 15.2) and do not function.

In thoracic, lumbar, and sacral regions, intermediate mesoderm *(a)* loses its contact with the coelomic cavity, *(b)* loses its segmentation, and *(c)* forms two, three, or even more excretory tubules per original segment (Fig. 15.2). As a result, the unsegmented mesoderm forms **nephrogenic tissue cords.** These cords give rise to excretory (renal) tubules and produce bilateral longitudinal ridges, the **urogenital ridges,** on the dorsal wall of the coelomic cavity (Fig. 15.3).

Kidney Systems

Three different, slightly overlapping kidney systems are formed in a cranial to caudal sequence during intrauterine life in humans: the **pronephros, mesonephros,** and **metanephros.** The first of these systems is rudimentary and nonfunctional; the second may function for a short time during the early fetal period; the third forms the permanent kidney.

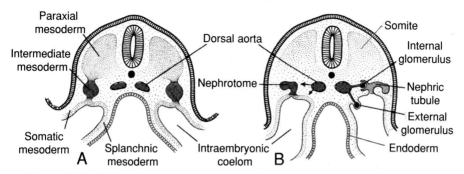

Figure 15.1. Schematic transverse sections through embryos at various stages of development to show formation of nephric tubules. **A.** 21 days. **B.** 25 days. Note formation of external and internal glomeruli and the open connection between the coelomic cavity and the nephric tubule.

PRONEPHROS

In the human embryo, the pronephros is represented by 7–10 solid cell groups in the cervical region (Fig. 15.2B). The first groups form vestigial nephrotomes that regress before more caudal ones are formed, and at the end of the 4th week, all indications of the pronephric system have disappeared.

MESONEPHROS

The mesonephros and mesonephric ducts are derived from intermediate mesoderm from upper thoracic to upper lumbar (L3) segments. Early in the 4th week of development, during regression of the pronephric system, the first excretory tubules of the mesonephros appear. They lengthen rapidly, form an S-shaped loop, and acquire a glomerulus at their medial extremity (Fig. 15.3A). Here, the tubules form **Bowman's capsule.** The capsule and glomerulus together form a **renal corpuscle.** Laterally, the tubule enters the longitudinal collecting duct known as the **mesonephric** or **wolffian duct** (Figs. 15.2 and 15.3).

In the middle of the 2nd month, the mesonephros forms a large ovoid organ on each side of the midline (Fig. 15.3). Since the developing gonad is located on its medial side, the ridge formed by both organs is known as the **urogenital ridge** (Fig. 15.3). While caudal tubules are still differentiating, cranial tubules and glomeruli show degenerative changes, and by the end of the 2nd month, the majority have disappeared. A few of the caudal tubules and the mesonephric duct, however, persist in the male to participate in formation of the genital system, but disappear in the female (see Genital System).

METANEPHROS OR PERMANENT KIDNEY

The third urinary organ, the **metanephros** or **permanent kidney,** appears in the 5th week. Its excretory units develop from **metanephric mesoderm** (Fig.

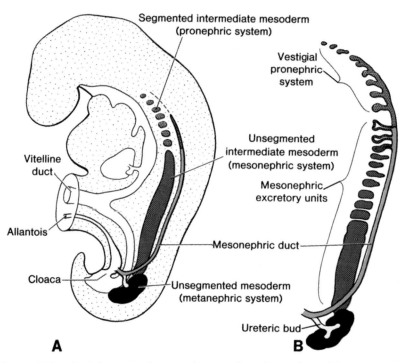

**Segmented intermediate mesoderm
(pronephric system)**

**Vestigial
pronephric
system**

**Unsegmented
intermediate mesoderm
(mesonephric system)**

**Mesonephric
excretory units**

**Vitelline
duct**

Allantois

Cloaca

Mesonephric duct

**Unsegmented mesoderm
(metanephric system)**

Ureteric bud

A

B

Figure 15.2. **A.** Schematic diagram showing the relationship of the intermediate mesoderm of the pronephric, mesonephric, and metanephric systems. In cervical and upper thoracic regions, intermediate mesoderm is segmented; in lower thoracic, lumbar, and sacral regions, it forms a solid, unsegmented mass of tissue, the nephrogenic cord. Note the longitudinal collecting duct, formed initially by the pronephros but later by the mesonephros. **B.** Schematic representation of excretory tubules of the pronephric and mesonephric systems in a 5-week-old embryo.

15.4) in the same manner as in the mesonephric system. The development of the duct system, however, differs from the other kidney systems.

Collecting System

Collecting ducts of the permanent kidney develop from the **ureteric bud,** an outgrowth of the mesonephric duct close to its entrance into the cloaca (Figs. 15.3 and 15.4). The bud penetrates the metanephric tissue, which, as a cap, is molded over its distal end (Fig. 15.4). Subsequently, the bud dilates, forming the primitive **renal pelvis,** and splits into cranial and caudal portions, the future **major calyces** (Fig. 15.5, *A* and *B*).

Each calyx, while penetrating into the metanephric tissue, forms two new buds. These buds continue to subdivide until 12 or more generations of tubules have been formed (Fig. 15.5). Meanwhile, at the periphery, more tubules are formed until the end of the 5th month. The tubules of the second order enlarge and absorb those of the third and fourth generations, thus forming the **minor**

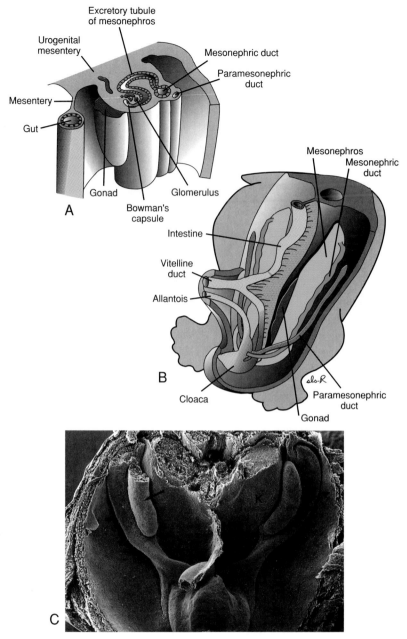

Figure 15.3. A. Transverse section through the urogenital ridge in the lower thoracic region of a 5-week embryo, showing formation of an excretory tubule of the mesonephric system. Note the appearance of Bowman's capsule and the gonadal ridge. The mesonephros and gonad are attached to the posterior abdominal wall by a broad urogenital mesentery. **B.** Drawing to show the relationship of the gonad and the mesonephros. Note the size of the mesonephros. The mesonephric duct (wolffian duct) runs along the lateral side of the mesonephros. **C.** Scanning electron micrograph of a mouse embryo, showing the genital ridge *(arrow)* and mesonephric duct *(arrowheads). K,* kidneys.

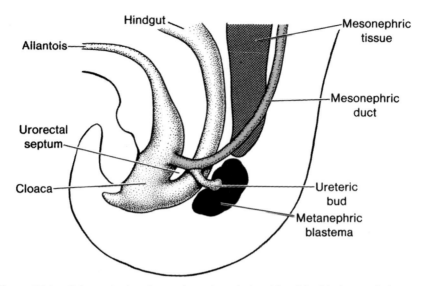

Figure 15.4. Schematic drawing to show the relationship of the hindgut and cloaca at the end of the 5th week. The ureteric bud penetrates the metanephric mesoderm (blastema).

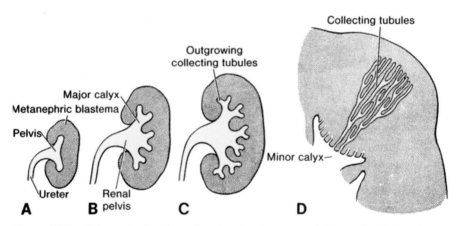

Figure 15.5. Schematic drawings showing development of the renal pelvis, calyces, and collecting tubules of the metanephros. **A.** 6 weeks. **B.** At the end of the 6th week. **C.** 7 weeks. **D.** In the newborn. Note the pyramid form of the collecting tubules entering the minor calyx.

calyces of the renal pelvis. During further development, collecting tubules of the 5th and successive generations elongate considerably and converge on the minor calyx, thereby forming the **renal pyramid** (Fig. 15.5D). Hence, **the ureteric bud gives rise to the ureter, the renal pelvis, the major and minor calyces, and approximately 1 million to 3 million collecting tubules.**

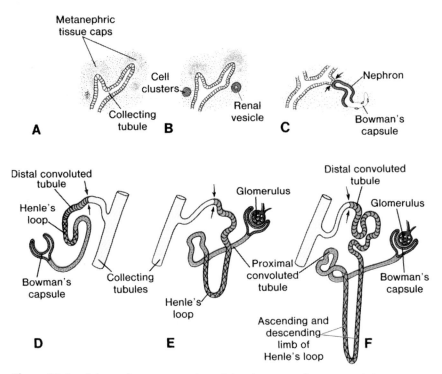

Figure 15.6. Schematic representation of development of a metanephric excretory unit. *Arrows* indicate the place where the excretory unit *(blue)* establishes an open communication with the collecting system *(yellow)*, thus allowing flow of urine from the glomerulus into the collecting ducts.

Excretory System

Each newly formed collecting tubule is covered at its distal end by a **metanephric tissue cap** (Fig. 15.6A). Under the inductive influence of the tubule, cells of the tissue cap form small vesicles, the **renal vesicles,** which, in turn, give rise to small tubules (Fig. 15.6, B and C). These tubules, together with tufts of capillaries known as **glomeruli,** form **nephrons** or **excretory units.** The proximal end of each nephron forms **Bowman's capsule,** which is deeply indented by a glomerulus (Fig. 15.6, C and D). The distal end forms an open connection with one of the collecting tubules, thus establishing a passageway from Bowman's capsule to the collecting unit. Continuous lengthening of the excretory tubule results in formation of the **proximal convoluted tubule, loop of Henle,** and **distal convoluted tubule** (Fig. 15.6, E and F). Hence, the kidney develops from two different sources: *(a)* metanephric mesoderm, which provides excretory units; and *(b)* the ureteric bud, which gives rise to the collecting system.

At birth, the kidneys have a lobulated appearance. During infancy, the lobulation disappears as a result of further growth of the nephrons. Their numbers, however, do not increase.

CLINICAL CORRELATES

There are a number of cystic diseases of the kidneys. **Congenital polycystic kidney** (Fig. 15.7) is a condition in which numerous cysts form, causing renal insufficiency and death unless a transplant is made. The disease may be inherited as an autosomal recessive or dominant disorder or may be caused by other factors. Evidence suggests that the initial defect lies in abnormal formation or function of the proximal convoluted tubules. Degenerative changes then occur, and multiple cysts form.

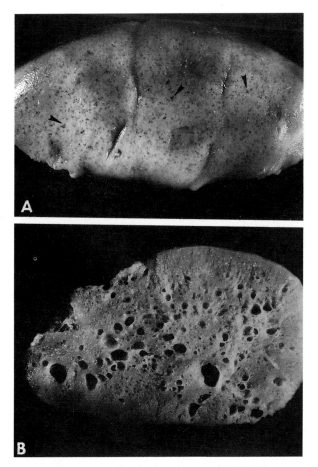

Figure 15.7. **A.** Surface view of a fetal kidney with multiple cysts *(arrowheads)* characteristic of polycystic kidney disease. **B.** Section of the kidney in **A,** showing multiple cysts.

Sometimes, one or more cysts are found close to the pelvis of the kidney. These cysts are thought to be remnants of 2nd-, 3rd-, or 4th-order nephrons. Another cause for cyst formation in the kidney is abnormal development of the collecting system. In some of these cases, cyst formation results from hyperplasia of the wall of the collecting tubules, while in others, abnormal differentiation of the ureteric bud, resulting in dilated, constricted, or sometimes atretic tubules, produces cysts.

Bilateral or unilateral renal agenesis is presumably caused by early degeneration of the ureteric bud. When the ureteric bud does not reach the metanephric tissue cap, the latter fails to proliferate. Unilateral renal agenesis occurs in 1 in 1000 individuals; bilateral agenesis occurs in 1 in 3000.

In the case of bilateral renal agenesis, severe **oligohydramnios** is present by 14 weeks gestation. This condition occurs because the fetus drinks amniotic fluid but cannot excrete it. The fetus will survive to birth, since kidneys are not necessary for exchange of waste products, but will die within a few days. Other severe defects accompany this condition in 85% of cases, including absence of or abnormalities of the vagina and uterus, vas deferens, and seminal vesicles. Defects in other systems are also common, including cardiac anomalies, tracheal and duodenal atresias, cleft lip and palate, and brain abnormalities.

Early splitting of the ureteric bud may result in partial or complete **duplication of the ureter** (Fig. 15.8). Metanephric tissue may then be divided into two parts, each with its own renal pelvis and ureter. More frequently, however, the two parts have a number of lobes in common, as a result of intermingling of collecting tubules. In rare cases, one ureter opens into the bladder, while the other is ectopic and enters the vagina, urethra, or vestibule (Fig. 15.8C). This abnormality results from development of two ureteric buds. One of the buds usually has a normal position, while the abnormal bud moves downward together with the mesonephric duct. Thus, it has a low, abnormal entrance in the bladder, urethra, vagina, or epididymal region.

POSITION OF KIDNEY

The kidney, initially located in the pelvic region, later shifts to a more cranial position in the abdomen. This **"ascent of the kidney"** is caused by diminution of body curvature as well as by growth of the body in the lumbar and sacral regions (Fig. 15.9). In the pelvis, the metanephros receives its arterial supply from a pelvic branch of the aorta. During its ascent to the abdominal level, it is vascularized by arteries that originate from the aorta at continuously higher levels. The lower vessels usually degenerate.

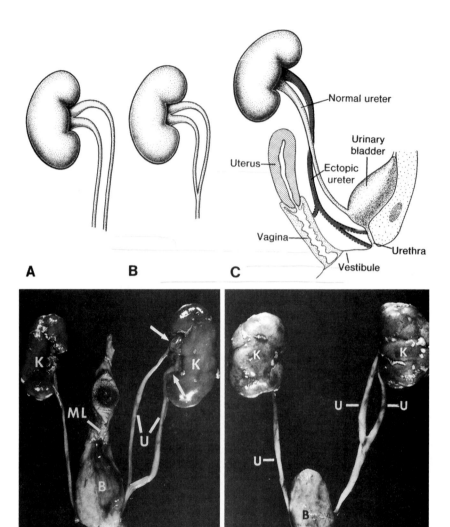

Figure 15.8. **A** and **B.** Drawings of a complete and a partial double ureter. **C.** Drawing showing possible sites of ectopic ureteral openings in the vagina, urethra, and vestibule. **D** and **E.** Photomicrographs of complete and partial duplications of the ureters *(U). Arrows,* duplicated hilum; *B,* bladder; *K,* kidneys; and *ML,* median umbilical ligament.

CLINICAL CORRELATES

   During their ascent, the kidneys pass through the arterial fork formed by the umbilical arteries, but occasionally one of them fails to do so. It then remains in the pelvis close to the common iliac artery

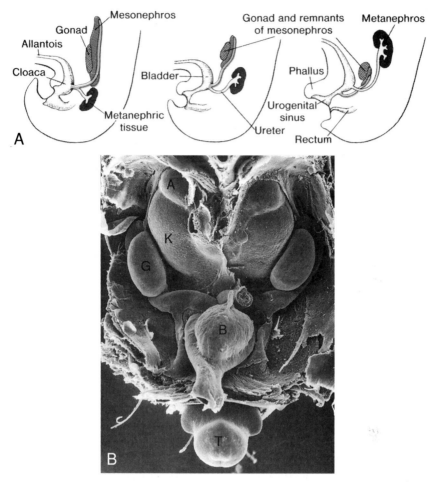

Figure 15.9. A. Drawings of ascent of the kidneys. Note the change in position between the mesonephric and metanephric systems. The mesonephric system degenerates almost entirely, and only a few remnants persist in close contact with the gonad. In both male and female embryos, the gonads descend from their original level to a much lower position. **B.** Scanning electron micrograph of a mouse embryo, showing the kidneys in the pelvis. *B,* bladder; *K,* kidney *A,* adrenal gland; *G,* gonad; *T,* tail.

and is known as a **pelvic kidney** (Fig. 15.10*A*). Sometimes, both kidneys are pushed so close together during their passage through the arterial fork that the lower poles fuse. This results in formation of a **horseshoe kidney** (Fig. 15.10, *B* and *C*). The horseshoe kidney is usually located at the level of the lower lumbar vertebrae, since its ascent is prevented by the root of the inferior mesenteric artery (Fig. 15.10*B*). The ureters arise from the anterior surface of the kidney and

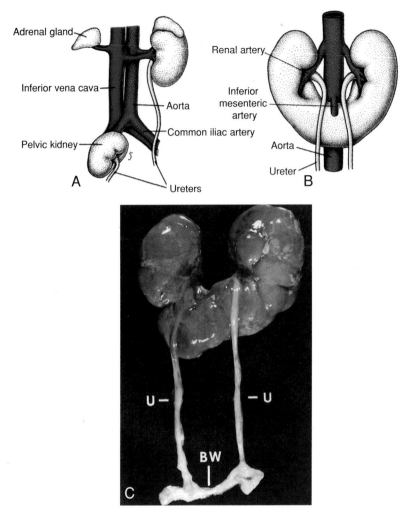

Figure 15.10. **A.** Drawing of a unilateral pelvic kidney. Note the position of the adrenal gland on the affected side. **B** and **C.** Drawing and photomicrograph, respectively, of horseshoe kidneys. Note the position of the inferior mesenteric artery. *BW,* bladder wall; and *U,* ureters.

pass ventral to the isthmus in a caudal direction. Horseshoe kidney is a common abnormality and is found in 1 in 600 people.

Accessory renal arteries are common and represent the persistence of embryonic vessels that formed during ascent of the kidneys. These arteries usually arise from the aorta and enter the superior or inferior poles of the kidneys.

FUNCTION OF THE KIDNEY

The metanephros or definitive kidney becomes functional at the end of the 1st trimester. Urine is passed into the amniotic cavity and mixes with amniotic fluid. This fluid is swallowed by the fetus and enters the intestinal tract, where it is absorbed into the bloodstream and passes through the kidneys to be once again excreted into the amniotic fluid. During fetal life, the kidneys are not responsible for excretion of waste products, since the placenta serves this function.

BLADDER AND URETHRA

During the 4th and 7th weeks of development, the **urorectal septum** divides the **cloaca** into the **anorectal canal** and primitive **urogenital sinus** (Fig. 15.11). The cloacal membrane itself is then divided into the **urogenital membrane,** anteriorly, and the **anal membrane,** posteriorly (Fig. 15.11C). Three portions of the primitive urogenital sinus can be distinguished:

① The upper and largest part is the **urinary bladder** (Fig. 15.12A). Initially, the bladder is continuous with the allantois, but when the lumen of the allantois is obliterated, a thick fibrous cord, the **urachus,** remains and

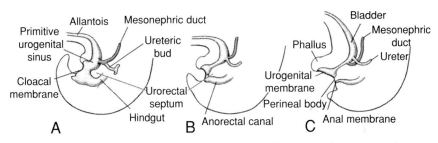

Figure 15.11. Diagrams showing divisions of the cloaca into the urogenital sinus and anorectal canal. Note that the mesonephric duct is gradually absorbed into the wall of the urogenital sinus and the ureters enter separately. **A.** At the end of the 5th week. **B.** 7 weeks. **C.** 8 weeks.

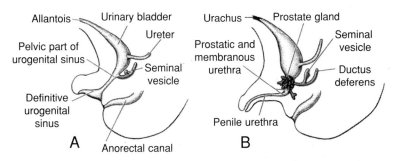

Figure 15.12. **A.** Diagram of development of the urogenital sinus into the urinary bladder and definitive urogenital sinus. **B.** In the male, the definitive urogenital sinus develops into the penile urethra. The prostate gland is formed by buds from the urethra, while seminal vesicles are formed by budding from the ductus deferens.

connects the apex of the bladder with the umbilicus (Fig. 15.12*B*). In the adult, the ligament is known as the **median umbilical ligament.**

② The next part is a rather narrow canal, the **pelvic part of the urogenital sinus,** which in the male gives rise to the **prostatic** and **membranous** parts of the **urethra.**

③ The last part is the definitive **urogenital sinus,** also known as the **phallic part** of the urogenital sinus. It is considerably flattened from side to side and is separated from the outside by the urogenital membrane (Fig. 15.12*A*). (Development of the definitive urogenital sinus differs greatly between the two sexes: see Genital System.)

During division of the cloaca, the caudal portions of the mesonephric ducts are absorbed into the wall of the urinary bladder (Fig. 15.13). Consequently, the ureters, initially outgrowths from the mesonephric ducts, enter the bladder separately (Fig. 15.13*B*). As a result of ascent of the kidneys, the orifices of the ureters move farther cranially; those of the mesonephric ducts move close together to enter the prostatic urethra and in the male become the **ejaculatory ducts** (Fig. 15.13, *C* and *D*). Since both the mesonephric ducts and ureters are of mesodermal origin, the mucosa of the bladder formed by incorporation of the ducts (the **trigone** of the bladder) is mesodermal in origin. With time, the mesodermal lining of the trigone is replaced by endodermal epithelium, so that, finally, the inside of the bladder is completely lined with epithelium of endodermal origin.

Urethra

The epithelium of the male urethra and the female urethra is of endodermal origin, while the surrounding connective and smooth muscle tissue is derived from splanchnic mesoderm. At the end of the 3rd month, epithelium of the prostatic urethra begins to proliferate and forms a number of outgrowths that penetrate the surrounding mesenchyme. In the male, these buds form the **prostate gland** (Fig. 15.12*B*). In the female, the cranial part of the urethra gives rise to the **urethral** and **paraurethral glands.**

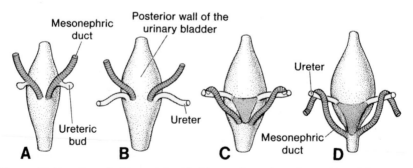

Figure 15.13. Dorsal views of the bladder to show the relationship of the ureters and mesonephric ducts during development. Initially, the ureters are formed by an outgrowth of the mesonephric duct, but with time they assume a separate entrance into the urinary bladder. Note the trigone of the bladder formed by incorporation of the mesonephric ducts.

CLINICAL CORRELATES

When the lumen of the intraembryonic portion of the allantois persists, urine may drain from the umbilicus (Fig. 15.14A). This abnormality is known as a **urachal fistula.** If only a localized area of the allantois persists, secretory activity of its lining results in a cystic dilatation, a **urachal cyst** (Fig. 15.14B). When the lumen in the upper part persists, it forms a **urachal sinus.** This sinus is usually continuous with the urinary bladder (Fig. 15.14C).

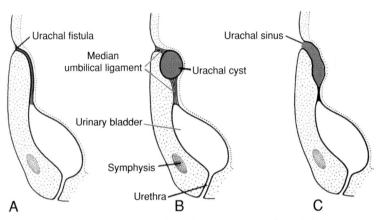

Figure 15.14. **A.** Diagram of urachal fistula. **B.** Diagram of urachal cyst. **C.** Diagram of urachal sinus. The sinus may or may not be in open communication with the urinary bladder.

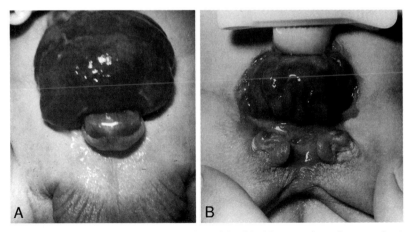

Figure 15.15. **A.** Patient with exstrophy of the bladder. **B.** Cloacal exstrophy in a newborn.

Exstrophy of the bladder (Fig. 15.15A) is a ventral body wall defect in which the bladder mucosa is exposed. Epispadias is a constant feature (see Fig. 15.32), and the open urinary tract extends along the dorsal aspect of the penis through the bladder to the umbilicus. The defect is caused by a lack of mesodermal migration into the region between the umbilicus and genital tubercle, followed by rupture of the thin layer of ectoderm. This anomaly is rare, occurring in 0.2/10,000 live births.

Exstrophy of the cloaca (Fig. 15.15B) represents a more severe ventral body wall defect in which migration of mesoderm to the midline is inhibited and the tail (caudal) fold fails to progress. As a result, there is an extended thin layer of ectoderm that ruptures. The defect includes exstrophy of the bladder, spinal defects with or without meningomyelo cele, imperforate anus, and usually omphalocele. Occurrence of the abnormality is rare (1 in 30,000), and causation has not been defined, although the defect is associated with early amniotic rupture.

Genital System

Sex differentiation is a complex process that involves many genes, including some that are autosomal. The key to sexual dimorphism is the Y chromosome, which contains the **testis-determining factor (TDF) gene** on its **sex-determining region (SRY).** The presence or absence of this factor has a direct effect on gonadal differentiation and also acts as a switch to initiate a cascade of many genes "downstream" from the Y chromosome that then determine the fate of rudimentary sexual organs. In the presence of the factor, male development occurs; in its absence, female development is established.

GONADS

Although the sex of the embryo is determined genetically at the time of fertilization, the gonads do not acquire male or female morphologic characteristics until the 7th week of development.

Gonads appear initially as a pair of longitudinal ridges, the **genital** or **gonadal ridges** (Fig. 15.16), and are formed by proliferation of the coelomic epithelium and a condensation of underlying mesenchyme. **Germ cells** do not appear in the genital ridges until the 6th week of development.

In human embryos, primordial germ cells appear at an early stage of development among endoderm cells in the wall of the yolk sac close to the allantois (Fig. 15.17A). They migrate by ameboid movement along the dorsal mesentery of the hindgut (Fig. 15.17, B and C), arriving at the primitive gonads at the beginning of the 5th week and invading the genital ridges in the 6th week of development. If they fail to reach the ridges, the gonads do not develop. Hence, the primordial germ cells have an inductive influence on development of the gonad into ovary or testis.

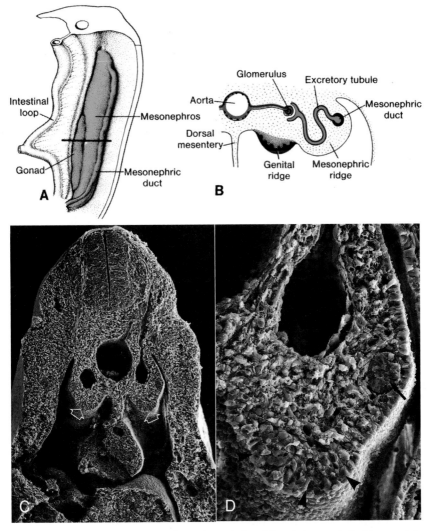

Figure 15.16. **A.** Drawing to show the relationship of the genital ridge and the mesonephros. Note the location of the mesonephric duct. **B.** Transverse section through the mesonephros and genital ridge at the level indicated in **A**. **C.** Scanning electron micrograph of a mouse embryo, showing the genital ridge *(arrows)*. **D.** High magnification of the genital ridge, showing the mesonephric duct *(arrow)* and the developing gonad *(arrowheads)*.

Indifferent Gonad

Shortly before and during arrival of primordial germ cells, the coelomic epithelium of the genital ridge proliferates, and epithelial cells penetrate the underlying mesenchyme. Here, they form a number of irregularly shaped cords, the **primitive sex cords** (Fig. 15.18). In both male and female embryos, these cords are

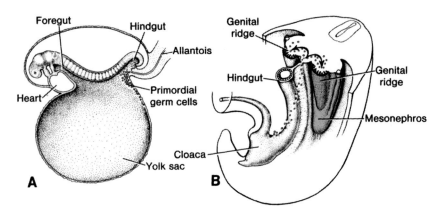

Figure 15.17. **A.** Schematic drawing of a 3-week-old embryo, showing the primordial germ cells in the wall of the yolk sac, close to the attachment of the allantois. **B.** Drawing to show the migrational path of the primordial germ cells along the wall of the hindgut and the dorsal mesentery into the genital ridge.

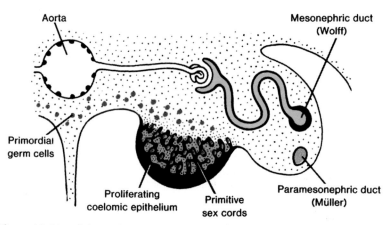

Figure 15.18. Schematic transverse section through the lumbar region of a 6-week embryo, showing the indifferent gonad with the primitive sex cords. Some of the primordial germ cells are surrounded by cells of the primitive sex cords.

connected to surface epithelium, and it is impossible to differentiate between the male and female gonad. Hence, the gonad is known as the **indifferent gonad.**

Testis

If the embryo is genetically male, the primordial germ cells carry an XY sex chromosome complex. Under influence of the Y chromosome, which encodes testis-determining factor, the primitive sex cords continue to proliferate and penetrate deep into the medulla to form the **testis** or **medullary cords** (Table 15.1) (Fig. 15.19A). Toward the hilum of the gland, the cords break up into a network of tiny cell strands, which later give rise to tubules of the **rete testis** (Fig. 15.19, *A* and *B*).

Table 15.1.
Influence of Primordial Germ Cells on Indifferent Gonad

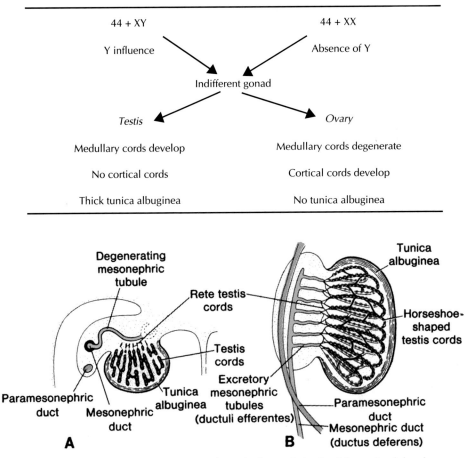

44 + XY		44 + XX
Y influence		Absence of Y
	Indifferent gonad	
Testis		*Ovary*
Medullary cords develop		Medullary cords degenerate
No cortical cords		Cortical cords develop
Thick tunica albuginea		No tunica albuginea

Figure 15.19. **A.** Transverse section through the testis in the 8th week of development. Note the tunica albuginea, testis cords, rete testis, and primordial germ cells. The glomerulus and Bowman's capsule of the mesonephric excretory tubule are degenerating. **B.** Schematic representation of the testis and genital duct in the 4th month of development. The horseshoe-shaped testis cords are continuous with the rete testis cords. Note the ductuli efferentes (excretory mesonephric tubules) that enter the mesonephric duct.

During further development, testis cords lose contact with the surface epithelium. They then become separated from the epithelium by a dense layer of fibrous connective tissue, the **tunica albuginea,** a characteristic feature of the testis (Fig. 15.19).

In the 4th month, the testis cords become horseshoe shaped, and their extremities are continuous with those of the rete testis (Fig. 15.19B). Testis cords are now composed of primitive germ cells and **sustentacular cells of Sertoli** derived from the surface epithelium of the gland (Fig. 1.17).

Interstitial cells of Leydig are derived from the original mesenchyme of the gonadal ridge. They lie between the testis cords and begin development shortly after onset of differentiation of these cords. By the 8th week of gestation, **testosterone** production by Leydig cells begins, and the testis is now able to influence sexual differentiation of the genital ducts and external genitalia.

Testis cords remain solid until puberty, when they acquire a lumen, thus forming the **seminiferous tubules.** Once the seminiferous tubules are canalized, they join the rete testis tubules, which, in turn, enter the **ductuli efferentes.** These efferent ductules are the remaining parts of the excretory tubules of the mesonephric system. They function as the link between the rete testis and the mesonephric or wolffian duct, which is known as the **ductus deferens** (Fig. 15.19*B*).

Ovary

In female embryos with an XX sex chromosome complement and an absence of the Y chromosome, primitive sex cords dissociate into irregular cell clusters (Fig. 15.20*A*). These clusters, containing groups of primitive germ cells, are located in the medullary part of the ovary. Later, they disappear and are replaced by a vascular stroma that forms the **ovarian medulla** (Table 15.1).

The surface epithelium of the female gonad, unlike that of the male, continues to proliferate. In the 7th week, it gives rise to a 2nd generation of cords, **cortical cords,** which penetrate the underlying mesenchyme but remain close to the surface (Fig. 15.20*A*). In the 4th month, these cords are split into isolated cell clusters, with each surrounding one or more primitive germ cells (Fig. 15.20*B*). Germ cells subsequently develop into oogonia, while the surrounding epithelial cells, descendants of the surface epithelium, form **follicular cells** (see Chapter 1).

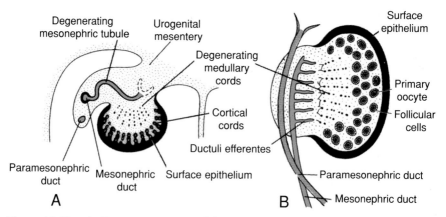

Figure 15.20. **A.** Transverse section of the ovary at the 7th week of development, showing degeneration of the primitive (medullary) sex cords and formation of the cortical cords. **B.** Drawing of the ovary and genital ducts in the 5th month of development. Note degeneration of the medullary cords. The excretory mesonephric tubules (efferent ductules) do not communicate with the rete. The cortical zone of the ovary contains groups of oogonia surrounded by follicular cells.

It may thus be stated that the sex of an embryo is determined at the time of fertilization and depends on whether the spermatocyte carries an X or a Y chromosome. In embryos with an XX sex chromosome configuration, medullary cords of the gonad regress, and a secondary generation of cortical cords develops (Fig. 15.20). In embryos with an XY sex chromosome complex, medullary cords develop into testis cords, and secondary cortical cords fail to develop (Fig. 15.19).

GENITAL DUCTS

Indifferent Stage

Initially, both male and female embryos have two pairs of genital ducts: **mesonephric ducts** and **paramesonephric ducts.** The paramesonephric duct arises as a longitudinal invagination of the coelomic epithelium on the antero-lateral surface of the urogenital ridge (Fig. 15.21). Cranially, the duct opens into the coelomic cavity with a funnel-like structure. Caudally, it first runs lateral to the mesonephric duct but then crosses it ventrally to grow in a caudomedial direction (Fig. 15.21). In the midline, it comes in close contact with the paramesonephric duct from the opposite side. The two ducts are initially separated by a septum but later fuse to form the **uterine canal** (Fig. 15.24A). The caudal tip of the combined ducts projects into the posterior wall of the urogenital sinus, where it causes a small swelling, the paramesonephric or müllerian tubercle (Fig. 15.24A). The mesonephric ducts open into the urogenital sinus on either side of the müllerian tubercle.

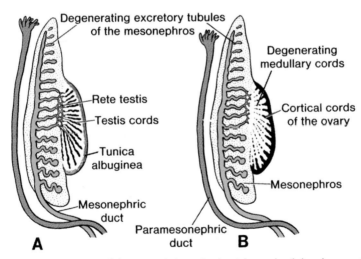

Figure 15.21. Diagram of the genital ducts in the 6th week of development in the male **(A)** and female **(B).** The mesonephric and paramesonephric ducts are present in both. Note the excretory tubules of the mesonephros and their relationship to the developing gonad in both sexes.

DIFFERENTIATION OF THE DUCT SYSTEM

Development of the genital duct system and external genitalia occurs under influence of hormones circulating in the fetus during intrauterine life. Also, Sertoli cells in the fetal testes produce a nonsteroidal substance known as **müllerian inhibiting substance (MIS)** or **antimüllerian hormone (AMH)** that causes regression of the paramesonephric duct. In addition to this inhibiting substance, the testes produce **testosterone** (the major **androgen** produced by the testes), which enters cells of target tissues. Here, it may be converted by a 5α-reductase enzyme to **dihydrotestosterone.** Testosterone and dihydrotestosterone bind to a specific high-affinity intracellular receptor protein, and ultimately this hormone-receptor complex binds to DNA to regulate transcription of tissue-specific genes and their protein products (Fig. 15.22). Testosterone-receptor complexes mediate virilization of the mesonephric ducts, whereas dihydrotestosterone-receptor complexes modulate differentiation of the male external genitalia (Table 15.2).

Table 15.2.
Influence of the Sex Glands on Further Sex Differentiation

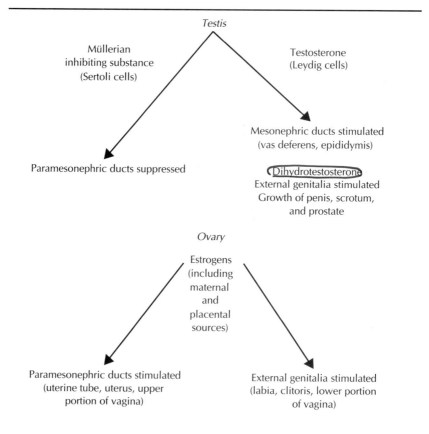

Testis

Müllerian inhibiting substance
(Sertoli cells)

Testosterone
(Leydig cells)

Mesonephric ducts stimulated
(vas deferens, epididymis)

Paramesonephric ducts suppressed

Dihydrotestosterone
External genitalia stimulated
Growth of penis, scrotum,
and prostate

Ovary

Estrogens
(including
maternal
and
placental
sources)

Paramesonephric ducts stimulated
(uterine tube, uterus, upper
portion of vagina)

External genitalia stimulated
(labia, clitoris, lower portion
of vagina)

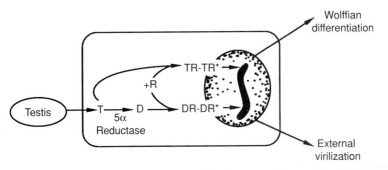

Figure 15.22. Schematic representation of androgen action at the cellular level. Receptor complexes with testosterone *(T)* and dihydrotestosterone *(D)* interact with DNA to control differentiation of the wolffian duct and external genitalia, respectively. *R,* androgen receptor; and *R**, transformed androgen receptor-hormone complex.

In the female, no MIS is produced, and in its absence the paramesonephric duct system is retained and develops into the uterine tubes and uterus. Controlling factors for this process are not clear but may involve estrogens produced by the maternal system, placenta, and fetal ovaries. Since the male inducer substance is absent, the mesonephric duct system regresses. In the absence of androgens, the indifferent external genitalia are stimulated by estrogens and differentiate into labia majora, labia minora, clitoris, and part of the vagina (Table 15.2).

Genital Ducts in the Male

As the mesonephros regresses, a few excretory tubules, the **epigenital tubules,** establish contact with cords of the rete testis and finally form the **efferent ductules** of the testis (Fig. 15.23). Excretory tubules along the caudal pole of the testis, the **paragenital tubules,** do not join the cords of the rete testis (Fig. 15.23*B*). Their vestiges are collectively known as the **paradidymis.**

The mesonephric ducts persist except for the most cranial portion, the **appendix epididymis,** and form the main genital ducts (Fig. 15.23). Immediately below the entrance of the efferent ductules, the mesonephric ducts elongate and become highly convoluted, thus forming the **(ductus) epididymis.** From the tail of the epididymis to the outbudding of the **seminal vesicle,** the mesonephric ducts obtain a thick muscular coat, and this region is known as the **ductus deferens.** The region of the ducts beyond the seminal vesicles is known as the **ejaculatory duct.** The paramesonephric ducts in the male degenerate except for a small portion at their cranial ends, the **appendix testis.**

Genital Ducts in the Female

The paramesonephric ducts develop into the main genital ducts of the female. Initially, three parts can be recognized in each duct: *(a)* a cranial vertical portion that opens into the coelomic cavity, *(b)* a horizontal part that crosses the mesonephric duct, and *(c)* a caudal vertical part that fuses with its partner from

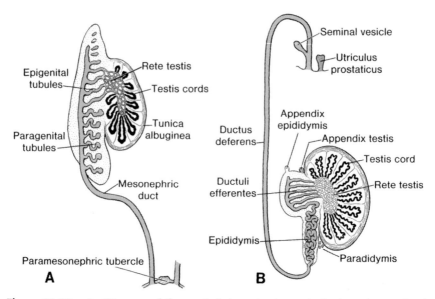

Figure 15.23. **A.** Diagram of the genital ducts in the male in the 4th month of development. Cranial and caudal (paragenital tubule) segments of the mesonephric system regress. **B.** Diagram of the genital ducts after descent of the testis. Note the horseshoe-shaped testis cords, rete testis, and efferent ductules entering the ductus deferens. The paradidymis is formed by remnants of the paragenital mesonephric tubules. The paramesonephric duct has degenerated except for the appendix testis. The prostatic utricle is an outpocketing from the urethra.

the opposite side (Fig. 15.24*A*). With descent of the ovary, the first two parts develop into the **uterine tube** (Fig. 15.24*B*), and the caudal parts fuse to form the **uterine canal.** When the second part of the paramesonephric ducts moves in a mediocaudal direction, the urogenital ridges gradually come to lie in a transverse plane (Fig. 15.25, *A* and *B*). After the ducts have fused in the midline, a broad transverse pelvic fold is established (Fig. 15.25*C*). This fold, which extends from the lateral sides of the fused paramesonephric ducts toward the wall of the pelvis, is known as **the broad ligament of the uterus.** In its upper border lies the uterine tube, and on its posterior surface lies the ovary (Fig. 15.23*C*). The uterus and broad ligaments divide the pelvic cavity into the **uterorectal pouch** and the **uterovesical pouch.** The fused paramesonephric ducts give rise to the **corpus** and **cervix** of the uterus. They are surrounded by a layer of mesenchyme that forms the muscular coat of the uterus, the **myometrium,** and its peritoneal covering, the **perimetrium.**

Vagina

Shortly after the solid tip of the paramesonephric ducts has reached the urogenital sinus (Figs. 15.26*A* and 15.27*A*), two solid evaginations grow out from the pelvic part of the sinus (Figs. 15.26*B* and 15.27*B*). These evaginations, the **sinovaginal bulbs,** proliferate and form a solid **vaginal plate.** Proliferation

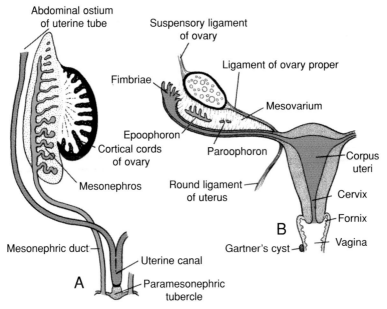

Figure 15.24. **A.** Drawing of the genital ducts in the female at the end of the 2nd month of development. Note the paramesonephric (müllerian) tubercle and formation of the uterine canal. **B.** Drawing of the genital ducts after descent of the ovary. The only parts remaining from the mesonephric system are the epoophoron, paroophoron, and Gartner's cyst. Note the suspensory ligament of the ovary, ligament of the ovary proper, and round ligament of the uterus.

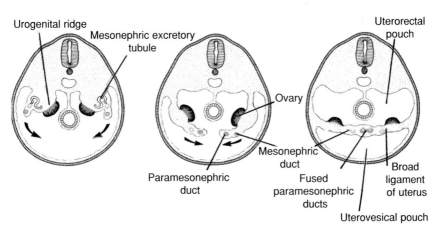

Figure 15.25. Transverse sections through the urogenital ridge at progressively lower levels. Note that the paramesonephric ducts approach each other in the midline to fuse. As a result of fusion, a transverse fold, the broad ligament of the uterus, is formed in the pelvis. The gonads come to lie at the posterior aspect of the transverse fold.

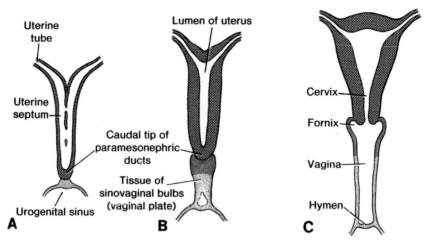

Figure 15.26. Schematic drawing showing formation of the uterus and vagina. **A.** 9 weeks. Note the disappearance of the uterine septum. **B.** At the end of the 3rd month. Note the tissue of the sinovaginal bulbs. **C.** In the newborn. The fornices and the upper portion of the vagina are formed by vacuolization of the paramesonephric tissue, and the lower portion of the vagina is formed by vacuolization of the sinovaginal bulbs.

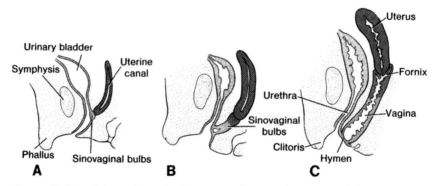

Figure 15.27. Schematic sagittal sections showing formation of the uterus and vagina at various stages of development.

continues at the cranial end of the plate, thus increasing the distance between the uterus and the urogenital sinus. By the 5th month, the vaginal outgrowth is entirely canalized. The wing-like expansions of the vagina around the end of the uterus, the **vaginal fornices,** are of paramesonephric origin (Fig. 15.27C). Thus, the vagina has a dual origin, with the upper portion derived from the uterine canal and the lower portion derived from the urogenital sinus.

The lumen of the vagina remains separated from that of the urogenital sinus by a thin tissue plate known as the **hymen** (Figs. 15.26C and 15.27C). It consists of the epithelial lining of the sinus and a thin layer of vaginal cells. It usually develops a small opening during perinatal life.

Some remnants of the cranial and caudal excretory tubules may remain in the female. They are located in the mesovarium, where they form the **epoophoron** and **paroophoron,** respectively (Fig. 15.24*B*). The mesonephric duct disappears except for a small cranial portion found in the epoophoron and, occasionally, a small caudal portion that may be found in the wall of the uterus or vagina. Later in life, it may form a cyst known as **Gartner's cyst** (Fig. 15.24*B*).

CLINICAL CORRELATES

Duplications of the uterus result from lack of fusion of the paramesonephric ducts in a localized area or throughout the length of the ducts. In its extreme form, the uterus is entirely double **(uterus didelphys)** (Fig. 15.28*A*); in the least severe form, it is only slightly indented in the middle **(uterus arcuatus)** (Fig. 15.28*B*). One of the more common anomalies is the **uterus bicornis,** in which the uterus has two horns entering a common vagina (Fig. 15.28*C*). This condition is normal in many mammals below the primates.

In patients with complete or partial atresia of one of the paramesonephric ducts, the rudimentary part lies as an appendage to the well-developed side. Since its lumen usually does not communicate with the vagina, however, complications are common (uterus bicornis

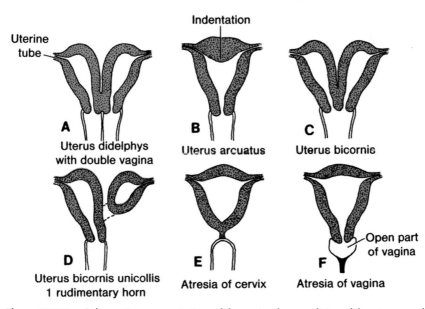

Figure 15.28. Schematic representation of the main abnormalities of the uterus and vagina, caused by persistence of the uterine septum or obliteration of the lumen of the uterine canal.

unicollis with one rudimentary horn) (Fig. 15.28*D*). If the atresia involves both sides, an atresia of the cervix may result (Fig. 15.26*E*). If the sinovaginal bulbs fail to fuse or do not develop at all, a double vagina or atresia of the vagina, respectively, results (Fig. 15.28, *A* and *F*). In the latter case, a small vaginal pouch originating from the paramesonephric ducts will usually surround the opening of the cervix.

EXTERNAL GENITALIA

Indifferent Stage

In the 3rd week of development, mesenchyme cells originating in the region of the primitive streak migrate around the cloacal membrane to form a pair of slightly elevated folds, the **cloacal folds** (Fig. 15.29*A*). Cranial to the cloacal membrane, the folds unite to form the **genital tubercle.** In the 6th week, the cloacal membrane is subdivided into urogenital and anal membranes. Cloacal folds are also subdivided into **urethral folds,** anteriorly, and **anal folds,** posteriorly (Fig. 15.29*B*).

In the meantime, another pair of elevations, the **genital swellings,** become visible on each side of the urethral folds. These swellings later form the **scrotal swellings** in the male (Fig. 15.30*A*) and the **labia majora** in the female (Fig. 15.33*B*). At the end of the 6th week, however, it is impossible to distinguish between the two sexes (Fig. 15.29*C*).

External Genitalia in the Male

Development of the external genitalia in the male is under the influence of androgens secreted by the fetal testes and is characterized by rapid elongation of the genital tubercle, which is now called the **phallus** (Figs. 15.30*A* and 15.31*A*). During this elongation, the phallus pulls the urethral folds forward so that they form the lateral walls of the **urethral groove.** This groove extends along the caudal aspect of the elongated phallus but does not reach the most distal part, known as the glans. The epithelial lining of the groove is of endodermal origin and forms the **urethral plate** (Fig. 15.30*B*).

At the end of the 3rd month, the two urethral folds close over the urethral plate, thus forming the **penile urethra** (Figs. 15.30*B* and 15.31*A*). This canal does not extend to the tip of the phallus. This most distal portion of the urethra is formed during the 4th month when ectodermal cells from the tip of the glans penetrate inward and form a short epithelial cord. This cord later obtains a lumen, thus forming the **external urethral meatus** (Fig. 15.30*C*).

The genital swellings, known in the male as the scrotal swellings, are initially located in the inguinal region. With further development they move caudally, and each swelling then makes up half of the scrotum. The two are separated from each other by the **scrotal septum** (Figs. 15.30*D* and 15.31*A*).

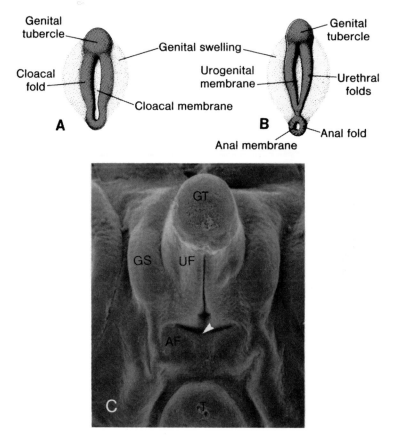

Figure 15.29. Schematic representations (**A** and **B**) of the indifferent stages of the external genitalia. **A.** Approximately 4 weeks. **B.** Approximately 6 weeks. **C.** Scanning electron micrograph of the external genitalia of a human embryo at approximately the 7th week of development. *AF,* anal fold; *arrowhead,* anal opening; *GS,* genital swelling; *GT,* genital tubercle; *T,* tail; and *UF,* urethral fold.

CLINICAL CORRELATES

Hypospadias is a condition in which fusion of the urethral folds is incomplete and abnormal openings of the urethra occur along the inferior aspect of the penis. The defect occurs in 3 in 1000 births, and abnormal orifices are usually near the glans, along the shaft, or near the base of the penis (Fig. 15.32). In rare cases, the urethral meatus extends along the scrotal raphe. When fusion of the urethral folds fails entirely, a wide sagittal slit is found along the entire length of the penis and the scrotum. The two scrotal swellings then closely resemble the labia majora.

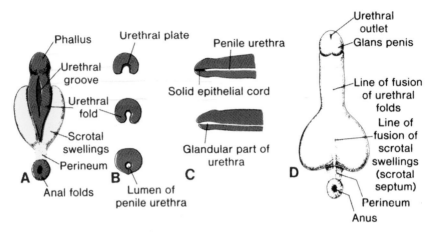

Figure 15.30. A. Schematic representation of the development of external genitalia in the male at 10 weeks. Note the deep urethral groove flanked by the urethral folds. **B.** Transverse sections through the phallus during formation of the penile urethra. The urogenital groove is bridged by the urethral folds. **C.** Development of the glandular portion of the penile urethra. **D.** In the newborn.

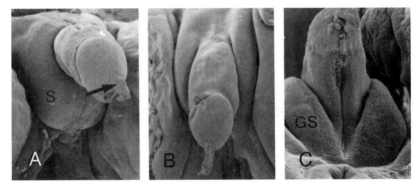

Figure 15.31. A. Genitalia of a male fetus at 14 weeks gestation, showing fusion of the scrotal swellings *(S)*. *Arrow,* epithelial tag. **B** and **C.** Dorsal and ventral views, respectively, of the genitalia of a female fetus at 11 weeks gestation. The genital tubercle at this stage is longer than in the male **(A),** and the genital swellings *(GS)* remain unfused.

Epispadias is a rare abnormality (1 in 30,000 births) in which the urethral meatus is found on the dorsum of the penis. Instead of having developed at the cranial margin of the cloacal membrane, the genital tubercle seems to have formed in the region of the urorectal septum. Hence, a portion of the cloacal membrane is then found cranial to the genital tubercle, and when this membrane ruptures, the outlet of the urogenital sinus comes to lie on the cranial aspect of the penis (Fig.

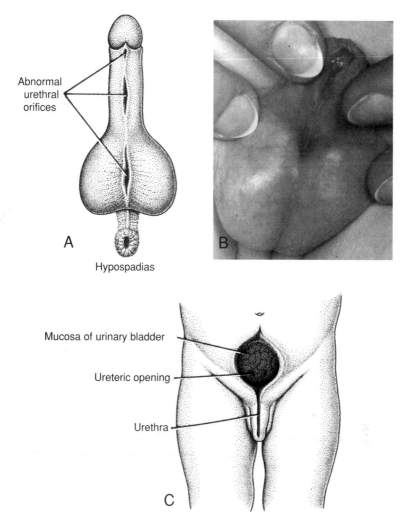

Abnormal urethral orifices

A

Hypospadias

B

Mucosa of urinary bladder

Ureteric opening

Urethra

C

Figure 15.32. A. Drawing of hypospadias, showing the various locations of abnormal urethral orifices. **B.** Patient with hypospadias. The urethra is open on the ventral surface of the penis. **C.** Drawing of epispadias combined with exstrophy of the bladder. Bladder mucosa is exposed to the surface.

15.32). Although the abnormality may occur as an isolated defect, it is most often associated with exstrophy of the bladder.

Exstrophy of the bladder, in which epispadias is a constant feature, is a condition in which the bladder mucosa is exposed to the outside (Figs. 15.15A and 15.32C). Normally, the abdominal wall in front of the bladder is formed by primitive streak mesoderm, which migrates around the cloacal membrane. When this migration does not occur, rupture of the cloacal membrane extends in a cranial direction, thereby creating exstrophy of the bladder.

Micropenis occurs when there is insufficient androgen stimulation for growth of the external genitalia. The condition is usually caused by primary hypogonadism or hypothalamic or pituitary dysfunction. By definition, the penis is 2.5 SD below the mean in length as measured along the dorsal surface from the pubis to the tip with the penis stretched to resistance.

Bifid penis and **double penis** may occur if the genital tubercle splits.

External Genitalia in the Female

Factors controlling development of external genitalia of the female are not clear, but estrogens play a role (see Table 15.2). The genital tubercle elongates only slightly and forms the **clitoris** (Figs. 15.31*B* and 15.33*A*); urethral folds do not fuse as in the male but develop into the **labia minora.** Genital swellings enlarge and form the **labia majora.** The urogenital groove is open and forms the **vestibule** (Figs. 15.31*C* and 15.33*B*). Although the genital tubercle does not elongate extensively in the female, it is larger than in the male during the early stages of development (Fig. 15.31, *A* and *B*). In fact, using tubercle length as a criterion (as monitored by ultrasound) has resulted in mistakes in identification of the sexes during the 3rd and 4th months of gestation.

CLINICAL CORRELATES

Klinefelter syndrome, with a karyotype of 47,XXY (or other variants, e.g., XXXY), is the most common major abnormality of sexual differ-

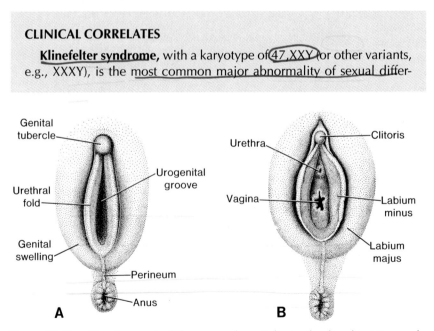

Genital tubercle
Urethral fold
Genital swelling
Urogenital groove
Perineum
Anus
A

Urethra
Vagina
Clitoris
Labium minus
Labium majus
B

Figure 15.33. Development of the external genitalia in the female at 5 months gestation (**A**) and in the newborn (**B**).

entiation, occurring with a frequency of 1 in 500 males. Patients are characterized by infertility, gynecomastia, varying degrees of impaired sexual maturation, and in some cases underandrogenization. Nondisjunction of the XX homologues is the most common causative factor.

Gonadal dysgenesis is a condition in which oocytes are absent and the ovaries appear as "streak" gonads. Individuals are phenotypically female but may have a variety of chromosomal complements, including XY. Those with an XY complement, however, do not produce testosterone. In most cases, individuals have a 45,X karyotype and characteristics of **Turner syndrome**, including short stature, high arched palate, webbed neck, shield-like chest, cardiac and renal anomalies, and inverted nipples (Fig. 15.34). Absence of oocytes in

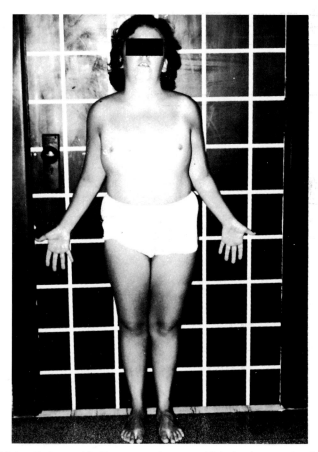

Figure 15.34. Patient with Turner syndrome, which is characterized by a 45,X chromosome complement. Note the absence of sexual maturation. Other typical features are webbed neck, broad chest with widely spaced nipples, and short stature.

45,X cases is due to increased oocyte loss and not to germ cell abnormalities. **Mixed gonadal dysgenesis** is a condition in which there is one streak gonad and one dysgenic testis. Individuals are mosaic with a 45X, 46XY karyotype. They have ambiguous genitalia and some müllerian duct derivatives, usually a uterus.

Since sexual development of males and females begins in an identical fashion, it is not surprising that abnormalities in differentiation and sex determination occur. In some cases, these abnormalities result in individuals with characteristics of both sexes, known as hermaphrodites. True hermaphrodites have both testicular and ovarian tissue usually combined as ovotestes. In 70% of cases the karyotype is 46,XX, and there is usually a uterus. External genitalia are ambiguous or predominantly female, and most of these individuals are raised as females.

In pseudohermaphrodites, the genotypic sex is masked by a phenotypic appearance that closely resembles the other sex. When the pseudohermaphrodite has a testis, the patient is called a male pseudohermpahrodite; when an ovary is present, the patient is called a female pseudohermaphrodite.

Female pseudohermaphroditism is most commonly caused by **congenital adrenal hyperplasia (CAH) (adrenogenital syndrome).** Biochemical abnormalities in the adrenal glands result in decreased steroid hormone production and an increase in adrenocorticotropic hormone (ACTH). In turn, ACTH produces adrenal hyperplasia and excessive production of androgens. Patients have a 46,XX chromosome complement, chromatin-positive nuclei, and ovaries, but excessive production of androgens causes the external genitalia to become masculinized. This masculinization may vary from enlargement of the clitoris to almost male genitalia (Fig. 15.35). Frequently, there is clitoral hypertrophy, partial fusion of the labia majora, giving the appearance of a scrotum, and a small persistent urogenital sinus. Although progestins administered to prevent abortion during pregnancy cause abnormalities similar to the adrenogenital syndrome, the syndrome itself causes most female pseudohermaphrodites.

Male pseudohermaphrodites have a 46,XY chromosome complement, and their cells are usually chromatin-negative. Reduced production of androgenic hormones and MIS are responsible for the condition. Internal and external sex characteristics may vary considerably, depending on the degree of development of external genitalia and the presence of paramesonephric derivatives.

Testicular feminization syndrome (androgen insensitivity syndrome) occurs in patients who have a 46,XY chromosome complement but have the external appearance of normal females (Fig. 15.36).

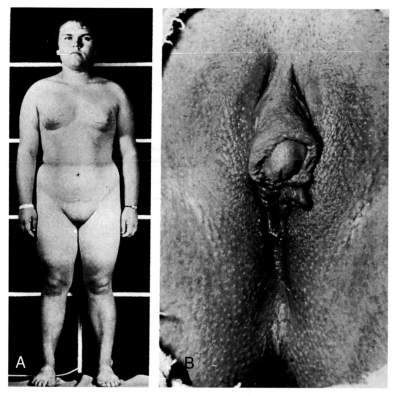

Figure 15.35. **A.** Patient with female pseudohermaphrodism caused by congenital adrenal hyperplasia (adrenogenital syndrome). **B.** External genitalia show fusion of the labia majora and enlargement of the clitoris.

Tissues of the external genitalia are unresponsive to androgens produced by the testes and develop and differentiate as in the normal female under the influence of estrogens. Since these patients have testes and MIS is present, the paramesonephric system is suppressed, and uterine tubes and uterus are absent. The vagina is short and ends blindly. The testes are frequently found in the inguinal or labial regions, but spermatogenesis does not occur. Furthermore, there is an increased risk of tumor formation in these structures, and 33% of these individuals will develop malignancies prior to age 50. The syndrome is rare, occurring in 1 in 20,000 live births.

DESCENT OF THE TESTIS

Toward the end of the 2nd month, the testis and mesonephros are attached to the posterior abdominal wall by the **urogenital mesentery** (Fig. 15.3A). With degeneration of the mesonephros the attachment serves as a mesentery for the

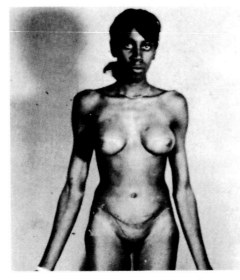

Figure 15.36. Patient with testicular feminization syndrome (androgen insensitivity syndrome), which is characterized by a 46,XY chromosome complement.

gonad (Fig. 15.25*B*). Caudally, it becomes ligamentous and is known as the **caudal genital ligament** (Fig. 15.37*A*). Also extending from the caudal pole of the testis is a mesenchymal condensation rich in extracellular matrices that is known as the **gubernaculum** (Fig. 15.37). Prior to descent of the testis, this band of mesenchyme terminates in the inguinal region between the differentiating internal and external abdominal oblique muscles. Later, as the testis begins to descend toward the inguinal ring, an extraabdominal portion of the gubernaculum is formed and grows from the inguinal region toward the scrotal swellings. At the time the testis passes through the inguinal canal, this extraabdominal portion contacts the scrotal floor (the gubernaculum forms in females also, but in normal cases it remains rudimentary).

Factors controlling descent of the testis are not entirely clear. It appears, however, that outgrowth of the extraabdominal portion of the gubernaculum produces intraabdominal migration, that an increase in intraabdominal pressure due to organ growth produces passage through the inguinal canal, and that regression of the extraabdominal portion of the gubernaculum completes movement of the testis into the scrotum (Fig. 15.37). The process is undoubtedly influenced by hormones and may involve androgens and MIS. During descent, blood supply to the testis from the aorta is retained, and testicular vessels extend from their original lumbar position to the testis in the scrotum.

Independently from descent of the testis, the peritoneum of the coelomic cavity forms an evagination on each side of the midline into the ventral abdominal wall. This evagination follows the course of the gubernaculum testis into the scrotal swellings (Fig. 15.37*B*) and is known as the **processus vaginalis.** Hence, the processus vaginalis, accompanied by the muscular and fascial layers

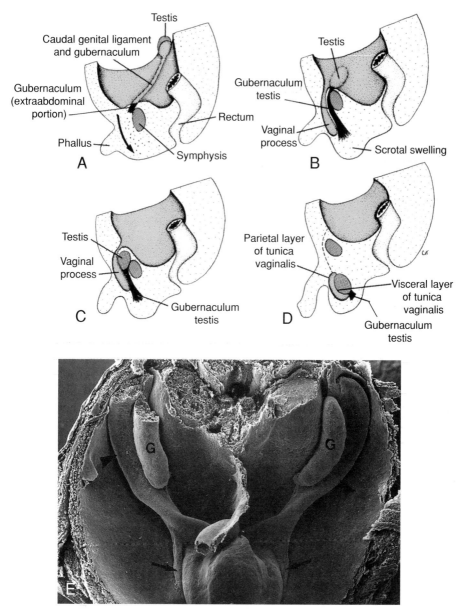

Figure 15.37. Schematic representation of descent of the testis. **A.** During the 2nd month. **B.** In the middle of the 3rd month. Note that peritoneum lining the coelomic cavity evaginates into the scrotal swelling, where it forms the vaginal process (tunica vaginalis). **C.** In the 7th month. **D.** Shortly after birth. **E.** Scanning electron micrograph of a mouse embryo, showing the primitive gonad *(G)*, mesonephric duct *(arrowheads)*, and gubernaculum *(arrows)*.

of the body wall, evaginates into the scrotal swelling, thus forming the **inguinal canal** (Fig. 15.38).

The testis descends through the inguinal ring and over the rim of the pubic bone into the scrotal swelling at the time of birth. The testis is then covered by a reflected fold of the processus vaginalis (Fig. 15.37D). The peritoneal layer covering the testis is known as the **visceral layer of the tunica vaginalis;** the remainder of the peritoneal sac forms the **parietal layer of the tunica vaginalis** (Fig. 15.37D). The narrow canal connecting the lumen of the vaginal process with the peritoneal cavity is obliterated at birth or shortly thereafter.

In addition to being covered by peritoneal layers derived from the processes vaginalis, the testis becomes ensheathed in layers derived from the anterior abdominal wall through which it passes. Thus, the **transversalis fascia** forms the **internal spermatic fascia,** the **internal abdominal oblique muscle** gives rise to the **cremasteric fascia and muscle,** and the **external abdominal oblique muscle** forms the **external spermatic fascia** (Fig. 15.36A). The transversus abdominis muscle does not contribute a layer, since it arches over this region and does not cover the path of migration.

CLINICAL CORRELATES

The connection between the abdominal cavity and the processus vaginalis in the scrotal sac normally closes in the 1st year after birth (Fig. 15.37D). If this passageway remains open, intestinal loops may descend into the scrotum, causing a **congenital inguinal hernia** (Fig. 15.38B). Sometimes, obliteration of this passageway is irregular, leaving small cysts along its course. Later, these cysts may secrete fluid, resulting in formation of a **hydrocele of the testis and/or spermatic cord.**

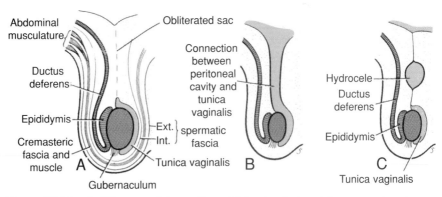

Figure 15.38. **A.** Diagram of the testis, epididymis, ductus deferens, and various layers of the abdominal wall that surround the testis in the scrotum. **B.** Vaginal process in open communication with the peritoneal cavity. In such a case, portions of the intestinal loops often descend toward and, occasionally, into the scrotum, causing an inguinal hernia. **C.** Hydrocele.

At about the time of birth, but with wide individual variation, the testes arrive in the scrotum. In certain cases, one or both testes may remain in the pelvic cavity or somewhere in the inguinal canal until puberty and then descend or remain indefinitely in the abnormal position. This condition is known as cryptorchism and seems to be due to abnormal androgen production. An undescended testis is unable to produce mature spermatozoa, most likely because of high temperature in the abdominal cavity.

DESCENT OF THE OVARY

In the female, descent of the gonad is considerably less than in the male, and the ovary is finally located just below the rim of the true pelvis. The cranial genital ligament forms the **suspensory ligament** of the ovary, whereas the caudal genital ligament forms the **ligament of the ovary proper** and the **round ligament of the uterus** (Fig. 15.24). The latter extends into the labia majora.

SUMMARY

The urinary and genital systems both develop from mesodermal tissue. The urinary system develops from three successive systems:

① The **pronephros** forms in the cervical region and is vestigial.

② The **mesonephros** forms in the thoracic and lumbar regions, is large, and is characterized by excretory units (nephrons) and its own collecting duct, the mesonephric or wolffian duct. In the human, it may function briefly, but most of the system disappears.

③ The **metanephros** or permanent kidney develops from two sources. It forms its own excretory tubules or nephrons like the other systems, but its collecting system originates from the **ureteric bud,** an outgrowth of the mesonephric duct. This bud gives rise to the ureter, renal pelvis, calyces, and the entire collecting system (Fig. 15.5).

Connection between the collecting and excretory tubule systems is essential for normal development (Fig. 15.6). Early division of the ureteric bud may lead to bifid or supernumerary kidneys with ectopic ureters (Fig. 15.8). Abnormal positions of the kidney, such as pelvic and horseshoe kidney, are also well known (Fig. 15.10).

The genital system consists of *(a)* gonads or primitive sex glands, *(b)* genital ducts, and *(c)* external genitalia. All three components go through an **indifferent stage** in which they may develop in either a male or a female direction. The Y chromosome is testis determining and causes *(a)* development of the medullary (testis) cords, *(b)* formation of the tunica albuginea, and *(c)* failure of the cortical (ovarian) cords to develop. Absence of the Y chromosome stimulates formation of the ovary with *(a)* its typical cortical cords, *(b)* disappearance of the medullary (testis) cords, and *(c)* failure of the tunica albuginea to develop (Table 15.1). When primordial germ cells fail to reach the indifferent gonad, the gonad remains indifferent or is absent.

The indifferent duct system and external genitalia develop under the influence of hormones. Testosterone produced by the testis stimulates the development of the mesonephric ducts (vas deferens-epididymis), while müllerian inhibiting substance (MIS) suppresses the paramesonephric ducts (female duct system). Dihydrotestosterone stimulates development of the external genitalia, penis, scrotum, and prostate (Table 15.2). Estrogens influence development of the paramesonephric female system, including the uterine tube, the uterus, and the upper portion of the vagina. They also stimulate the external genitalia, including the clitoris, labia, and lower portion of the vagina (Table 15.2). Errors in production of or sensitivity to hormones of the testes lead to a predominance of female characteristics under influence of the maternal and placental estrogens.

PROBLEMS TO SOLVE

1. During development of the urinary system, three different systems form. What are these three systems, and what parts of each, if any, remain in the newborn?

2. At birth, an apparently male baby has no testicles in the scrotum. Later, it is determined that both are located in the abdominal cavity. What is the term given to this condition, and can you explain the origin of this defect from the embryology involved?

3. It is said that male and female external genitalia have homologies. What are they, and what are their embryological origins?

4. After several years of trying to become pregnant a young woman seeks consultation. Examination reveals the presence of a bicornate uterus. How could such an abnormality occur?

SUGGESTED READINGS

Byskov AG: Differentiation of mammalian embryonic gonad. *Physiol Rev* 66:71, 1986.
George FW, Wilson JD: Sex determination and differentiation. *In* Knobil E, et al (eds): *The Physiology of Reproduction.* New York, Raven Press, 1988:3.
Griffin JE, Wildon JD: Disorders of sexual differentiation. *In* Walsh PC, et al (eds): *Campbell's Urology.* Philadelphia, WB Saunders, 1986:1819–1855.
Josso N, Picard JY, Tran D: The antimüllerian hormone. *Recent Prog Horm Res* 37:117, 1977.
Jost A, Magre S: Control mechanisms of testicular differentiation. *Philos Trans R Soc Lond Biol* 322:55, 1988.
McElreavey K, Vilain E, Abbas N, Herskowitz I, Fellows M: A regulatory cascade hypothesis for mammalian sex determination: SRY represses a negative regulator of male development. *Proc Natl Acad Sci* 90:3368, 1993.
Mittwoch U: Sex determination and sex reversal: genotype, phenotype, dogma and semantics. *Hum Genet* 89:467, 1992.
Nidess R, Koch WE, Fried FA, McFarland E, Mandell J: Development of the embryonic murine kidney in normal and congenital polycystic kidney disease: characterization of a proximal tubular degenerative process as the first observable light microscopic defect. *J Urol* 131:156–162, 1984.
O'Rahilly R: The development of the vagina in the human. *In* Blandau RJ, Bergsma D (eds): *Morphogenesis and Malformation of the Genital Systems.* New York, Alan R Liss, 1977:123–136.

Page DC, et al: The sex determining region of the human Y chromosome encodes a finger protein. *Cell* 51:1091–1104, 1987.

Persuad TVN: Embryology of the female genital tract and gonads. *In* Copeland LJ, Jarrell J, McGregor J (eds): *Textbook of Gynecology.* Philadelphia, WB Saunders, 1992.

Saxen L: Embryonic induction. *Clin Obstet Gynecol* 18:149, 1975.

Saxen L, Sariola H, Lehtonen E: Sequential cell and tissue interactions governing organogenesis of the kidney. *Anat Embryol* 175:1, 1986.

Stevenson RE, Hall JG, Goodman RM (eds): *Human Malformations and Related Anomalies.* New York, Oxford University Press, 1993, vol II.

Swan DA, Donahoe PK, Ito Y, Morkawa Y, Hendren WH: Extraction of müllerian inhibiting substance from newborn calf testes. *Dev Biol* 69:73, 1977.

Vilain E, Jaubert F, Fellows M, McElreavey K: Pathology of 46,XY pure gonadal dysgenesis: absence of testes differentiation associated with mutations in the testes determining factor. *Differentiation* 52:151, 1993.

Wensing CJG, Colenbrander B: Normal and abnormal testicular descent. *Oxf Rev Reprod Biol* 130–164, 1986.

chapter 16

Head and Neck

Mesenchyme for formation of the head region is derived from **paraxial** and **lateral plate mesoderm, neural crest,** and thickened regions of ectoderm known as **ectodermal placodes.** Paraxial mesoderm (**somites** and **somitomeres**) forms the floor of the brain case and a small portion of the occipital region (Fig. 16.1; see Chapter 9), all voluntary muscles of the craniofacial region (see Chapter 10), the dermis and connective tissues in the dorsal region of the head, and the meninges caudal to the prosencephalon. Lateral plate mesoderm forms the laryngeal cartilages (arytenoid and cricoid) and connective tissue in this region. Neural crest cells originate in the neuroectoderm of forebrain, midbrain, and hindbrain regions and migrate ventrally into the pharyngeal arches and rostrally around the forebrain and optic cup into the facial region (Fig. 16.2). In these locations, they form midfacial and pharyngeal arch skeletal structures (Fig. 16.1) and all other tissues in these regions, including cartilage, bone, dentin, tendon, dermis, pia and arachnoid, sensory neurons, and glandular stroma. Cells from **ectodermal placodes,** together with neural crest, form neurons of the 5th, 7th, 9th, and 10th cranial sensory ganglia.

The most typical feature in development of the head and neck is formed by the **pharyngeal** or **branchial arches.** These arches appear in the 4th and 5th weeks of development and contribute to the characteristic external appearance of the embryo (Table 16.1 and Fig. 16.3). Initially, they consist of bars of mesenchymal tissue separated by deep clefts known as **pharyngeal** or **branchial clefts** (Figs. 16.3C and 16.6). Simultaneously, with development of the arches and clefts, a number of outpocketings, the **pharyngeal pouches,** appear along the lateral walls of the pharyngeal gut, the most cranial part of the foregut (Figs. 16.4 and 16.6). The pouches penetrate the surrounding mesenchyme but do not establish an open communication with the external clefts (Fig. 16.6). Hence, although development of pharyngeal arches, clefts, and pouches resembles formation of gills in fishes and amphibia, in the human embryo real gills (branchia) are never formed. Therefore, the term **pharyngeal** (arches, clefts, and pouches) has been adopted for the human embryo.

Pharyngeal arches not only contribute to formation of the neck but also play an important role in formation of the face. At the end of the 4th week, the center of the face is formed by the stomodeum, surrounded by the first pair of pharyngeal arches (Fig. 16.5). When the embryo is 4½ weeks old, five mesenchymal prominences can be recognized: the **mandibular prominences**

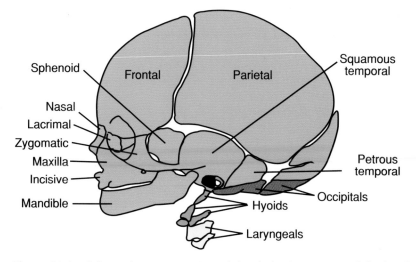

Figure 16.1. Schematic representation of the skeletal structures of the head and face. Mesenchyme for these structures is derived from neural crest *(blue)*, lateral plate mesoderm *(yellow)*, and paraxial mesoderm (somites and somitomeres) *(red)*.

(1st pharyngeal arch), caudal to the stomodeum; the **maxillary prominences** (dorsal portion of the 1st pharyngeal arch), lateral to the stomodeum; and the **frontonasal prominence,** a slightly rounded elevation cranial to the stomodeum. Development of the face is later complemented by formation of the **nasal prominences** (Fig. 16.5).

Pharyngeal Arches

Each pharyngeal arch consists of a core of mesenchymal tissue covered on the outside by surface ectoderm and on the inside by epithelium of endodermal origin (Fig. 16.6). In addition to mesenchyme derived from paraxial and lateral plate mesoderm, the core of each arch receives substantial numbers of **neural crest cells,** which migrate into the arches to contribute to **skeletal components** of the face. The original mesoderm of the arches gives rise to the musculature of the face and neck. Thus, each pharyngeal arch is characterized by its own **muscular components** (Fig. 10.3). The muscular components of each arch carry their own nerve, and wherever the muscle cells migrate, they carry their **cranial nerve component** with them (Figs. 16.6 and 16.7). In addition, each arch has its own **arterial component** (Figs. 16.4 and 16.6). (Derivatives of the pharyngeal arches and their nerve supply are summarized in Table 16.1.)

FIRST PHARYNGEAL ARCH

The **1st pharyngeal arch** consists of a dorsal portion, known as the **maxillary process,** which extends forward beneath the region of the eye, and a ventral portion, the **mandibular process,** which contains **Meckel's cartilage** (Figs. 16.5 and 16.8*A*). During further development, Meckel's cartilage disappears except

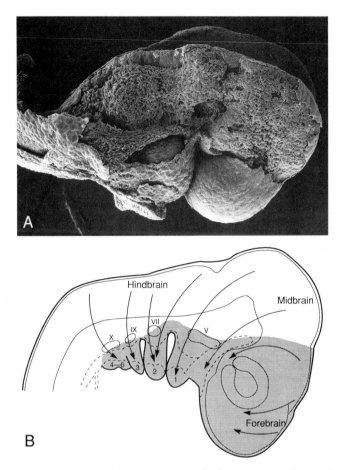

A

B

Figure 16.2.   A. Scanning electron micrograph showing cranial neural crest cells migrating into the facial region beneath the ectoderm that has been removed. **B.** Schematic representation of the migration pathways of neural crest cells from forebrain, midbrain, and hindbrain regions into their final locations *(shaded areas)* in the pharyngeal arches and face. Regions of ectodermal thickenings (placodes), which will assist crest cells in formation of the 5th (V), 7th (VII), 9th (IX), and 10th (X) cranial sensory ganglia, are also illustrated.

for two small portions at its dorsal end that persist and form the **incus** and **malleus** (Figs. 16.8*B* and 16.9). Mesenchyme of the maxillary process gives rise to the **premaxilla, maxilla, zygomatic bone,** and part of the **temporal bone** through membranous ossification (Fig. 16.8*B*). The **mandible** is also formed by membranous ossification of mesenchymal tissue surrounding Meckel's cartilage. In addition, the 1st arch contributes to formation of the bones of the middle ear (Chapter 17).

Musculature of the 1st pharyngeal arch includes the **muscles of mastication** (temporal, masseter, and pterygoids), **anterior belly of the digastric, mylohy-**

Table 16.1.
Derivatives of the Pharyngeal Arches and Their Innervation

Pharyngeal Arch	Nerve	Muscles	Skeleton
1 Mandibular	V. Trigeminal mandibular division	Muscles of mastication (temporal, masseter, medial and lateral pterygoids) Mylohyoid Anterior belly of digastric Tensor palatine and tensor tympani	Quadrate cartilage, incus Meckel's cartilage, malleus, anterior ligament of malleus, sphenomandibular ligament, portion of mandible
2 Hyoid	VII. Facial	Muscles of facial expression (buccinator, auricularis, frontalis, platysma, orbicularis oris and oculi) Posterior belly of digastric Stylohyoid Stapedius	Stapes Styloid process Stylohyoid ligament Lesser horn and upper portion of body of hyoid bone
3	IX. Glossopharyngeal	Stylopharyngeus	Greater horn and lower porton of body of hyoid bone
4–6	X. Vagus Superior laryngeal branch (nerve to 4th arch) Recurrent laryngeal branch (nerve to 6th arch)	Cricothyroid Levator palatine Constrictors of pharynx Intrinsic muscles of larynx	Laryngeal cartilages (thyroid, cricoid, arytenoid, corniculate, and cuneiform)

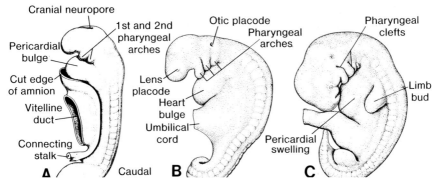

Figure 16.3. Series of human embryos to show development of the pharyngeal arches. **A.** Approximately 25 days. **B.** 28 days. **C.** 5 weeks.

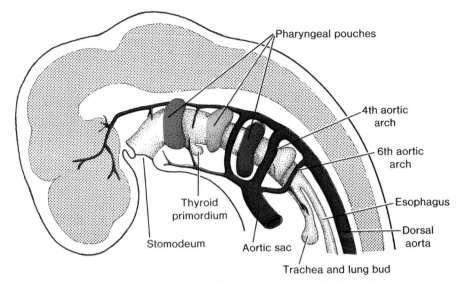

Figure 16.4. Drawing of the pharyngeal pouches as outpocketings of the foregut. Note also the primordium of the thyroid gland and the aortic arches.

oid, tensor tympani, and **tensor palatini.** The **nerve** supply to the muscles of the 1st arch is provided by the **mandibular branch of the trigeminal nerve** (Fig. 16.7). Since mesenchyme from the 1st arch also contributes to the dermis of the face, sensory supply to the skin of the face is provided by **ophthalmic, maxillary,** and **mandibular branches of the trigeminal nerve.**

Muscles of the different arches do not always attach to the bony or cartilaginous components of their own arch but sometimes migrate into surrounding regions. The origin of these muscles, however, can always be traced, since their nerve supply is derived from the arch of origin.

SECOND PHARYNGEAL ARCH

The cartilage of the **2nd** or **hyoid arch (Reichert's cartilage)** (Fig. 16.8*B*) gives rise to the **stapes, styloid process of the temporal bone, stylohyoid ligament,** and, ventrally, the **lesser horn** and **upper part of the body of the hyoid bone** (Fig. 16.9). Muscles of the hyoid arch are the **stapedius, stylohyoid, posterior belly of the digastric, auricular,** and **muscles of facial expression.** The **facial nerve,** the nerve of the 2nd arch, supplies all these muscles.

THIRD PHARYNGEAL ARCH

The **cartilage** of the 3rd pharyngeal arch produces the **lower part of the body** and **greater horn of the hyoid bone** (Fig. 16.9). The **musculature** is limited to the **stylopharyngeus muscle.** These muscles are innervated by the **glossopharyngeal nerve,** the nerve of the 3rd arch (Fig. 16.7).

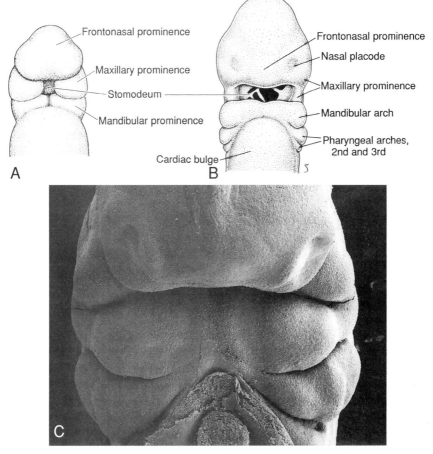

A

Frontonasal prominence

Maxillary prominence

Stomodeum

Mandibular prominence

B

Frontonasal prominence

Nasal placode

Maxillary prominence

Mandibular arch

Pharyngeal arches,
2nd and 3rd

Cardiac bulge

C

Figure 16.5. **A.** Frontal view of an embryo of approximately 24 days. The stomodeum, temporarily closed by the buccopharyngeal membrane, is surrounded by five mesenchymal prominences. **B.** Frontal view of a slightly older embryo, showing rupture of the buccopharyngeal membrane and formation of the nasal placodes on the frontonasal prominence. **C.** Scanning electron micrograph of a human embryo similar to that shown in **B.**

FOURTH AND SIXTH PHARYNGEAL ARCHES

Cartilaginous components of the 4th and 6th pharyngeal arches fuse to form the **thyroid, cricoid, arytenoid, corniculate, and cuneiform cartilages** of the **larynx** (Fig. 16.9). **Muscles** of the 4th arch (**cricothyroid, levator palatini,** and **constrictors of the pharynx**) are innervated by the **superior laryngeal branch of the vagus,** the nerve of the 4th arch. Intrinsic muscles of the larynx, however, are supplied by the **recurrent laryngeal branch of the vagus,** the nerve of the 6th arch.

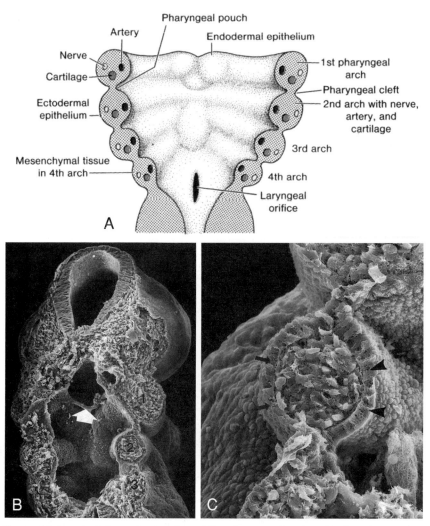

Figure 16.6. **A.** Schematic drawing of the pharyngeal arches. Each arch contains a cartilaginous component, a nerve, an artery, and a muscular component. **B.** Scanning electron micrograph of the pharyngeal region of a mouse embryo, showing the pharyngeal arches, pouches, and clefts. The first three arches (I, II, and III) are visible. A remnant of the buccopharyngeal membrane *(arrow)* is present at the entrance to the oral cavity. **C.** Higher magnification of the pharyngeal arches of a mouse embryo. Pharyngeal arches consist of a core of mesoderm lined by endoderm internally *(arrowheads)* and ectoderm externally *(arrows)*. Pouches and clefts occur between the arches where endoderm and ectoderm appose each other.

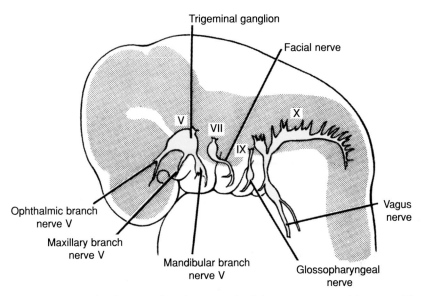

Figure 16.7. Each pharyngeal arch is supplied by its own cranial nerve. The trigeminal nerve supplying the 1st pharyngeal arch has three branches: the ophthalmic, maxillary, and mandibular branches. The nerve of the 2nd arch is the facial nerve; that of the 3rd, the glossopharyngeal nerve. The musculature of the 4th arch is supplied by the superior laryngeal branch of the vagus nerve, and that of the 6th arch, by the recurrent branch of the vagus nerve.

Pharyngeal Pouches

The human embryo has five pairs of pharyngeal pouches (Figs. 16.6 and 16.10). The last one of these is atypical and often considered as part of the 4th. Since the **epithelial endodermal lining** of the pouches gives rise to a number of important organs, the fate of each pouch is discussed separately.

FIRST PHARYNGEAL POUCH

The 1st pharyngeal pouch forms a stalk-like diverticulum, the **tubotympanic recess,** that comes in contact with the epithelial lining of the 1st pharyngeal cleft, the future **external auditory meatus** (Fig. 16.10, *A* and *B*). The distal portion of the diverticulum widens into a sac-like structure, the **primitive tympanic** or **middle ear cavity,** whereas the proximal part remains narrow, forming the **auditory (eustachian) tube.** The lining of the tympanic cavity later aids in formation of the **tympanic membrane** or **eardrum** (see Chapter 17).

SECOND PHARYNGEAL POUCH

The epithelial lining of the 2nd pharyngeal pouch proliferates and forms buds that penetrate into the surrounding mesenchyme. The buds are secondarily invaded by mesodermal tissue, thus forming the primordium of the **palatine tonsil** (Fig. 16.10, *A* and *B*). During the 3rd and 5th months, the tonsil is

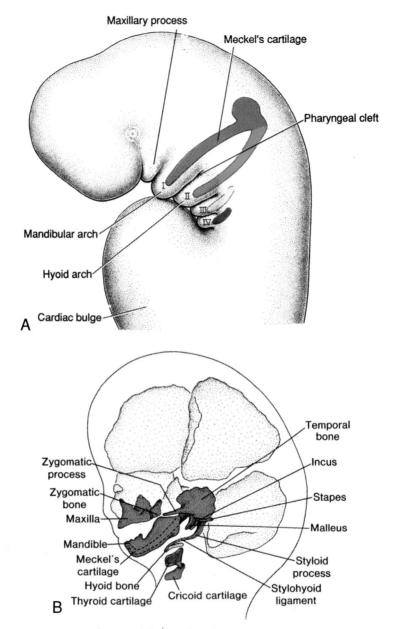

Figure 16.8. **A.** Lateral view of the head and neck region of a 4-week embryo to demonstrate the cartilages of the pharyngeal arches participating in formation of the bones of the face and neck. **B.** Drawing showing various components of the pharyngeal arches at a later stage of development. Some of the components ossify, while others disappear or become ligamentous. The maxillary process and Meckel's cartilage are replaced by the maxilla and mandible, respectively, which develop by membranous ossification.

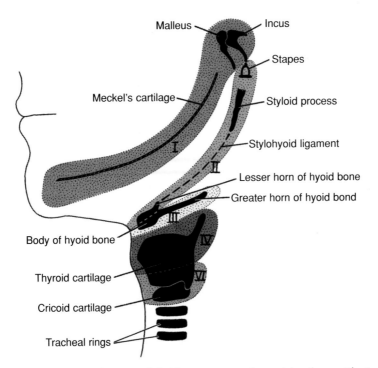

Figure 16.9. Drawing showing definitive structures formed by the cartilaginous components of the various pharyngeal arches.

infiltrated by lymphatic tissue. Part of the pouch remains and is found in the adult as the **tonsillar fossa.**

THIRD PHARYNGEAL POUCH

The 3rd and 4th pouches are characterized at their distal extremity by a dorsal and a ventral wing (Fig. 16.10). In the 5th week, epithelium of the dorsal wing of the 3rd pouch differentiates into the **inferior parathyroid gland,** while the ventral wing forms the **thymus** (Fig. 16.10, *A* and *B*). Both gland primordia lose their connection with the pharyngeal wall, and the thymus then migrates in a caudal and a medial direction, pulling the **inferior parathyroid** with it (Fig. 16.11). Although the main portion of the thymus moves rapidly to its final position in the thorax (where it fuses with its counterpart from the opposite side), its tail portion sometimes persists either embedded in the thyroid gland or as isolated thymic nests.

Growth and development of the thymus continue after birth until puberty. In the young child, the gland occupies considerable space in the thorax and lies behind the sternum and anterior to the pericardium and great vessels. In older persons, the gland is difficult to recognize, since it is atrophied and replaced by fatty tissue.

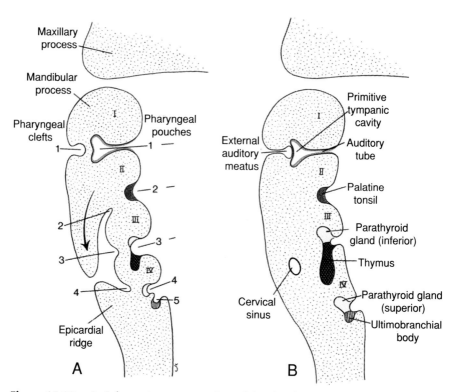

Figure 16.10. **A.** Schematic representation of the development of the pharyngeal clefts and pouches. Note that the 2nd arch grows over the 3rd and 4th arches, thereby burying the 2nd, 3rd, and 4th pharyngeal clefts. **B.** Remnants of the 2nd, 3rd, and 4th pharyngeal clefts form the cervical sinus, which is normally obliterated. Note the structures formed by the various pharyngeal pouches.

The parathyroid tissue of the 3rd pouch finally comes to rest on the dorsal surface of the thyroid gland and forms the **inferior parathyroid gland** (Fig. 16.11).

FOURTH PHARYNGEAL POUCH

Epithelium of the dorsal wing of this pouch forms the **superior parathyroid gland.** When the parathyroid gland loses contact with the wall of the pharynx, it attaches itself to the caudally migrating thyroid and, finally, is located on the dorsal surface of this gland as the **superior parathyroid gland** (Fig. 16.11).

FIFTH PHARYNGEAL POUCH

The 5th pharyngeal pouch is the last of the pharyngeal pouches to develop and is usually considered to be a part of the 4th pouch. It gives rise to the **ultimobranchial body,** which is later incorporated into the thyroid gland. Cells of the ultimobranchial body give rise to the **parafollicular** or **C cells** of the

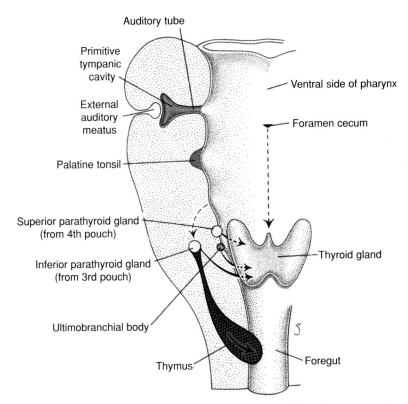

Auditory tube

Primitive
tympanic
cavity

External
auditory
meatus

Palatine tonsil

Superior parathyroid gland
(from 4th pouch)

Inferior parathyroid gland
(from 3rd pouch)

Ultimobranchial body

Thymus

Ventral side of pharynx

Foramen cecum

Thyroid gland

Foregut

Figure 16.11. Schematic representation of migration of the thymus, parathyroid glands, and ultimobranchial body. The thyroid gland originates in the midline at the level of the foramen cecum and descends to the level of the 1st tracheal rings.

thyroid gland. These cells secrete **calcitonin,** a hormone involved in regulation of the calcium level in the blood.

Pharyngeal Clefts

The 5-week embryo is characterized by the presence of four pharyngeal clefts (Fig. 16.6), of which only one contributes to the definitive structure of the embryo. The dorsal part of the 1st cleft penetrates the underlying mesenchyme and gives rise to the **external auditory meatus** (Figs. 16.10 and 16.11). The epithelial lining at the bottom of the meatus participates in formation of the **eardrum** (see Chapter 17).

Active proliferation of mesenchymal tissue in the 2nd arch causes it to overlap the 3rd and 4th arches. Finally, it merges with the **epicardial ridge** in the lower part of the neck (Fig. 16.10, *A* and *B*), and the 2nd, 3rd, and 4th clefts lose contact with the outside (Fig. 16.10*B*). Temporarily, the clefts form a cavity lined with ectodermal epithelium, the **cervical sinus,** but with further development this sinus disappears.

CLINICAL CORRELATES

Since glandular tissue derived from the pouches undergoes migration, it is not unusual for accessory glands or remnants of tissue to persist along the pathway. This is particularly true for thymic tissue, which may remain in the neck, and for the parathyroid glands. The inferior parathyroids are more variable in position than the superior ones and are sometimes located at the bifurcation of the common carotid artery.

Branchial fistulas occur when the 2nd pharyngeal arch fails to grow caudally over the 3rd and 4th arches, leaving remnants of the 2nd, 3rd, and 4th clefts in contact with the surface by a narrow canal (Fig. 16.12*A*). Such a fistula, found on the lateral aspect of the neck directly anterior to the **sternocleidomastoid muscle,** usually provides drainage for a **lateral cervical cyst** (Fig. 16.12*B*). These cysts are remnants of the cervical sinus and are most often located just below the angle of the jaw (Fig. 16.13). They may, however, be found anywhere along the anterior border of the sternocleidomastoid muscle. Frequently, a lateral cervical cyst is not visible at birth but becomes evident as the result of enlargement during childhood.

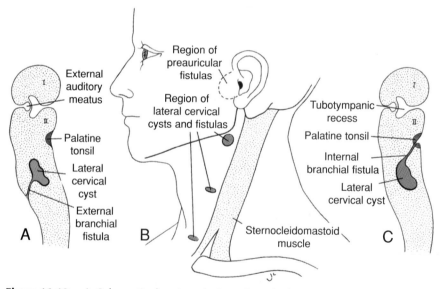

Figure 16.12. **A.** Schematic drawing of a lateral cervical cyst opening at the side of the neck by way of a fistula. **B.** Localization of lateral cervical cysts and fistulas in front of the sternocleidomastoid muscle. Note also the region of localization of preauricular fistulas. **C.** A lateral cervical cyst opening into the pharynx at the level of the palatine tonsil.

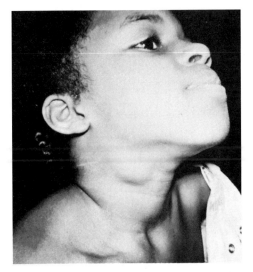

Figure 16.13. Photograph of a patient with a lateral cervical cyst. These cysts are always located on the lateral side of the neck in front of the sternocleidomastoid muscle. Frequently, they are located under the angle of the mandible and do not enlarge until later in life.

Internal branchial fistulas are rare and occur when the cervical sinus is connected to the lumen of the pharynx by a small canal, which usually opens in the tonsillar region (Fig. 16.12*C*). Such a fistula results from a rupture of the membrane between the 2nd pharyngeal cleft and pouch at some time during development.

Neural crest cells (Fig. 16.2) are essential for formation of much of the craniofacial region. Consequently, disruption of crest cell development results in severe craniofacial malformations. Since crest cells also contribute to **septation of the outflow tract of the heart** into pulmonary and aortic channels, many infants with craniofacial defects also suffer from cardiac abnormalities, including persistent truncus arteriosus and transposition of the great vessels. Unfortunately, crest cells appear to be a particularly vulnerable cell population and are easily killed by compounds such as alcohol and retinoic acid. One reason for this vulnerability may be that they are deficient in superoxide dismutase (SOD) and catalase enzymes that are responsible for scavenging free radicals that damage cells. Examples of craniofacial defects involving crest cells include:

① **Treacher Collins syndrome (mandibulofacial dysostosis)** is characterized by malar hypoplasia (due to underdevelopment of the zygomatic bones), mandibular hypoplasia, downslanting palpebral fissures, lower eyelid colobomas, and malformed external ears (Fig.

16.14*A*). The syndrome is inherited as an autosomal dominant trait, with 60% arising as new mutations. Phenocopies of the syndrome can be produced in laboratory animals following exposure to teratogenic doses of retinoic acid, however, suggesting that some cases in humans may be caused by teratogens.

② **Robin sequence** may occur independently or in association with other syndromes and malformations. Like Treacher Collins syndrome, Robin sequence alters 1st arch structures, with development of the mandible most severely affected. Infants usually have a triad of micrognathia, cleft palate, and glossoptosis (posteriorly placed tongue) (Fig. 16.14*B*). The defect may be due to genetic and/or environmental factors. It may also occur as a deformation, as, for example, when the chin is compressed against the chest in cases of oligohydramnios. The primary defect involves decreased growth of the mandible and, as a result, a posteriorly placed tongue that does not drop from between the palatal shelves, thereby preventing their fusion. The defect occurs in approximately 1 in 8500 births.

③ **DiGeorge sequence (3rd and 4th pharyngeal pouch syndrome)** includes hypoplasia or absence of the thymus (crest cells contribute the connective tissue stroma of the gland) and/or parathyroid glands with or without cardiovascular defects (persistent truncus arteriosus, interrupted aortic arch), abnormal external ears, micrognathia, and hypertelorism (widely spaced eyes) (Fig. 16.14*C*). Patients with complete DiGeorge sequence have immunologic problems, hypocalcemia, and a poor prognosis. The sequence occurs sporadically and may involve teratogens.

④ **Hemifacial microsomia (oculoauriculovertebral spectrum, Goldenhar syndrome)** includes a number of craniofacial abnormalities that usually involve the maxillary, temporal, and zygomatic bones, which are reduced in size and flattened. Ear (anotia, microtia), eye (tumors and dermoids in the eyeball), and vertebral (fused and hemivertebrae, spina bifida) defects are commonly observed in these patients (Fig. 16.14*D*). Asymmetry is present in 65% of the cases, which occur in 1 in 5600 births. Other malformations occur in 50% of cases, including cardiac abnormalities such as tetralogy of Fallot and ventricular septal defects. Causes for the disorder are unknown.

Tongue

The tongue appears in embryos of approximately 4 weeks in the form of two **lateral lingual swellings** and one **medial swelling,** the **tuberculum impar** (Fig. 16.15*A*). These three swellings originate from the 1st pharyngeal arch. A second median swelling, the **copula** or **hypobranchial eminence,** is formed by

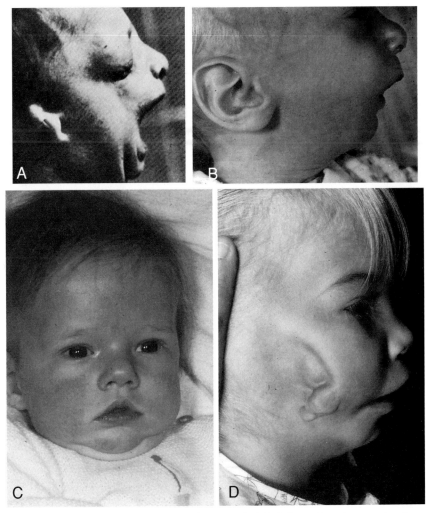

Figure 16.14. Series of patients with craniofacial defects thought to arise from insults to neural crest cells. **A.** Treacher Collins syndrome (mandibulofacial dysostosis). Note underdevelopment of the zygomatic bones, small mandible, and malformed ears. **B.** Robin sequence. Note the very small mandible (micrognathia). **C.** DiGeorge sequence. In addition to craniofacial defects, such as hypertelorism and microstomia, these individuals have partial or complete absence of the thymus. **D.** Hemifacial microsomia (oculoauriculovertebral spectrum, Goldenhar syndrome).

mesoderm of the 2nd, 3rd, and part of the 4th arch. Finally, a third median swelling, formed by the posterior part of the 4th arch, marks development of the epiglottis. Immediately behind this swelling is the **laryngeal orifice,** which is flanked by the **arytenoid swellings** (Fig. 16.15*A*).

As the lateral lingual swellings increase in size, they overgrow the tuberculum impar and merge with each other, thus forming the anterior two-thirds or body of

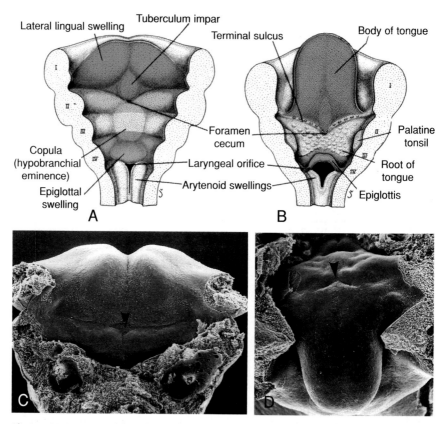

Figure 16.15. Ventral portion of the pharyngeal arches seen from above, to show development of the tongue. *I–IV* indicate the cut pharyngeal arches. **A.** 5 weeks (approximately 6 mm). **B.** 5 months. Note the foramen cecum, site of origin of the thyroid primordium. **C** and **D.** Scanning electron micrographs of similar stages of tongue development in human embryos. A depression marks the location of the foramen cecum *(arrowheads).*

the tongue (Fig. 16.15, *B* and *D*). Since the mucosa covering the body of the tongue originates from the 1st pharyngeal arch, **sensory innervation** to this area is by the **mandibular branch of the trigeminal nerve.** The anterior two-thirds or body of the tongue is separated from the posterior third by a V-shaped groove, the **terminal sulcus** (Fig. 16.15, *B* and *D*).

The posterior part or root of the tongue originates from the 2nd, 3rd, and part of the 4th pharyngeal arch. That **sensory innervation** to this part of the tongue is supplied by the **glossopharyngeal nerve** indicates that tissue of the 3rd arch overgrows that of the 2nd.

The epiglottis and the extreme posterior part of the tongue are innervated by the **superior laryngeal nerve,** reflecting their development from the 4th arch. Some of the tongue muscles probably differentiate in situ, but most are derived from myoblasts originating in **occipital somites.** Thus, tongue musculature is innervated by the **hypoglossal nerve.**

The general sensory innervation of the tongue is easy to understand. The anterior two-thirds are supplied by the trigeminal nerve, the nerve of the 1st arch; that of the posterior third is supplied by the glossopharyngeal and vagus nerves, the nerves of the 3rd and 4th arches, respectively. **Special sensory innervation (taste) to the anterior two-thirds of the tongue is provided by the chorda tympani branch of the facial nerve.**

CLINICAL CORRELATES

Ankyloglossia (tongue-tie) refers to the case where the tongue is not freed from the floor of the mouth. Normally, extensive cell degeneration occurs, and the frenulum is the only tissue persisting, tying the tongue to the floor of the mouth. In the most common form of ankyloglossia, the frenulum extends to the tip of the tongue.

Thyroid Gland

The thyroid gland appears as an epithelial proliferation in the floor of the pharynx between the tuberculum impar and the copula, at a point later indicated by the **foramen cecum** (Figs. 16.15 and 16.16*A*). Subsequently, the thyroid descends in front of the pharyngeal gut as a bilobed diverticulum (Fig. 16.16). During this migration, the gland remains connected to the tongue by a narrow canal, the **thyroglossal duct.** This duct later becomes solid and finally disappears.

With further development, the thyroid gland descends in front of the hyoid bone and the laryngeal cartilages. It reaches its final position in front of the trachea in the 7th week (Fig. 16.16*B*). By then, it has acquired a small median

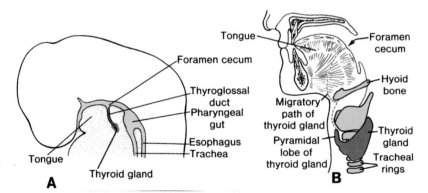

Figure 16.16. **A.** The thyroid primordium arises as an epithelial diverticulum in the midline of the pharynx immediately caudal to the tuberculum impar. **B.** Position of the thyroid gland in the adult. *Broken line* indicates the path of migration.

isthmus and two lateral lobes. The thyroid begins to function at approximately the end of the 3rd month, at which time the first follicles containing colloid become visible. **Follicular cells** produce the colloid that serves as a source of **thyroxine** and **triiodothyronine. Parafollicular** or **C cells** derived from the **ultimobranchial body** (Fig. 16.10) serve as a source of calcitonin.

CLINICAL CORRELATES

A **thyroglossal cyst** may be located at any point along the migratory pathway of the thyroid gland but is always located near or in the midline of the neck. As indicated by its name, it is a cystic remnant of the thyroglossal duct. Although approximately 50% of these cysts are located close to or just inferior to the body of the hyoid bone (Figs. 16.17 and 16.18), they may also be found at the base of the tongue or close to the thyroid cartilage. Sometimes, a thyroglossal cyst is connected to the outside by a fistulous canal, a **thyroglossal fistula.** Such a fistula usually arises secondarily after rupture of a cyst but may be present at birth.

Aberrant thyroid tissue may be found anywhere along the path of descent of the thyroid gland. It is commonly found in the base of the tongue, just behind the foramen cecum, and is subject to the same diseases as the gland itself.

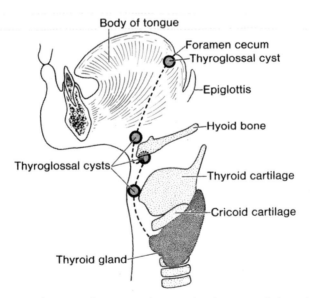

Figure 16.17. Schematic drawing indicating localization of thyroglossal cysts. These cysts, most frequently found in the hyoid region, are always located close to the midline.

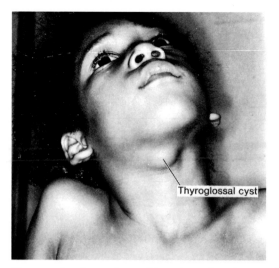

Figure 16.18. Photograph of a patient with a thyroglossal cyst. These cysts are remnants of the thyroglossal duct and may be located at any place along the migration pathway of the thyroid gland. They are frequently located behind the arch of the hyoid bone. An important diagnostic characteristic is their midline location.

Face

At the end of the 4th week, **facial prominences** consisting primarily of neural crest-derived mesenchyme and formed mainly by the first pair of pharyngeal arches appear. **Maxillary prominences** can be distinguished lateral to the stomodeum, and **mandibular prominences** can be distinguished caudal to this structure (Fig. 16.19). The **frontonasal prominence,** formed by proliferation of mesenchyme ventral to the brain vesicles, constitutes the upper border of the stomodeum. On both sides of the frontonasal prominence, local thickenings of the surface ectoderm, the **nasal (olfactory) placodes,** originate under inductive influence of the ventral portion of the forebrain (Fig. 16.19).

During the 5th week, the nasal placodes invaginate to form **nasal pits.** In so doing, they create a ridge of tissue that surrounds each pit and forms the **nasal prominences.** Those prominences on the outer edge of the pits are the **lateral nasal prominences;** those on the inner edge are the **medial nasal prominences** (Fig. 16.20).

During the following 2 weeks, the maxillary prominences continue to increase in size. Simultaneously, they grow in a medial direction, thereby compressing the medial nasal prominences toward the midline. Subsequently, the cleft between the medial nasal prominence and the maxillary prominence is lost, and the two fuse (Fig. 16.21). Hence, the upper lip is formed by the two medial nasal prominences and the two maxillary prominences. The lateral nasal prominences do not participate in formation of the upper lip. The lower lip and jaw are formed from the mandibular prominences that merge across the midline.

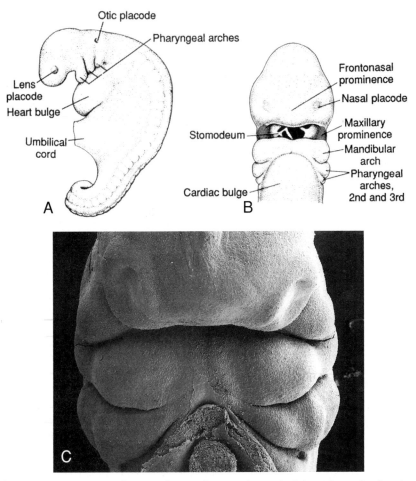

Figure 16.19. **A.** Lateral view of an embryo at the end of the 4th week, showing position of the pharyngeal arches. **B.** Frontal view of a 4½-week embryo. Note the location of the mandibular and maxillary prominences. The nasal placodes are visible on either side of the frontonasal prominence. **C.** Scanning electron micrograph of a human embryo at a stage similar to that of **B.**

Initially, the maxillary and lateral nasal prominences are separated by a deep furrow, the **nasolacrimal groove** (Figs. 16.20 and 16.21). Ectoderm in the floor of this groove forms a solid epithelial cord that detaches from the overlying ectoderm. After canalization, the cord forms the **nasolacrimal duct;** its upper end widens to form the **lacrimal sac.** Following detachment of the cord, the maxillary and lateral nasal prominences merge with each other. The nasolacrimal duct then runs from the medial corner of the eye to the inferior meatus of the nasal cavity. The maxillary prominences then enlarge to form the **cheeks** and **maxillae.**

The **nose** is formed from five facial prominences (Fig. 16.21): the frontal prominence gives rise to the bridge; the merged medial nasal prominences

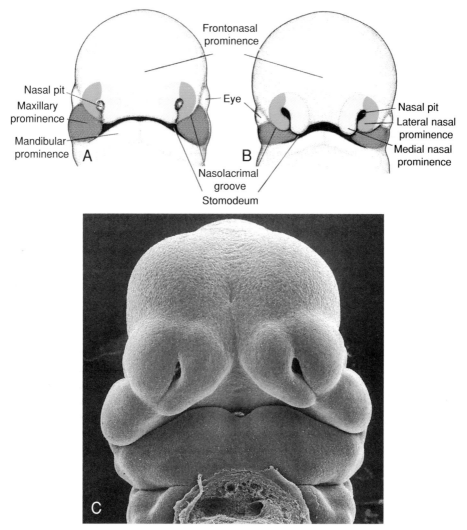

Figure 16.20. Frontal aspect of the face. **A.** Five-week embryo. **B.** Six-week embryo. The nasal prominences are gradually separated from the maxillary prominence by deep furrows. **C.** Scanning electron micrograph of a mouse embryo at a stage similar to that of **B.**

provide the crest and tip; and the lateral nasal prominences form the sides (alae) (Table 16.2).

Intermaxillary Segment

As a result of medial growth of the maxillary prominences, the two medial nasal prominences merge not only at the surface but also at a deeper level. The structure formed by the two merged prominences is known as the **intermaxillary**

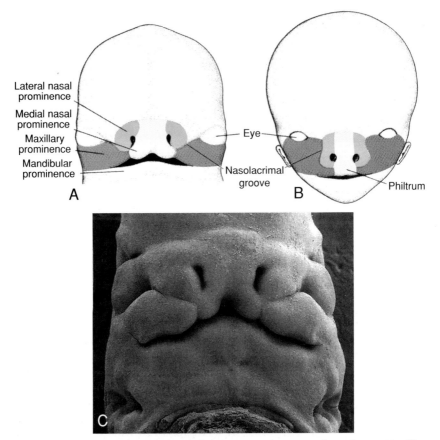

Labels (Figure A):
- Lateral nasal prominence
- Medial nasal prominence
- Maxillary prominence
- Mandibular prominence
- Eye
- Nasolacrimal groove
- Philtrum

A   B   C

Figure 16.21. Frontal aspects of the face. **A.** Seven-week embryo. Maxillary prominences have fused with the medial nasal prominences. **B.** Ten-week embryo. **C.** Scanning electron micrograph of a human embryo at a stage similar to that of **A.**

Table 16.2.
Structures Contributing to Formation of the Face

Prominence	Structures Formed
Frontonasal[a]	Forehead, bridge of nose, medial and lateral nasal prominences
Maxillary	Cheeks, lateral portion of upper lip
Medial nasal	Philtrum of upper lip, crest and tip of nose
Lateral nasal	Alae of nose
Mandibular	Lower Lip

[a] The frontonasal prominence represents a single unpaired structure, whereas the other prominences are paired.

segment. It is composed of *(a)* a **labial component,** which forms the philtrum of the upper lip; *(b)* an **upper jaw component,** which carries the four incisor teeth; and *(c)* a **palatal component,** which forms the triangular primary palate (Fig. 16.22). Cranially, the intermaxillary segment is continuous with the rostral portion of the **nasal septum,** which is formed by the frontal prominence.

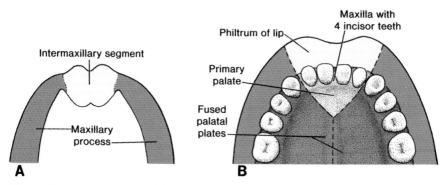

Figure 16.22. **A.** Drawing of the intermaxillary segment and maxillary processes. **B.** The intermaxillary segment gives rise to the philtrum of the upper lip, the median part of the maxillary bone and its four incisor teeth, and the triangular primary palate.

Secondary Palate

Although the primary palate is derived from the intermaxillary segment (Fig. 16.22), the main part of the definitive palate is formed by two shelf-like outgrowths from the maxillary prominences. These outgrowths, the **palatine shelves,** appear in the 6th week of development and are directed obliquely downward on each side of the tongue (Fig. 16.23). In the 7th week, however, the palatine shelves ascend to attain a horizontal position above the tongue and fuse with each other, thus forming the secondary palate (Figs. 16.24 and 16.25).

Anteriorly, the shelves fuse with the triangular primary palate, and the **incisive foramen** is the midline landmark between the primary and secondary palates (Fig. 16.24*B*). At the same time as the palatine shelves fuse, the nasal septum grows down and joins with the cephalic aspect of the newly formed palate (Fig. 16.25).

CLINICAL CORRELATES

Cleft lip and cleft palate are common defects that result in abnormal facial appearance and defective speech. The **incisive foramen** is considered the dividing landmark between the **anterior** and **posterior** cleft deformities. Those anterior to the incisive foramen include **lateral cleft lip, cleft upper jaw,** and **cleft** between the **primary and secondary palates** (Figs. 16.26, *B* and *D,* and 16.27, *A* and *B*). Such defects are due to a partial or complete lack of fusion of the maxillary prominence with the medial nasal prominence on one or both sides. Those that lie posterior to the incisive foramen include **cleft (secondary) palate** and **cleft uvula** (Figs. 16.26*E* and 16.27, *C* and *D*). Cleft palate results from a lack of fusion of the palatine shelves, which may be due to decreased size of the shelves, failure of the shelves to elevate, inhibition of the fusion process itself, or failure of the tongue to drop from between the shelves due to micrognathia. The third

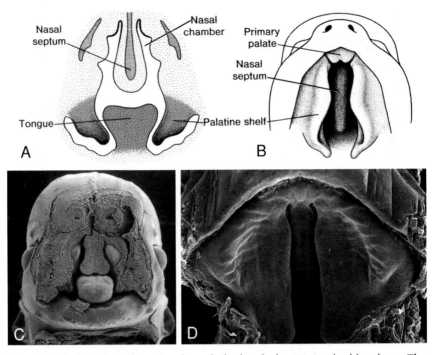

Figure 16.23.   A. Frontal section through the head of a 6½-week-old embryo. The palatine shelves are located in the vertical position on each side of the tongue. **B.** Ventral view of the palatine shelves after removal of the lower jaw and the tongue. Note the clefts between the primary triangular palate and the palatine shelves, which are still in a vertical position. **C.** Scanning electron micrograph of a mouse embryo at a stage similar to that of **A. D.** Palatal shelves at a stage slightly older than those in **B.** The shelves have elevated, but they are widely separated. The primary palate has fused with the secondary palatal shelves.

category is formed by a combination of clefts lying anterior as well as posterior to the incisive foramen (Fig. 16.26F). Anterior clefts may vary in severity from a barely visible defect in the vermilion of the lip to clefts extending into the nose (Fig. 16.27A). In more severe cases, the cleft extends to a deeper level, thereby forming a cleft of the upper jaw. The maxilla is then split between the lateral incisor and the canine tooth. Frequently, such a cleft extends to the incisive foramen (Fig. 16.26, C and D). Likewise, posterior clefts may vary in severity from clefts involving the entire secondary palate (Fig. 16.27D) to clefts of the uvula only.

Oblique facial clefts are produced by failure of the maxillary prominence to merge with its corresponding lateral nasal prominence. When this occurs, the nasolacrimal duct is usually exposed to the surface (Fig. 16.27E).

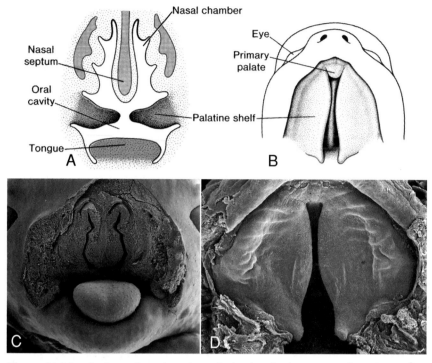

Figure 16.24. **A.** Frontal section through the head of a 7½-week embryo. The tongue has moved downward, and the palatine shelves have reached a horizontal position. **B.** Ventral view of the palatine shelves after removal of the lower jaw and tongue. The shelves are in a horizontal position. Note the nasal septum. **C.** Scanning electron micrograph of a mouse embryo at a stage similar to that of **A.** **D.** Palatal shelves at a stage similar to **B.**

Median cleft lip, a rare abnormality, is caused by incomplete merging of the two medial nasal prominences in the midline. This anomaly is usually accompanied by a deep groove between the right and left sides of the nose (Fig. 16.27*F*). Infants with midline clefts are often **mentally retarded** and may have brain abnormalities that include varying degrees of loss of midline structures **(holoprosencephaly).** Loss of midline tissue may be so extensive that fusion of the lateral ventricles occurs. These defects are induced very early in development at the beginning of neurulation (days 19–21) when the midline of the forebrain is being established.

Most cases of cleft lip and cleft palate are multifactorial in origin. Cleft lip (approximately 1:1000 births) occurs more frequently in males (80%) than females; its incidence is slightly higher with increasing maternal age; and it varies in different populations.

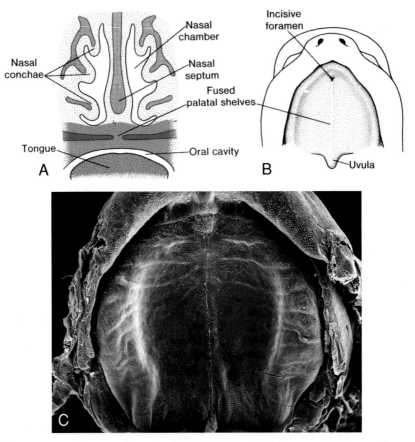

Figure 16.25. A. Frontal section through the head of a 10-week embryo. The two palatine shelves have fused with each other and with the nasal septum. **B.** Ventral view of the palate. The incisive foramen forms the midline landmark between the primary and secondary palate. **C.** Scanning electron micrograph of the palatal shelves of a mouse embryo at a stage similar to that of **B.**

If the parents are normal and have had one child with a cleft lip, the chance that the next baby will have the same defect is 4%. If two siblings are affected, the risk for the next child increases to 9%. If, however, one of the parents has a cleft lip, and they have one child with the same defect, the probability that the next baby will be affected rises to 17%.

The frequency of **cleft palate** is much lower than that of cleft lip (1:2500 births), occurs more often in females (67%) than males, and is not related to maternal age. If the parents are normal and have one child with a cleft palate, the probability of the next child being affected

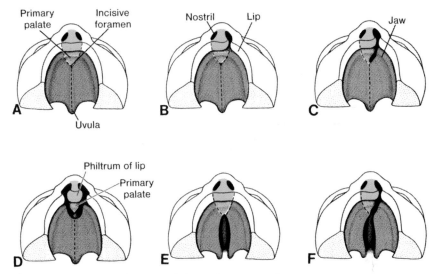

Figure 16.26. Ventral view of the palate, gum, lip, and nose. **A.** Normal. **B.** Unilateral cleft lip extending into the nose. **C.** Unilateral cleft involving the lip and jaw and extending to the incisive foramen. **D.** Bilateral cleft involving the lip and jaw. **E.** Isolated cleft palate. **F.** Cleft palate combined with unilateral anterior cleft.

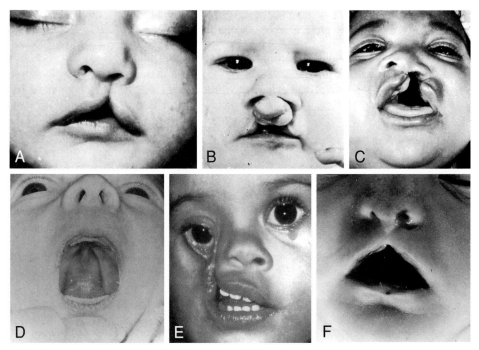

Figure 16.27. Photographs of incomplete cleft lip (**A**), bilateral cleft lip (**B**), cleft lip, cleft jaw, and cleft palate (**C**), isolated cleft palate (**D**), oblique facial cleft (**E**), and midline cleft lip (**F**).

is about 2%. If, however, there is a similarly affected relative or parent and child with a cleft palate, the probability increases to 7% and 15%, respectively. It has been shown that in females the palatal shelves fuse approximately 1 week later than in the male. This may explain why isolated cleft palate occurs more frequently in the female than in the male. Anticonvulsant drugs, such as **phenobarbital and diphenylhydantoin,** given during pregnancy increase the risk of cleft palate.

Nasal Cavities

During the 6th week, the nasal pits deepen considerably, partly because of growth of the surrounding nasal prominences and partly because of their penetration into the underlying mesenchyme (Fig. 16.28A). At first, the **oronasal membrane** separates the pits from the primitive oral cavity by way of the newly formed foramina, the **primitive choanae** (Fig. 16.28C). These choanae are located on each side of the midline and immediately behind the primary palate. Later, with formation of the secondary palate and further development of the

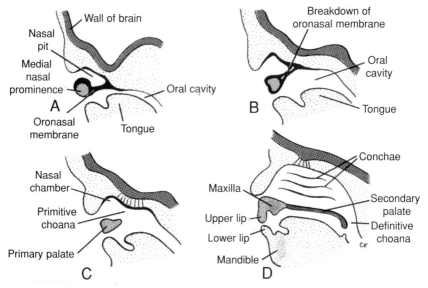

Figure 16.28. **A.** Drawing of a sagittal section through the nasal pit and lower rim of the medial nasal prominence of a 6-week embryo. The primitive nasal cavity is separated from the oral cavity by the oronasal membrane. **B.** Similar section as in **A,** showing the oronasal membrane breaking down. **C.** Drawing of a 7-week embryo with a primitive nasal cavity in open connection with the oral cavity. **D.** Sagittal section through the face of a 9-week embryo, showing separation of the definitive nasal and oral cavities by the primary and secondary palate. Definitive choanae are located at the junction of the oral cavity and the pharynx.

primitive nasal chambers (Fig. 16.28D), the **definitive choanae** are located at the junction of the nasal cavity and the pharynx.

Paranasal air sinuses develop as diverticula of the lateral nasal wall and extend into the maxilla, ethmoid, frontal, and sphenoid bones. They reach their maximum size during puberty and contribute to the definitive shape of the face.

Teeth

The shape of the face is determined not only by expansion of the paranasal sinuses but also by growth of the mandible and maxilla to accommodate the teeth. By the 6th week of development, the basal layer of the epithelial lining of the oral cavity forms a C-shaped structure, the **dental lamina,** along the length of the upper and lower jaws. This lamina subsequently gives rise to a number of **dental buds** (Fig. 16.29A), 10 in each jaw, which form the primordia of the ectodermal components of the teeth. Soon, the deep surface of the buds invaginates, resulting in the **cap stage of tooth development** (Fig. 16.29B). Such a cap consists of an outer layer, the **outer dental epithelium,** an inner layer, the **inner dental epithelium,** and a central core of loosely woven tissue, the **stellate reticulum.** The **mesenchyme,** which is of **neural crest** origin, located in the indentation, forms the **dental papilla** (Fig. 16.29B).

As the dental cap grows and the indentation deepens, the tooth takes on the appearance of a bell (**bell stage**) (Fig. 16.29C). Mesenchyme cells of the papilla

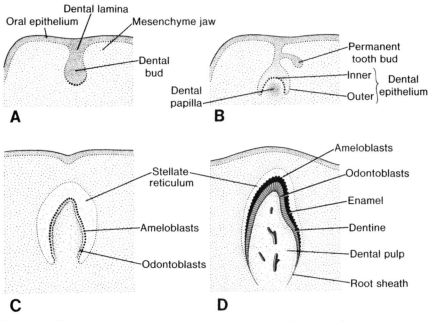

Figure 16.29. Schematic representation of formation of the tooth at successive stages of development. **A.** 8 weeks. **B.** 10 weeks. **C.** 3 months. **D.** 6 months.

adjacent to the inner dental layer then differentiate into **odontoblasts,** which later produce **dentin.** With thickening of the dentin layer, odontoblasts retreat into the dental papilla, thereby leaving a thin cytoplasmic process **(dental process)** behind in the dentin (Fig. 16.29*D*). The odontoblast layer persists throughout the life of the tooth and continuously provides predentin, which is subsequently transformed into **dentin.** The remaining cells of the dental papilla form the **pulp** of the tooth (Fig. 16. 29*D*).

In the meantime, epithelial cells of the outer dental epithelium differentiate into **ameloblasts (enamel formers).** These cells produce long enamel prisms that are deposited over the dentin (Fig. 16.29*D*). The contact layer between the enamel and dentin layers is known as the **enamel dentin junction.**

Enamel is first laid down at the apex of the tooth and from here spreads toward the neck. When the enamel thickens, the ameloblasts retreat into the stellate reticulum. Here they regress, temporarily leaving a thin membrane **(dental cuticle)** on the surface of the enamel. After eruption of the tooth, this membrane gradually sloughs off.

Formation of the root of the tooth begins when the dental epithelial layers penetrate into the underlying mesenchyme and form the **epithelial root sheath** (Fig. 16.29*D*). Cells of the dental papilla lay down a layer of dentin continuous with that of the crown (Fig. 16.30, *A* and *B*). As more and more dentin is deposited, the pulp chamber narrows and finally forms a canal containing blood vessels and nerves of the tooth.

Mesenchymal cells located on the outside of the tooth and in contact with dentin of the root differentiate into **cementoblasts** (Fig. 16.30*A*). These cells produce a thin layer of specialized bone, the **cementum.** Outside the cement layer, mesenchyme gives rise to the **periodontal ligament** (Fig. 16.30, *A* and *B*), which holds the tooth firmly in position and simultaneously functions as a shock absorber.

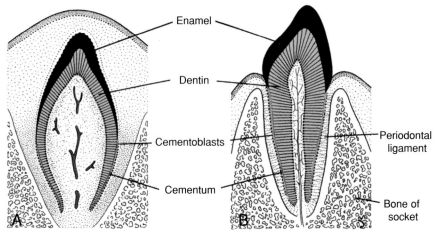

Figure 16.30. The tooth just before birth **(A)** and after eruption **(B).**

With further lengthening of the root, the crown is gradually pushed through the overlying tissue layers into the oral cavity (Fig. 16.30*B*). The eruption of **deciduous** or **milk teeth** occurs 6–24 months after birth.

Buds for the **permanent teeth** are located on the lingual aspect of the milk teeth and are formed during the 3rd month of development. These buds remain dormant until approximately the 6th year of postnatal life (Fig. 16.31). Then they begin to grow, thereby pushing against the underside of the corresponding milk teeth and aiding in their shedding. As a permanent tooth grows, the root of the overlying deciduous tooth is resorbed by osteoclasts.

CLINICAL CORRELATES

Natal teeth are those that have erupted by the time of birth. Usually, they involve the mandibular incisors that may be abnormally formed and have little enamel.

Teeth may be abnormal in number, shape, and size. They may be discolored by foreign substances, such as tetracyclines, or be deficient in enamel, a condition often caused by **vitamin D deficiency (rickets).** Many factors affect tooth development, including genetic and environmental influences.

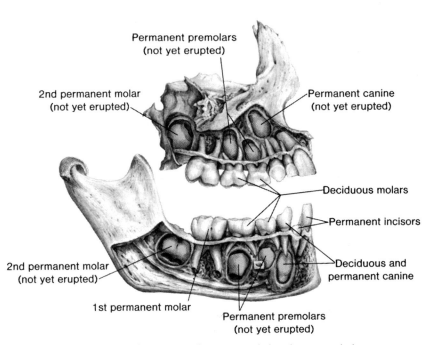

Figure 16.31. Drawing showing replacement of deciduous teeth by permanent teeth in a child of 8–9 years.

SUMMARY

Pharyngeal (branchial) arches, consisting of bars of mesenchymal tissue and separated from each other by pharyngeal pouches and clefts, initially give the head and neck their typical appearance (Fig. 16.3). Postnatally, the appearance of teeth and paranasal sinuses provides the face with its own personal characteristics.

Each arch contains its own artery (Fig. 16.4), nerve (Fig. 16.7), muscle element (Fig. 10.3), and cartilage bar or skeletal element (Figs. 16.8 and 16.9; see Table 16.1 for summary). Endoderm of the **pharyngeal pouches** gives rise to a number of endocrine glands and part of the middle ear. In subsequent order the pouches give rise to *(a)* the **middle ear cavity** and **auditory tube** (pouch 1), *(b)* the stroma of the **palatine tonsil** (pouch 2), *(c)* the **inferior parathyroid glands** and **thymus** (pouch 3), and *(d)* the **superior parathyroid glands** and **ultimobranchial body** (pouches 4 and 5) (Fig. 16.10).

Pharyngeal clefts give rise to only one structure: the **external auditory meatus.**

The **thyroid gland** originates from an epithelial proliferation in the floor of the tongue and descends to its level in front of the tracheal rings in the course of development.

The paired **maxillary** and **mandibular** prominences and the **frontonasal prominence** are the first prominences of the facial region. Later, medial and lateral nasal prominences form around the nasal placodes on the frontonasal prominence. All of these structures are important in that they determine, through fusion and specialized growth, the size and integrity of the mandible, upper lip, palate, and nose (Table 16.2). Formation of the upper lip occurs by fusion of the two maxillary prominences with the two medial nasal prominences (Figs. 16.20 and 16.21). The intermaxillary segment is formed by merging of the two medial nasal prominences in the midline. This segment is composed of *(a)* the **philtrum,** *(b)* the **upper jaw component,** which carries the four incisor teeth, and *(c)* the **palatal component,** which forms the triangular primary palate. The nose is derived from *(a)* the **frontonasal prominence,** which forms the **bridge,** *(b)* the **medial nasal prominences,** which provide the **crest and tip,** and *(c)* the **lateral nasal prominences,** which form the **alae** (Fig. 16.21). Fusion of the **palatal shelves,** which form from the **maxillary prominences,** creates the **hard (secondary)** and **soft palate.** A series of cleft deformities may result from partial or incomplete fusion of these mesenchymal tissues, which may be caused by hereditary factors and drugs (diphenylhydantoin).

The adult form of the face is influenced by development of **paranasal sinuses, nasal conchae,** and **teeth.** Teeth develop from ectodermal and mesodermal components. **Enamel** is made by **ameloblasts** (Figs. 16.29 and 16.30). It lies on a thick layer of **dentin** produced by **odontoblasts,** a neural crest derivative. **Cementum** is formed by **cementoblasts,** another mesenchymal derivative found in the root of the tooth. Although the first teeth (**deciduous** or **milk teeth**) appear 6–24 months after birth, the definitive or **permanent teeth,** which appear postnatally, are formed during the 3rd month of development (Fig. 16.31).

PROBLEMS TO SOLVE

1. Why are neural crest cells considered such an important cell population for craniofacial development?

2. You are called as a consultant for a child with a very small mandible and ears that are represented by small protuberances, bilaterally. The baby has had numerous episodes of pneumonia and is small for its age. What might your diagnosis be, and what might have caused these abnormalities?

3. A child is born with a median cleft lip. Should you be concerned about any other abnormalities?

4. A child presents with a midline swelling beneath the arch of the hyoid bone. What might this swelling be, and what is its basis embryologically?

SUGGESTED READINGS

Ballabio M, Nicolini U, Jowett T, et al: Maturation of thyroid function in normal human fetuses. *Clin Endocrinol* 31:565, 1989.

Bockman DE, Kirby ML: Neural crest interactions in the development of the immune system. *J Immunol* 135:766, 1985.

Burdi AR: Sexual differences in closure of the human palatal shelves. *Cleft Palate J* 6:1, 1969.

Couly GF, Coltey PM, LeDouarin NM: The triple origin of skull in higher vertebrates: a study of quail-chick chimeras. *Development* 117:409, 1993.

Ferguson MWJ: Palate development. *Dev Suppl* 103:41, 1988.

Fraser FC: Genetics and congenital malformations. *In* Steinberg AG (ed): *Progress in Medical Genetics.* New York, Grune & Stratton, 1961:38.

Freidberg J: Pharyngeal cleft sinuses and cysts, and other benign neck lesions. *Pediatr Clin North Am* 36:1451, 1989.

Gorlin RJ, Cervenka J, Pruzansky S: Facial clefting and its syndromes. *Birth Defects* 8:3, 1971.

Gorlin RJ, Cohen MM, Levin LS (eds): *Syndromes of the Head and Neck.* New York, Oxford University Press, 1990.

Kirby M: Plasticity and predetermination of mesencephalic and trunk neural crest transplanted into the region of the cardiac neural crest. *Dev Biol* 134:402, 1989.

Lobach DF, Haynes BF: Ontogeny of the human thymus during fetal development. *J Clin Immunol* 7:81, 1987.

Merida-Velasco JA, Garcia-Garcia JD, Espin-Ferra J, Linares J: Origin of the ultimobranchial body and its colonizing cells in human embryos. *Acta Anat* 136:325, 1989.

Noden DM: Interactions and fates of avian craniofacial mesenchyme. *Development* 103:121, 1988.

Nichols DH: Mesenchyme formation from the trigeminal placodes of the mouse embryo. *Am J Anat* 176:19–31, 1986.

Poswillo D: The aetiology and pathogenesis of craniofacial deformity. *Dev Suppl* 103:207, 1988.

Shepard TH: Development of the thyroid gland. *In* Gardner LI (ed): *Endocrine and Genetic Diseases of Childhood and Adolescence.* 2nd ed. Philadelphia, WB Saunders, 1975.

Sperber GH, Honoré LH, Machin GA: Microscopic study of holoprosencephalic facial anomalies in trisomy 13 fetuses. *Am J Med Genet* 32:443, 1989.

Sulik KK, Cook CS, Webster WS: Teratogens and craniofacial malformations: relationships to cell death. *Dev Suppl* 103:213, 1988.

Sulik KK, Johnston MC, Daft PA, et al: Fetal alcohol syndrome and DiGeorge anomaly: critical ethanol exposure periods for craniofacial malformation as illustrated in an animal model. *Am J Med Genet* 2(suppl):97, 1986.

Sulik KK, Johnston MC, Smiley SJ, et al: Mandibulofacial dysostosis (Treacher Collins syndrome): a new proposal for pathogenesis. *Am J Med Genet* 27:359, 1987.

Sulik KK, Schoenwokf GC: Highlights of craniofacial morphogenesis in mammalian embryos, as revealed by scanning electron microscopy. *Scanning Electron Microsc* 4:1735, 1985.

Webster WS, Johnston MC, Lammer EJ, Sulik KK: Isotretinoin embryopathy and the cranial neural crest: an in vivo and in vitro study. *J Craniofac Genet Dev Biol* 6:211, 1986.

Webster WS, Lipson AH, Sulik KK: Interference with gastrulation during the third week of pregnancy as a cause of some facial abnormalities and CNS defects. *Am J Med Genet* 31:505, 1988.

chapter 17

Ear

In the adult, the ear forms one anatomical unit serving both hearing and equilibrium. In the embryo, however, it develops from three distinctly different parts: *(a)* the **external ear,** which serves as the sound-collecting organ; *(b)* the **middle ear,** which functions as a sound conductor from the external to the internal ear; and *(c)* the **internal ear,** which converts sound waves into nerve impulses and registers changes in equilibrium.

Internal Ear

OTIC VESICLE

The first indication of the developing ear can be found in embryos of approximately 22 days as a thickening of the surface ectoderm on each side of the rhombencephalon (Fig. 17.1, *A* and *B*). These thickenings, the **otic placodes,** invaginate rapidly and form the **otic** or **auditory vesicles (otocysts)** (Fig. 17.2). During later development, each vesicle divides into *(a)* a ventral component that gives rise to the **saccule** and **cochlear duct** and *(b)* a dorsal component that forms the **utricle, semicircular canals,** and **endolymphatic duct** (Figs. 17.3–17.6). The epithelial structures so formed are known collectively as the **membranous labyrinth.**

SACCULE, COCHLEA, AND ORGAN OF CORTI

In the 6th week of development, the saccule forms a tubular-shaped outpocketing at its lower pole (Fig. 17.3, *C–E* and *G*). This outgrowth, the **cochlear duct,** penetrates the surrounding mesenchyme in a spiral fashion until, at the end of the 8th week, it has completed 2.5 turns (Fig. 17.3, *D* and *E*). Its connection with the remaining portion of the saccule is then confined to a narrow pathway, the **ductus reuniens** (Fig. 17.3*E*).

Mesenchyme surrounding the cochlear duct soon differentiates into cartilage (Fig. 17.4*A*). In the 10th week, this cartilaginous shell undergoes vacuolization, and two perilymphatic spaces, the **scala vestibuli** and **scala tympani,** are formed (Fig. 17.4, *B* and *C*). The cochlear duct is then separated from the scala vestibuli by the **vestibular membrane** and from the scala tympani by the **basilar membrane** (Fig. 17.4*C*). The lateral wall of the cochlear duct remains attached to the surrounding cartilage by the **spiral ligament,** whereas its median angle is connected to, and partly supported by, a long cartilaginous process, the **modiolus,** the future axis of the bony cochlea (Fig. 17.4*B*).

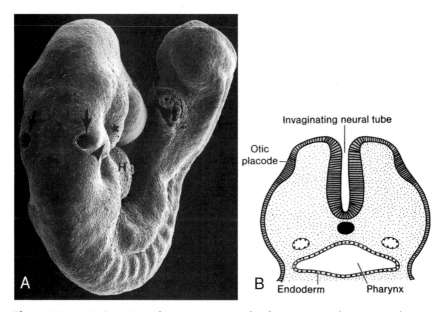

Figure 17.1. **A.** Scanning electron micrograph of a mouse embryo equivalent to approximately 28 days of human development. The otic placodes, as shown in **B,** are invaginating to form the otic pits *(arrows)*. *Arrowhead,* 2nd arch; *H,* heart; and *star,* mandibular prominence. **B.** Schematic section through the region of the rhombencephalon to show the otic placodes in a 22-day embryo.

Initially, epithelial cells of the cochlear duct are alike (Fig. 17.4*A*). With further development, however, they form two ridges: the **inner ridge,** the future **spiral limbus,** and the **outer ridge** (Fig. 17.4*B*). The latter forms one row of inner and three or four rows of outer **hair cells,** the sensory cells of the auditory system (Fig. 17.5). They are covered by the **tectorial membrane,** a fibrillar gelatinous substance that is attached to the spiral limbus and rests with its tip on the hair cells (Fig. 17.5). The sensory cells and tectorial membrane together are known as the **organ of Corti.** Impulses received by this organ are transmitted to the spiral ganglion and then to the nervous system by the **auditory fibers of cranial nerve VIII** (Figs. 17.4 and 17.5).

UTRICLE AND SEMICIRCULAR CANALS

During the 6th week of development, **semicircular canals** appear as flattened outpocketings of the utricular part of the otic vesicle (Fig. 17.6, *A* and *B*). Central portions of the walls of these outpocketings eventually become apposed to each other (Fig. 17.6, *C* and *D*) and disappear, thus giving rise to three semicircular canals (Fig. 17.6, *E* and *F*). Whereas one end of each canal dilates to form the **crus ampullare,** the other does not widen and is known as the **crus nonampullare** (Fig. 17.6*E*). Since two of the latter type fuse, however, only five crura enter the utricle, three with an ampulla and two without.

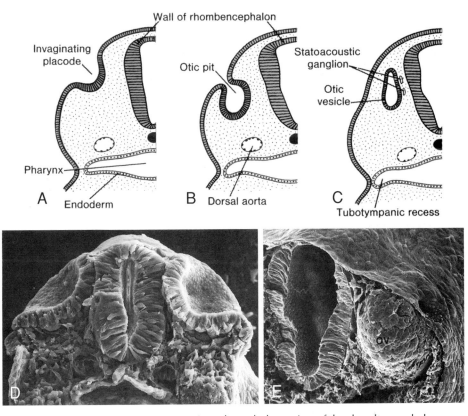

Figure 17.2. **A–C.** Transverse sections through the region of the rhombencephalon, showing formation of the otic vesicles: **A,** 24 days; **B,** 27 days; and **C,** 4.5 weeks. Note the appearance of the statoacoustic ganglia. **D** and **E.** Scanning electron micrographs of mouse embryos equivalent to stages depicted in **A** and **B** showing development of the otic vesicles *(OV)*.

Cells in the ampullae form a crest, the **crista ampullaris,** containing sensory cells for maintenance of equilibrium. Similar sensory areas develop in the walls of the utricle and saccule, where they are known as **maculae acusticae.** Impulses generated in sensory cells of the cristae and maculae as a result of a change in position of the body are carried to the brain by **vestibular fibers of cranial nerve VIII.**

During formation of the otic vesicle, a small group of cells breaks away from its wall and forms the **statoacoustic ganglion** (Fig. 17.2*C*). Other cells of this ganglion are derived from the neural crest. The ganglion subsequently splits into **cochlear** and **vestibular** portions, which supply sensory cells of the organ of Corti and those of the saccule, utricle, and semicircular canals, respectively (Fig. 17.2).

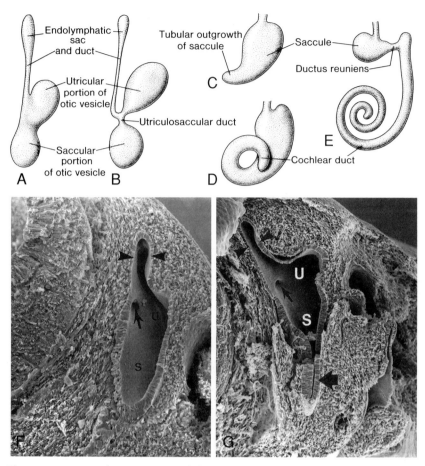

Figure 17.3. **A** and **B.** Drawings of development of the otocyst, showing a dorsal utricular portion with the endolymphatic duct and a ventral saccular portion. **C–E.** Drawings of the cochlear duct at 6, 7, and 8 weeks, respectively. Note formation of the ductus reuniens and the utriculosaccular duct. **F** and **G.** Scanning electron micrographs of mouse embryos, showing similar stages of development of the otocyst as depicted in **A** and **B.** *Arrowheads,* endolymphatic duct; *S,* saccule; *small arrow,* opening of a semicircular canal; and *U,* utricle. **G** also shows initial stages of cochlear duct formation *(large arrow).*

Middle Ear

TYMPANIC CAVITY AND EUSTACHIAN TUBE

The **tympanic cavity** is of endodermal origin. It is derived from the 1st pharyngeal pouch (Figs. 17.2 and 17.7). This pouch grows rapidly in a lateral direction and comes in contact with the floor of the 1st pharyngeal cleft. The distal part of the pouch, the **tubotympanic recess,** widens and gives rise to the primitive tympanic cavity, while the proximal part remains narrow and forms the

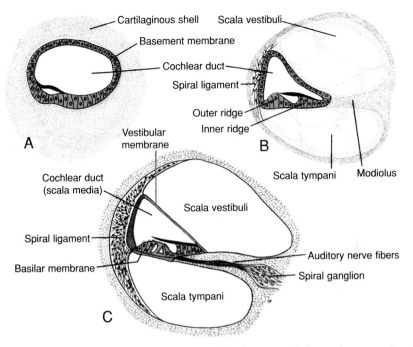

Figure 17.4. Schematic representation of development of the scala tympani and scala vestibuli. **A.** The cochlear duct is surrounded by a cartilaginous shell. **B.** During the 10th week, large vacuoles appear in the cartilaginous shell. **C.** The cochlear duct (scala media) is separated from the scala tympani and the scala vestibuli by the basilar and vestibular membranes, respectively. Note the auditory nerve fibers and the spiral (cochlear) ganglion.

auditory or eustachian tube (Fig. 17.7*B*). The latter is the channel through which the tympanic cavity communicates with the nasopharynx.

OSSICLES

The **malleus** and **incus** are derived from cartilage of the 1st pharyngeal arch, and the **stapes** is derived from that of the 2nd arch (Fig. 17.8*A*). Although the ossicles appear during the first half of fetal life, they remain embedded in mesenchyme until the 8th month (Fig. 17.7*B*), then the surrounding tissue dissolves (Fig. 17.8*B*). The endodermal epithelial lining of the primitive tympanic cavity then extends along the wall of the newly developing space. The tympanic cavity is now at least twice as large as before. When the ossicles are entirely free of surrounding mesenchyme, the endodermal epithelium connects them in a mesentery-like fashion to the wall of the cavity (Fig. 17.8*B*). The supporting ligaments of the ossicles develop later within these mesenteries.

Since the malleus is derived from the 1st pharyngeal arch, its muscle, the **tensor tympani,** is innervated by the **mandibular branch of the trigeminal nerve.** Similarly, the **stapedius muscle,** which is attached to the stapes, is innervated by the **facial nerve,** the nerve to the 2nd pharyngeal arch.

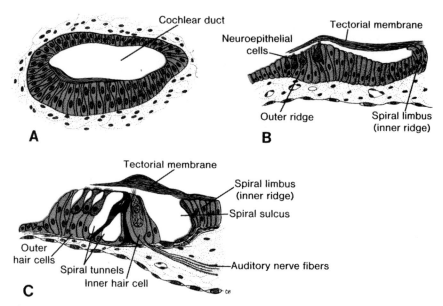

Figure 17.5. Drawings of development of the organ of Corti. **A.** 10 weeks. **B.** Approximately 5 months. **C.** In the full-term infant. Note the appearance of the spiral tunnels in the organ of Corti.

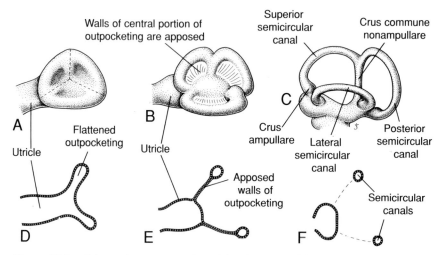

Figure 17.6. Schematic representation of development of the semicircular canals. **A.** 5 weeks. **C.** 6 weeks. **E.** 8 weeks. **B, D,** and **F.** Diagrammatic illustrations of the apposition, fusion, and disappearance, respectively, of the central portions of the walls of the semicircular outpocketings. Note the ampullae in the semicircular canals.

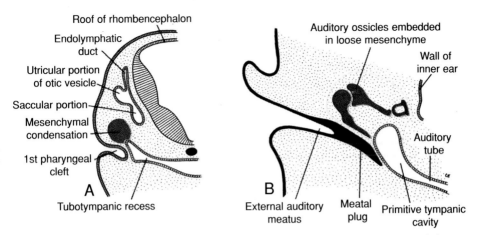

Figure 17.7. A. Transverse section of a 7-week embryo in the region of the rhombencephalon, showing the tubotympanic recess, the 1st pharyngeal cleft, and mesenchymal condensation, foreshadowing development of the ossicles. **B.** Schematic representation of the middle ear, showing the cartilaginous precursors of the auditory ossicles. *Thin yellow line* in mesenchyme indicates future expansion of the primitive tympanic cavity. Note the meatal plug extending from the primitive auditory meatus to the tympanic cavity.

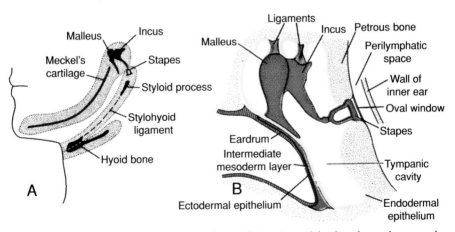

Figure 17.8. A. Schematic representation of derivatives of the first three pharyngeal arches. Note the malleus and incus at the dorsal tip of the 1st arch and the stapes at that of the 2nd arch. **B.** Schematic representation of the middle ear, showing the handle of the malleus in contact with the eardrum. The stapes will establish contact with the membrane in the oval window. The wall of the tympanic cavity is lined with epithelium of endodermal origin.

During late fetal life, the tympanic cavity expands dorsally by vacuolization of surrounding tissue to form the **tympanic antrum.** After birth, bone of the developing **mastoid process** is also invaded by epithelium of the tympanic cavity, and epithelial lined air sacs are formed **(pneumatization).** Later, most of the mastoid air sacs come in contact with the antrum and tympanic cavity. Expansion of inflammations of the middle ear into the antrum and mastoid air cells is a rather common complication of middle ear infections.

External Ear

EXTERNAL AUDITORY MEATUS

The **external auditory meatus** develops from the dorsal portion of the 1st pharyngeal cleft (Fig. 17.7A). At the beginning of the 3rd month, epithelial cells at the bottom of the meatus proliferate, thereby forming a solid epithelial plate, the meatal plug (Fig. 17.7B). In the 7th month, this plug dissolves, and the epithelial lining of the floor of the meatus then participates in formation of the definitive eardrum. Occasionally, the meatal plug persists until birth, resulting in congenital deafness.

EARDRUM OR TYMPANIC MEMBRANE

The eardrum is made up of (a) ectodermal epithelial lining at the bottom of the auditory meatus, (b) endodermal epithelial lining of the tympanic cavity, and (c) an intermediate layer of connective tissue (Fig. 17.8B) that forms the fibrous stratum. The major part of the eardrum is firmly attached to the handle of the malleus (Fig. 17.8B), while the remaining portion forms the separation between the external auditory meatus and the tympanic cavity.

AURICLE

The **auricle** develops from six mesenchymal proliferations located at the dorsal ends of the **1st** and **2nd pharyngeal arches,** surrounding the 1st pharyngeal cleft (Fig. 17.9A). These swellings **(auricular hillocks),** three on each side of the external meatus, later fuse and form the definitive auricle. As fusion of the auricular hillocks is rather complicated, developmental abnormalities of the auricle are common. Initially, the external ears are located in the lower neck region, but with development of the mandible, they ascend to the side of the head at the level of the eyes.

CLINICAL CORRELATES

Congenital deafness, usually associated with deaf-mutism, may be caused by abnormal development of the membranous and bony labyrinths, as well as by malformations of the auditory ossicles and eardrum. In the most extreme cases, the tympanic cavity and external meatus are absent.

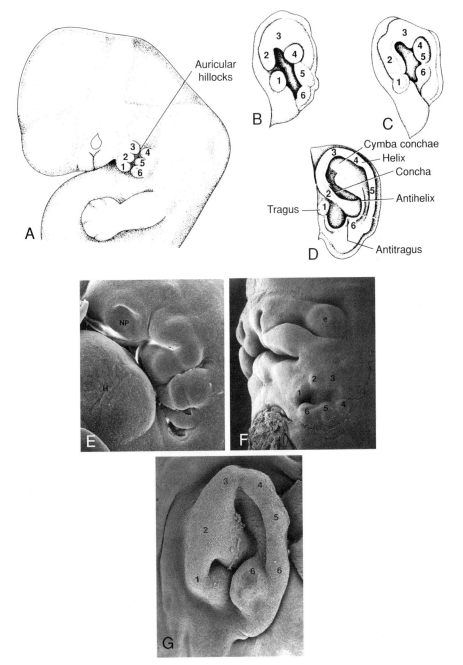

Figure 17.9. **A.** Lateral view of the head of an embryo, showing the six auricular hillocks surrounding the dorsal end of the 1st pharyngeal cleft. **B–D** illustrate fusion and progressive development of the hillocks into the adult auricle. **E–G.** Scanning electron micrographs showing development of human embryos: **E,** the six auricular hillocks from the 1st and 2nd pharyngeal arches; **F,** the hillocks becoming more defined; and **G,** the external ear nearly completed. Note the position of the ears with respect to the mouth and eyes *(e)* in **F.** Growth of the mandible and neck region places the ears in their permanent position. *H,* heart; and *NP,* nasal placode.

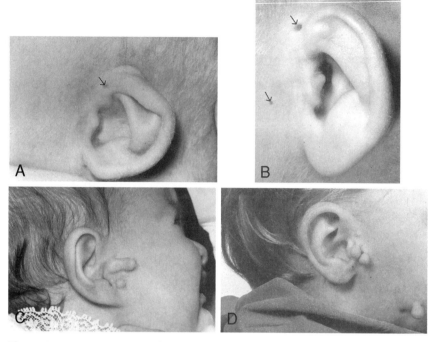

Figure 17.10. **A.** Microtia with preauricular pit *(arrow).* **B.** Preauricular pits *(arrows).*
C and **D.** Preauricular appendages (skin tags). Note the low position of the tag in **D.**

Most forms of congenital deafness are caused by genetic factors, but environmental factors may also interfere with normal development of the internal and middle ear. Rubella virus, affecting the embryo in the 7th or 8th week, may cause severe damage to the organ of Corti. It has also been suggested that poliomyelitis, erythroblastosis fetalis, diabetes, hypothyroidism, and toxoplasmosis cause congenital deafness.

External ear defects are common and include minor and severe abnormalities (Fig. 17.10). They are significant from the standpoint of the psychological and emotional trauma they may cause and for the fact they are often associated with other malformations. Thus, they serve as clues to examine infants carefully for other abnormalities. In this regard, **all of the frequently occurring chromosomal syndromes and most of the less common ones have ear anomalies as one of their characteristics.**

Preauricular appendages and pits (Fig. 17.10) are skin tags and shallow depressions, respectively, that occur anterior to the ear. Pits may represent abnormal development of the auricular hillocks, whereas appendages may be due to accessory hillocks. Like other external ear defects, both are associated with other malformations.

SUMMARY

The ear consists of three parts that have different origins but function as one unit. The **internal ear** originates from the **otic vesicle,** which in the 4th week of development detaches from surface ectoderm. This vesicle divides into a ventral component, which gives rise to the **saccule** and **cochlear duct,** and a dorsal component, which gives rise to the **utricle, semicircular canals,** and **endolymphatic duct** (Figs. 17.3–17.6). The epithelial structures thus formed are known collectively as the **membranous labyrinth.** Except for the **cochlear duct** that forms the **organ of Corti,** all structures derived from the membranous labyrinth are involved with equilibrium.

The **middle ear,** consisting of the **tympanic cavity** and **auditory tube,** is lined with epithelium of endodermal origin and is derived from the 1st pharyngeal pouch. The auditory tube extends between the tympanic cavity and nasopharynx. The **ossicles,** which transfer sound vibrations from the tympanic membrane to the oval window, are derived from the 1st (**malleus** and **incus**) and 2nd (**stapes**) pharyngeal arches.

The **external auditory meatus** develops from the 1st pharyngeal cleft and is separated from the tympanic cavity by the tympanic membrane (eardrum). The eardrum consists of *(a)* an ectodermal epithelial lining, *(b)* an intermediate layer of mesenchyme, and *(c)* an endodermal lining from the 1st pharyngeal pouch.

The **auricle** develops from six mesenchymal hillocks (Fig. 17.9) located along the 1st and 2nd pharyngeal arches. Defects in the auricle are often associated with other congenital malformations.

PROBLEMS TO SOLVE

1. A newborn has bilateral microtia. Should you be concerned about the presence of other malformations? What cell population might be involved in the embryological origin of the defect?

SUGGESTED READINGS

Ars B: Organogenesis of the middle ear structures. *J Laryngol Otol* 103:16, 1989.
McPhee JR, Van De Water TR: Epithelial mesenchymal tissue interactions guiding otic capsule formation: the role of the otocyst. *J Embryol Exp Morphol* 97:1, 1986.
Michaels L: Evolution of the epidermoid formation and its role in the development of the middle ear and tympanic membrane during the first trimester. *J Otolaryngol* 17:22, 1988.
Michaels L, Soucek S: Auditory epithelial migration on the human tympanic membrane. II. The existence of two discrete migratory pathways and their embryological correlates. *Am J Anat* 189:189, 1990.
O'Rahilly R: The early development of the otic vesicle in staged human embryos. *J Embryol Exp Morphol* 11:741, 1963.

chapter 18

Eye

Optic Cup and Lens Vesicle

The developing eye appears in the 22-day embryo as a pair of shallow grooves on each side of the forebrain (Fig. 18.1). With closure of the neural tube, these grooves form outpocketings of the forebrain, the optic vesicles. These vesicles subsequently come in contact with the surface ectoderm and induce changes in the ectoderm necessary for lens formation (Fig. 18.1). Shortly thereafter, the optic vesicle begins to invaginate and forms the double-walled optic cup (Figs. 18.1 and 18.2A). The inner and outer layers of this cup are initially separated by a lumen, the intraretinal space (Figs. 18.2B and 18.4A), but soon this lumen disappears, and the two layers are then opposed to each other (Fig. 18.4). Invagination is not restricted to the central portion of the cup but also involves a part of the inferior surface (Fig. 18.2A) that forms the choroid fissure. Formation of this fissure allows the hyaloid artery to reach the inner chamber of the eye (Figs. 18.3, 18.4, and 18.8). During the 7th week, the lips of the choroid fissure fuse, and the mouth of the optic cup then becomes a round opening, the future pupil.

While these events are occurring, cells of the surface ectoderm, initially in contact with the optic vesicle, begin to elongate and form the lens placode (Fig. 18.1). This placode subsequently invaginates and develops into the lens vesicle. During the 5th week, the lens vesicle loses contact with the surface ectoderm and is then located in the mouth of the optic cup (Figs. 18.2C, 18.3, and 18.4)

Retina, Iris, and Ciliary Body

The outer layer of the optic cup is characterized by the appearance of small pigment granules and is known as the pigment layer of the retina (Figs. 18.3, 18.4, and 18.7).

Development of the inner layer of the optic cup is more complicated. The posterior four-fifths, known as the **pars optica retinae,** contains cells bordering the intraretinal space that differentiate into light-receptive elements, **rods** and **cones** (Fig. 18.5). Adjacent to this photoreceptive layer is the mantle layer, which, as in the brain, gives rise to neurons and supporting cells. In the adult, the **outer nuclear layer,** the **inner nuclear layer,** and the **ganglion cell layer** can be distinguished (Fig. 18.5). On the surface is a fibrous layer that contains axons of nerve cells of the deeper layers. Nerve fibers in this zone converge toward the

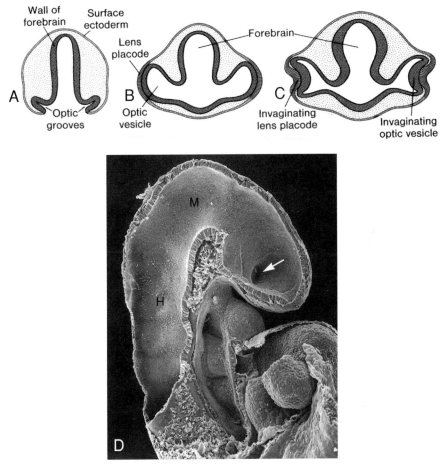

Figure 18.1. **A.** Transverse section through the forebrain of a 22-day embryo (approximately 14 somites), showing the optic grooves. **B.** Transverse section through the forebrain of a 4-week embryo, showing the optic vesicles in contact with the surface ectoderm. Note the slight thickening of the ectoderm (lens placode). **C.** Transverse section through the forebrain of a 5-mm embryo, showing invagination of the optic vesicle and the lens placode. **D.** Scanning electron micrograph of a mouse embryo during optic vesicle formation. The embryo has been cut sagittally to reveal the inside of the brain vesicles and outpocketing of the optic vesicle *(arrow)* from the forebrain. *H,* hindbrain; and *M,* midbrain.

optic stalk, which develops into the optic nerve (Figs. 18.3 and 18.7). Hence, light impulses pass through most layers of the retina before they reach the rods and cones.

The anterior one-fifth of the inner layer, known as the **pars ceca retinae,** remains one cell layer thick. It is later divided into the **pars iridica retinae,** which forms the inner layer of the iris, and the **pars ciliaris retinae,** which participates in formation of the **ciliary body** (Fig. 18.6).

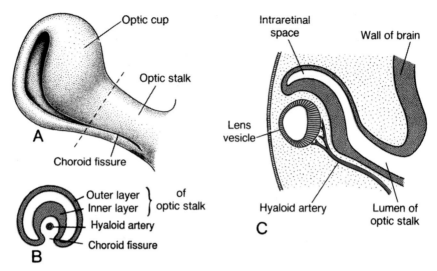

Figure 18.2. **A.** Ventrolateral view of the optic cup and optic stalk of a 6-week embryo. The choroid fissure located on the undersurface of the optic stalk gradually tapers off. **B.** Transverse section through the optic stalk as indicated in **A**, showing the hyaloid artery in the choroid fissure. **C.** Section through the lens vesicle, the optic cup, and optic stalk at the plane of the choroid fissure.

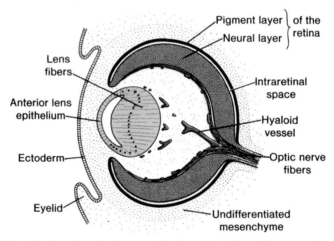

Figure 18.3. Section through the eye of a 7-week embryo. The eye primordium is completely embedded in mesenchyme. Fibers of the neural retina converge toward the optic nerve.

Meanwhile, the region between the optic cup and the overlying surface epithelium is filled with loose mesenchyme (Figs. 18.3, 18.4, and 18.7). In this tissue, the **sphincter** and **dilator pupillae** muscles are formed (Fig. 18.6). These muscles develop from the underlying ectoderm of the optic cup. In the adult, the iris is formed by the pigment-containing external layer and the unpigmented

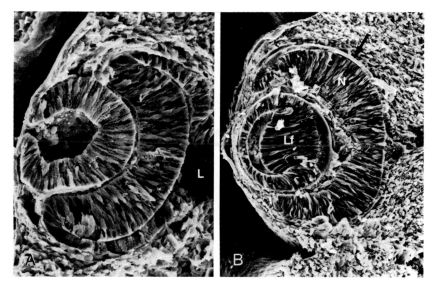

Figure 18.4. Scanning electron micrographs of sections through the eyes of mouse embryos at stages equivalent to 6 weeks **(A)** and 7 weeks **(B)** in the human. **A.** Note the forming lens vesicle that has not entirely closed, the two layers of the optic cup, and the lumen *(L)* of the optic stalk. (Compare with Fig. 18.2*C*.) **B.** By this stage, lens fibers *(Lf)* are forming, as are the neural *(N)* and pigment layers *(arrow)*. (Compare with Fig. 18.3.)

internal layer of the optic cup as well as by a layer of richly vascularized connective tissue, which contains the pupillary muscles (Fig. 18.6).

The **pars ciliaris retinae** is easily recognized by its marked folding (Figs. 18.6*B* and 18.7). Externally, it is covered by a layer of mesenchyme that forms the **ciliary muscle;** on the inside, it is connected to the lens by a network of elastic fibers, the **suspensory ligament** or zonula (Fig. 18.7). Contraction of the ciliary muscle changes tension in the ligament and controls curvature of the lens.

Lens

Shortly after formation of the lens vesicle (Fig. 18.2*C*), cells of the posterior wall begin to elongate in an anterior direction and form long fibers that gradually fill the lumen of the vesicle (Figs. 18.3 and 18.4*B*). By the end of the 7th week, these **primary lens fibers** reach the anterior wall of the lens vesicle. Growth of the lens is not finished at this stage, however, since new (secondary) lens fibers are continuously added to the central core.

Choroid, Sclera, and Cornea

At the end of the 5th week, the eye primordium is completely surrounded by loose mesenchyme (Fig. 18.3). This tissue soon differentiates into an inner layer, comparable to the pia mater of the brain, and an outer layer, comparable to the

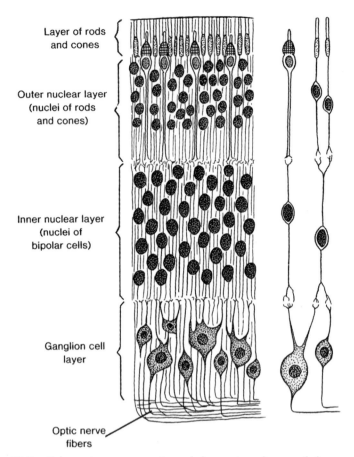

Layer of rods
and cones

Outer nuclear layer
(nuclei of rods
and cones)

Inner nuclear layer
(nuclei of
bipolar cells)

Ganglion cell
layer

Optic nerve
fibers

Figure 18.5. Schematic representation of the various layers of the pars optica retinae in a fetus of approximately 25 weeks.

dura mater. Whereas the inner layer later forms a highly vascularized pigmented layer known as the **choroid,** the outer layer develops into the sclera and is continuous with the dura mater around the optic nerve (Fig. 18.7).

Differentiation of mesenchymal layers overlying the anterior aspect of the eye is different. Through vacuolization, a space is formed known as the **anterior chamber,** which splits the mesenchyme into an inner layer in front of the lens and iris, the **iridopupillary membrane,** and an outer layer continuous with the sclera, the **substantia propria** of the **cornea** (Fig. 18.7). The anterior chamber itself is lined by flattened mesenchymal cells. Hence, the cornea is formed by (*a*) an epithelial layer derived from the surface ectoderm, (*b*) the **substantia propria** or **stroma,** which is continuous with the sclera, and (*c*) an epithelial layer, which borders the anterior chamber. The iridopupillary membrane in front of the lens disappears completely, thus providing a communication between the anterior and posterior eye chambers. Sometimes, resorption of the **iridopupillary membrane** is not complete, and connective tissue fibers are suspended in front of the pupil (Fig. 18.9*B*).

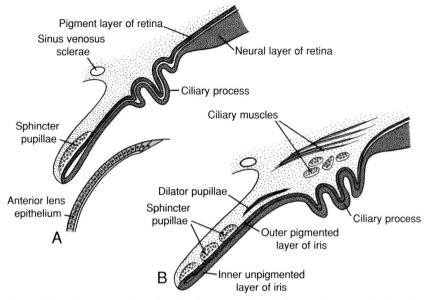

Figure 18.6. Drawings showing development of the iris and ciliary body. The rim of the optic cup is covered by mesenchyme, in which the sphincter and dilator pupillae develop from the underlying ectoderm.

Vitreous Body

Mesenchyme not only surrounds the eye primordium from the outside but also invades the inside of the optic cup by way of the choroid fissure. Here, it forms the hyaloid vessels, which, during intrauterine life, supply the lens and form the vascular layer located on the inner surface of the retina (Fig. 18.7). In addition, it forms a delicate network of fibers between the lens and retina. The interstitial spaces of this network are later filled with a transparent gelatinous substance, thus forming the vitreous body (Fig. 18.7). The hyaloid vessels in this region are obliterated and disappear during fetal life, leaving behind the hyaloid canal.

Optic Nerve

The optic cup is connected to the brain by the optic stalk, which, on its ventral surface, has a groove, the **choroid fissure** (Figs. 18.2 and 18.3). In this groove are the hyaloid vessels. The nerve fibers of the retina returning to the brain lie among cells of the inner wall of the stalk (Fig. 18.8). During the 7th week, the choroid fissure closes, and a narrow tunnel is formed inside the optic stalk (Fig. 18.8*B*). As a result of the continuously increasing number of nerve fibers, the inner wall of the stalk increases in size, and the inside and outside walls of the stalk fuse (Fig. 18.8*C*). Cells of the inner layer provide a network of neuroglia that support the optic nerve fibers.

The optic stalk is thus transformed into the **optic nerve.** In its center, it contains a portion of the hyaloid artery, which is later called the **central artery**

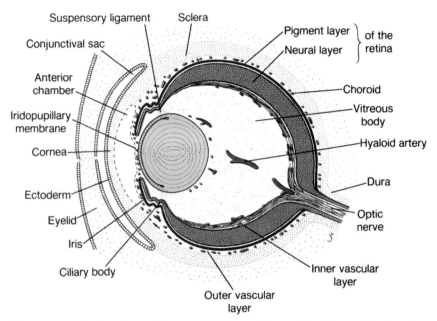

Figure 18.7. Section through the eye of a 15-week fetus. Note the anterior chamber, iridopupillary membrane, inner and outer vascular layers, choroid, and sclera.

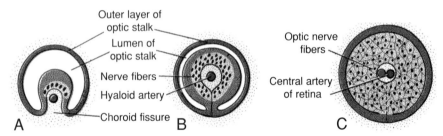

Figure 18.8. Diagrams showing transformation of the optic stalk into the optic nerve. **A.** Sixth week (9 mm). **B.** Seventh week (15 mm). **C.** Ninth week. Note the central artery of the retina in the optic nerve.

of the retina. On the outside, the optic nerve is surrounded by a continuation of the choroid and sclera, which are known as the **pia arachnoid** and **dura** layer of the nerve, respectively.

CLINICAL CORRELATES

Coloboma iridis may occur if closure of the choroid fissure fails to occur. Normally, this fissure closes during the 7th week of development (Fig. 18.8). When this fails to occur, a cleft persists. Although such a cleft is usually located in the iris only and is known as **coloboma iridis** (Fig. 18.9*A*), it may extend into the ciliary body, the retina, the choroid, and the optic nerve. This malformation is a common eye abnormality and frequently occurs in combination with other eye defects. Colobomas (clefts) of the eyelids may also occur.

Congenital cataracts are a condition in which the lens becomes opaque during intrauterine life. Although this anomaly is usually genetically determined, in 1941, Gregg observed that children of mothers who suffered from German measles (rubella) between the 4th and 7th weeks of pregnancy often had cataracts. If, however, the mother was infected after the 7th week of pregnancy, then the lens escaped damage, but the child was often deaf as a result of abnormalities of the cochlea.

The **hyaloid artery** may persist to form a cord or cyst. Normally, the distal portion of this vessel degenerates, leaving the proximal part to form the central artery of the retina.

Microphthalmia is a condition in which the eye is too small, and the eyeball may be reduced to two-thirds of its normal volume. Usually, it is associated with other ocular abnormalities. Microphthalmia frequently results from intrauterine infections such as cytomegalovirus and toxoplasmosis.

Anophthalmia is an absence of the eyeball. In some cases, histological analysis reveals some ocular tissues. The defect is usually accompanied by severe cranial abnormalities.

Congenital aphakia (absence of the lens) and **aniridia** (absence of the iris) are rare anomalies that are due to disturbances in induction and formation of tissues responsible for formation of these structures.

Cyclopia (single eye) and **synophthalmia** (fusion of the eyes) involve a spectrum of defects in which the eyes are partially or completely fused (Fig. 18.10). The defects are due to a loss of midline tissue near

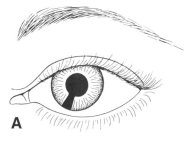
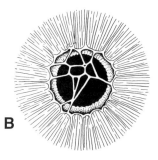

Figure 18.9. **A.** Coloboma iridis. **B.** Congenital cataract.

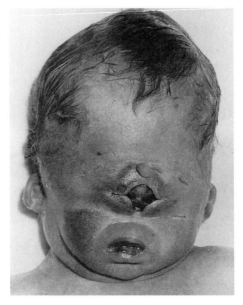

Figure 18.10. Synophthalmia. The eyes are fused, and the baby has severe cranial defects from the loss of midline structures.

days 19–21 of gestation, resulting in underdevelopment of the forebrain and frontonasal prominence. These defects are invariably associated with cranial defects such as holoprosencephaly in which the cerebral hemispheres are partially or completely fused (see Chapter 20).

SUMMARY

The eyes begin to develop as a pair of outpocketings that will become the **optic vesicles** on each side of the forebrain at the end of the 4th week of development. The optic vesicles contact the surface ectoderm and induce lens formation. When the optic vesicle begins to invaginate to form the pigment and neural layer of the retina, the lens placode invaginates to form the lens vesicle. Through a groove at the inferior aspect of the optic vesicle, i.e., the choroid fissure, the hyaloid artery (later the central artery of the retina) enters the eye (Figs. 18.2 and 18.3). Nerve fibers of the eye also occupy this groove to reach the optic areas of the brain. The cornea is formed by *(a)* a layer of surface ectoderm, *(b)* the stroma, which is continuous with the sclera, and *(c)* an epithelial layer bordering the anterior chamber (Fig. 18.7).

PROBLEMS TO SOLVE

1. A newborn has unilateral aphakia (absent lens). What is the embryological origin of this defect?

2. In taking a history of a young woman in her 10th week of gestation you become concerned that she may have contracted rubella sometime during the 4th to 8th weeks of her pregnancy. What types of defects might be produced in her offspring?

3. Physical examination of a newborn reveals clefts in the lower portion of the iris, bilaterally. What is the embryological basis for this defect? What other structures might be involved?

SUGGESTED READINGS

O'Rahilly R: The early development of the eye in staged embryos. *Contrib Embryol* 38:1, 1966.
O'Rahilly R: The timing and sequence of events in the development of the human eye and ear during the embryonic period proper. *Anat Embryol (Berl)* 168:87, 1983.
Saha MS, Spann C, Grainger RM: Embryonic lens induction: more than meets the optic vesicle. *Cell Differ Dev* 28:153, 1989.
Stromland K, Miller M, Cook C: Ocular teratology. *Surv Ophthalmol* 35:429, 1991.
Tamura T, Smelser JK: Development of the sphincter and dilator muscles of the iris. *Arch Ophthalmol* 89:332, 1973.
Tripathi BJ, Tripathi RC, Livingston AM, Borisuth NSC: The role of growth factors in the embryogenesis and differentiation of the eye. *Am J Anat* 192:442, 1991.

chapter 19

Integumentary System

Skin

The skin has a twofold origin: *(a)* a superficial layer, the **epidermis,** which develops from the surface ectoderm, and *(b)* a deep layer, the **dermis,** which develops from the underlying mesenchyme.

EPIDERMIS

Initially, the embryo is covered by a single layer of ectodermal cells (Fig. 19.1*A*). In the beginning of the 2nd month, this epithelium divides, and a layer of flattened cells, the **periderm** or **epitrichium,** is laid down on the surface (Fig. 19.1*B*). With further proliferation of cells in the basal layer, a third, intermediate zone is formed (Fig. 19.1*C*). Finally, at the end of the 4th month, the epidermis acquires its definitive arrangement, and four layers can be distinguished (Fig. 19.1*D*):

① The basal layer, known as the **germinative layer,** is responsible for production of new cells. This layer later forms ridges and hollows, which are reflected on the surface of the skin in the fingerprint.

② A thick **spinous layer** consisting of large polyhedral cells containing fine tonofibrils.

③ The **granular layer,** the cells of which contain small keratohyalin granules.

④ The **horny layer,** forming the tough scale-like surface of the epidermis, is made up of closely packed dead cells loaded with keratin.

Cells of the periderm are usually cast off during the second part of intrauterine life and can be found in the amniotic fluid.

During the first 3 months of development, the epidermis is invaded by cells of **neural crest** origin. These cells synthesize **melanin** pigment, which can be transferred to other cells of the epidermis by way of dendritic processes. They are known as **melanocytes** and after birth cause pigmentation of the skin (Fig. 19.1*D*).

CLINICAL CORRELATES

The epidermal ridges, which produce typical patterns on the surface of the fingertips, palms of the hand, and soles of the feet, are

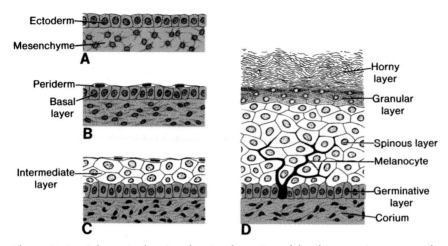

Figure 19.1. Schematic drawing showing formation of the skin at various stages of development. **A.** 5 weeks. **B.** 7 weeks. **C.** 4 months. **D.** At birth.

genetically determined. They form the basis for many studies in medical genetics and criminal investigations **(dermatoglyphics).** In children with chromosomal abnormalities, the epidermal pattern on the hand and fingers is sometimes used as a diagnostic tool.

DERMIS

The **dermis** is derived from mesenchyme. During the 3rd and 4th months, this tissue, the **corium** (Fig. 19.1*D*), forms many irregular papillary structures, the **dermal papillae,** which project upward into the epidermis. These papillae usually contain a small capillary or sensory nerve end organ. The deeper layer of the dermis, the **subcorium,** contains large amounts of fatty tissue.

At birth, the skin is covered by a whitish paste, the **vernix caseosa,** formed by secretions from sebaceous glands and degenerated epidermal cells and hairs. It protects the skin against the macerating action of amniotic fluid.

CLINICAL CORRELATES

Ichthyosis refers to excessive keratinization of the skin and is characteristic of a group of hereditary disorders that are usually inherited as an autosomal recessive trait but may also be X-linked. In severe cases, the disorder may result in a grotesque appearance of an infant, such as in the case of a harlequin fetus (Fig. 19.2).

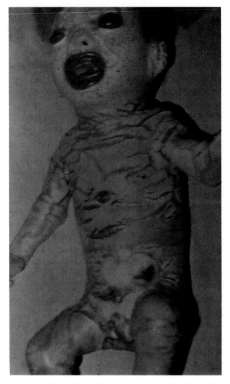

Figure 19.2. Photograph of ichthyosis in a harlequin fetus. There is massive thickening of the keratin layer, which cracks to form fissures between thickened plaques.

Hair

Hairs appear as solid epidermal proliferations penetrating the underlying dermis (Fig. 19.3*A*). At their terminal ends, hair buds invaginate. The invaginations, the **hair papillae,** are rapidly filled with mesoderm in which vessels and nerve endings develop (Fig. 19.3, *B* and *C*).

Soon, cells in the center of the hair buds become spindle-shaped and keratinized, forming the **hair shaft,** while peripheral cells become cuboidal, giving rise to the **epithelial hair sheath** (Fig. 19.3, *B* and *C*).

The **dermal root sheath** is formed by the surrounding mesenchyme. A small smooth muscle, also derived from mesenchyme, is usually attached to the dermal root sheath. The muscle is known as an **arrector pili muscle.** Continuous proliferation of epithelial cells at the base of the shaft pushes the hair upward, and by the end of the 3rd month, the first hairs appear on the surface in the region of the eyebrow and upper lip. The first hair that appears, **lanugo hair,** is shed at about the time of birth and is later replaced by coarser hairs arising from new hair follicles.

The epithelial wall of the hair follicle usually shows a small bud penetrating the surrounding mesoderm (Fig. 19.3*C*). Cells in the center of these buds, the

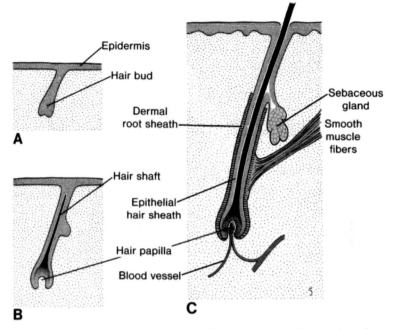

Figure 19.3. Schematic representation of development of a hair and a sebaceous gland. **A.** 4 months. **B.** 6 months. **C.** In a newborn.

sebaceous glands, degenerate, thereby forming a fat-like substance secreted into the hair follicle, from where it reaches the skin.

CLINICAL CORRELATES

Hypertrichosis (excessive hairiness) is caused by increased formation of hair follicles, may be localized in certain areas of the body (dorsal midline region), or may be general over the whole body.

Atrichia, the congenital absence of hair, is usually associated with abnormalities of other ectodermal derivatives, such as teeth and nails.

Mammary Glands

The first indication of mammary glands is found in the form of a band-like thickening of the epidermis, the **mammary line** or **ridge.** In a 7-week embryo, this line extends on each side of the body from the base of the forelimb to the region of the hindlimb (Fig. 19.4C). Although the major part of the mammary line disappears shortly after its formation, a small portion in the thoracic region persists and penetrates the underlying mesenchyme (Fig. 19.4A). Here, it forms 16–24 sprouts, which, in turn, give rise to small, solid buds. By the end of

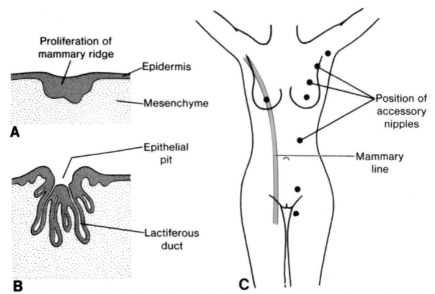

Figure 19.4. **A** and **B.** Sections through the developing mammary gland at the 3rd and 8th months, respectively. **C.** Diagram showing positions of accessory nipples (*blue line* indicates position of mammary line).

prenatal life, the epithelial sprouts are canalized and form the **lactiferous ducts,** whereas the buds form small ducts and alveoli of the gland. Initially, the **lactiferous ducts** open into a small epithelial pit (Fig. 19.3*B*). Shortly after birth, this pit is transformed into the **nipple** by proliferation of the underlying mesenchyme.

CLINICAL CORRELATES

Polythelia is a condition where accessory nipples have formed due to the persistence of fragments of the mammary line (Fig. 19.4). Accessory nipples may develop anywhere along the original mammary line but usually appear in the axillary region.

Polymastia occurs when a remnant of the mammary line develops into a complete breast.

Inverted nipple is a condition in which the lactiferous ducts open into the original epithelial pit that has failed to evert.

SUMMARY

The skin and its associated structures, the hair, nails, and glands, are derived from surface ectoderm. **Melanocytes,** which give the skin its color, are derived from **neural crest cells,** which migrate into the epidermis. The production of new cells occurs in the **germinative** layer. After moving to the surface, cells are sloughed off in the horny layer (Fig. 19.1). The dermis, the deep layer of the skin, is of mesenchymal origin.

Hairs develop from downgrowth of epidermal cells in the underlying dermis. By about 20 weeks, the fetus is covered by downy hair, **lanugo hair,** which is shed at the time of birth. **Sebaceous glands, sweat glands,** and **mammary glands** all develop from epidermal proliferations. Supernumerary nipples **(polythelia)** and breasts **(polymastia)** are relatively common (see Fig. 19.4).

PROBLEMS TO SOLVE

1. A woman appears to have accessory nipples in her axilla and on her abdomen, bilaterally. What is the embryological basis for these additional nipples, and why do they occur in these locations?

SUGGESTED READINGS

Beller F: Development and anatomy of the breast. *In* Mitchell GW Jr, Bassett LW (eds): *The Female Breast and Its Disorders.* Baltimore, Williams & Wilkins, 1990.

Fuchs E: Epidermal differentiation: the bare essential. *J Cell Biol* 111:2807, 1990.

Hirschhorn K: Dermatoglyphics. *In* Behrman RE (ed): *Nelson Textbook of Pediatrics.* 14th ed. Philadelphia, WB Saunders, 1992.

Newman M: Supernumerary nipples. *Am Fam Physician* 38:183, 1988.

Nordlund JJ, Abdel-Malek ZA, Boissy R, Rheins LA: Pigment cell biology: an historical review. *J Invest Dermatol* 92:53S, 1989.

Opitz JM: Pathogenetic analysis of certain developmental and genetic ectodermal defects. *Birth Defects* 24:75, 1988.

Smith LT, Holbrook KA: Embryogenesis of the dermis in human skin. *Pediatr Dermatol* 3:271, 1986.

chapter 20

Central Nervous System

The central nervous system (CNS) appears at the beginning of the 3rd week as a slipper-shaped plate of thickened ectoderm, the **neural plate.** This plate is located in the middorsal region in front of the **primitive pit.** Its lateral edges soon become elevated to form the **neural folds** (Fig. 20.1).

With further development, the neural folds become more elevated, approach each other in the midline, and finally fuse, thus forming the **neural tube** (Figs. 20.2 and 20.3). Fusion begins in the cervical region and proceeds in cephalic and caudal directions (Fig. 20.3*A*). At the cranial and caudal ends of the embryo, however, fusion is delayed, and the **cranial** and **caudal neuropores** temporarily form open connections between the lumen of the neural tube and the amniotic cavity (Fig. 20.3*B*). Closure of the cranial neuropore is bidirectional, proceeding from the initial closure site in the cervical region as well as from a later-forming site in the forebrain that also proceeds in cranial and caudal directions. Final closure of the cranial neuropore occurs at the 18–20-somite stage (25th day); closure of the caudal neuropore occurs about 2 days later.

The cephalic end of the neural tube shows three dilations, i.e., the **primary brain vesicles:** *(a)* the **prosencephalon** or **forebrain,** *(b)* the **mesencephalon** or **midbrain,** and *(c)* the **rhombencephalon** or **hindbrain** (Fig. 20.4). Simultaneously, it forms two flexures: *(a)* the **cervical flexure,** at the junction of the hindbrain and the spinal cord, and *(b)* the **cephalic flexure,** located in the midbrain region (Fig. 20.4).

When the embryo is 5 weeks old, the prosencephalon consists of two parts: *(a)* the **telencephalon,** formed by a midportion and two lateral outpocketings, the **primitive cerebral hemispheres,** and *(b)* the **diencephalon,** characterized by outgrowth of the optic vesicles (Fig. 20.5). The mesencephalon is separated from the rhombencephalon by a deep furrow, the **rhombencephalic isthmus.**

The rhombencephalon also consists of two parts: *(a)* the **metencephalon,** which later forms the **pons** and **cerebellum,** and *(b)* the **myelencephalon.** The boundary between these two portions is marked by a flexure known as the **pontine flexure** (Fig. 20.5).

The lumen of the spinal cord, the **central canal,** is continuous with that of the brain vesicles. The cavity of the rhombencephalon is known as the **4th ventricle,** that of the diencephalon is known as the **3rd ventricle,** and those of the cerebral hemispheres are known as the **lateral ventricles** (Fig. 20.5). The 3rd and 4th ventricles are connected to each other through the lumen of the mesencephalon.

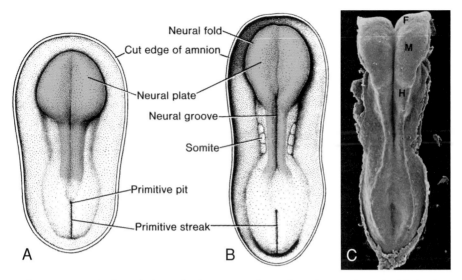

Figure 20.1. **A.** Dorsal view of a late presomite embryo (approximately 18 days). The amnion has been removed, and the neural plate is clearly visible. **B.** Dorsal view at approximately 20 days. Note the somites and the neural groove and neural folds. **C.** Scanning electron micrograph of a mouse embryo at a stage similar to that in **B.** **F,** forebrain; **M,** midbrain; and **H,** hindbrain.

This lumen becomes very narrow and is then known as the **aqueduct of Sylvius.** The lateral ventricles communicate with the 3rd ventricle through the **interventricular foramina of Monro** (Fig. 20.5).

Spinal Cord

NEUROEPITHELIAL, MANTLE, AND MARGINAL LAYERS

The wall of a recently closed neural tube consists of **neuroepithelial cells.** These cells extend over the entire thickness of the wall and form a thick pseudostratified epithelium (Fig. 20.6). They are connected to each other by junctional complexes at the lumen. During the neural groove stage and immediately after closure of the tube, they divide rapidly, resulting in production of more and more neuroepithelial cells. Collectively, they are referred to as the **neuroepithelial layer** or **neuroepithelium.**

Once the neural tube is closed, neuroepithelial cells begin to give rise to another cell type, which is characterized by a large round nucleus with pale nucleoplasm and a dark-staining nucleolus. These cells are the primitive nerve cells or **neuroblasts** (Fig. 20.7). They form a zone around the neuroepithelial layer, known as the **mantle layer** (Fig. 20.8). The mantle layer later forms the **gray matter of the spinal cord.**

The outermost layer of the spinal cord contains nerve fibers emerging from neuroblasts in the mantle layer and is known as the **marginal layer.** As a result

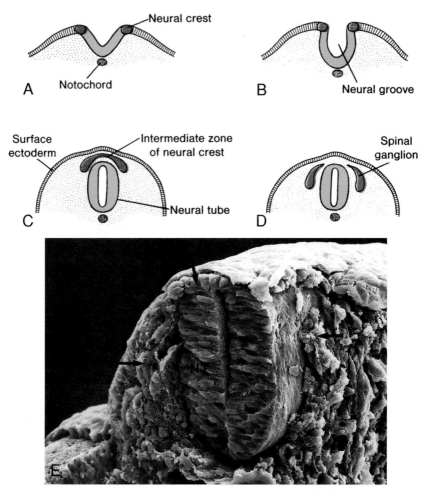

Figure 20.2. A–D. Transverse sections through successively older embryos, showing formation of the neural groove, neural tube, and neural crest. Cells of the neural crest, initially forming an intermediate zone between the neural tube and surface ectoderm **(C),** develop into spinal and cranial sensory ganglia **(D). E.** Scanning electron micrograph of a mouse embryo, showing the neural tube *(NT)* and neural crest cells *(arrows)* migrating from the dorsal region (compare with **C** and **D**).

of myelination of nerve fibers, this layer obtains a white appearance and is therefore referred to as the **white matter of the spinal cord** (Fig. 20.8).

BASAL, ALAR, ROOF, AND FLOOR PLATES

As a result of continuous addition of neuroblasts to the mantle layer, each side of the neural tube shows a ventral and a dorsal thickening. The ventral thickenings, the **basal plates,** contain ventral motor horn cells and form the motor areas of the spinal cord; the dorsal thickenings, the **alar plates, form the sensory areas** (Fig. 20.8*A*). A longitudinal groove, the **sulcus limitans,** marks the boundary between

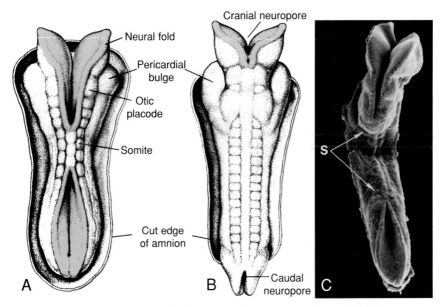

Figure 20.3. A. Dorsal view of a human embryo at approximately day 22. Seven distinct somites are visible on each side of the neural tube. **B.** Dorsal view of a human embryo at approximately day 23. The nervous system is in connection with the amniotic cavity through the cranial and caudal neuropores. **C.** Scanning electron micrograph of a mouse embryo at a stage similar to that in **A.** *S,* somites.

the two. The dorsal and ventral midline portions of the neural tube, known as the **roof** and **floor plates,** respectively, do not contain neuroblasts and serve primarily as pathways for nerve fibers crossing from one side to the other.

In addition to the ventral motor horn and the dorsal sensory horn, a group of neurons accumulates between the two areas and causes formation of a small **intermediate horn** (Fig. 20.8*B*). This horn contains neurons of the sympathetic portion of the autonomic nervous system and is present only at thoracic and upper lumbar levels (L2-L3) of the spinal cord.

HISTOLOGICAL DIFFERENTIATION

Nerve Cells

Neuroblasts or primitive nerve cells arise exclusively by division of the neuroepithelial cells. Initially, they have a central process extending to the lumen **(transient dendrite),** but when they migrate into the mantle layer, this process disappears, and neuroblasts are temporarily round and **apolar** (Fig. 20.9*A*). With further differentiation, two new cytoplasmic processes appear on opposite sides of the cell body, thus forming the **bipolar neuroblast** (Fig. 20.9*B*). The process at one end of the cell elongates rapidly to form the **primitive axon,** while the process at the other end shows a number of cytoplasmic arborizations, the **primitive dendrites** (Fig. 20.9*C*). The cell is then known as a **multipolar**

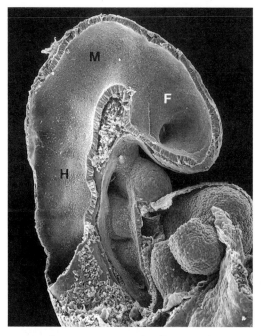

Figure 20.4. Scanning electron micrograph of a sagittal section through a mouse embryo at approximately 27 days of human development. Three brain vesicles representing the forebrain *(F)*, midbrain *(M)*, and hindbrain *(H)* are represented.

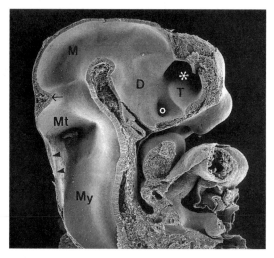

Figure 20.5. Scanning electron micrograph of a sagittal section through a mouse embryo at approximately 27 days of human development. The three brain vesicles have segregated into the telencephalon *(T)*, diencephalon *(D)*, mesencephalon *(M)*, metencephalon *(Mt)*, and myelencephalon *(My)*. *Asterisk,* outpocketing of the telencephalon; *arrow,* rhombencephalic isthmus; *arrowheads,* roof of the 4th ventricle; and *o,* optic stalk.

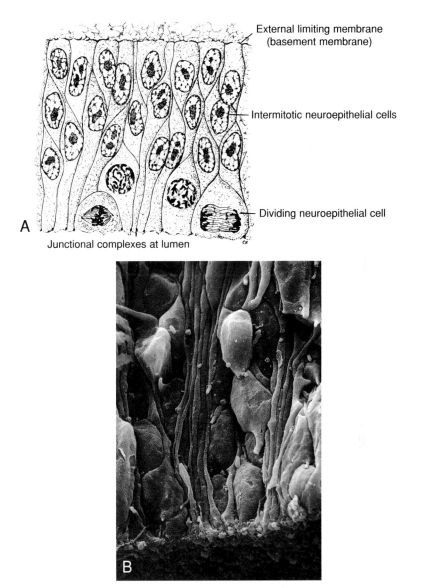

External limiting membrane (basement membrane)

Intermitotic neuroepithelial cells

Dividing neuroepithelial cell

A

Junctional complexes at lumen

B

Figure 20.6. **A.** Drawing of a section of the wall of the recently closed neural tube. Neuroepithelial cells, which form a pseudostratified epithelium extending over the full width of the wall, can be recognized. Note the dividing cells at the lumen of the tube. **B.** Scanning electron micrograph of a section of the neural tube of a mouse embryo similar to that in **A.**

neuroblast and with further development becomes the adult nerve cell or **neuron.** Once neuroblasts are formed, they lose their ability to divide. Axons of neurons in the basal plate break through the marginal zone and become visible on the ventral aspect of the cord. They are known collectively as the **ventral motor**

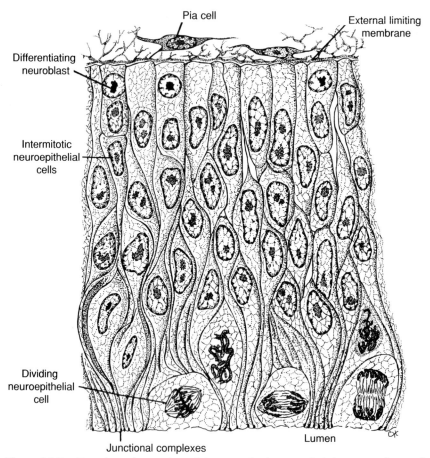

Figure 20.7. Drawing of a section of the neural tube at a slightly more advanced stage than that represented in Figure 20.6. The major portion of the wall consists of neuroepithelial cells. On the periphery, however, immediately adjacent to the external limiting membrane, neuroblasts form. These cells, which are produced by the neuroepithelial cells in ever-increasing numbers, will form the mantle layer.

root of the spinal nerve and conduct motor impulses from the spinal cord to the muscles (Fig. 20.10). Axons of neurons in the dorsal sensory horn (alar plate) behave differently from those in the ventral horn. They penetrate into the marginal layer of the cord, where they ascend to either higher or lower levels to form **association neurons.**

Glial Cells

The majority of primitive supporting cells, the **gliablasts,** are formed by neuroepithelial cells after production of neuroblasts has ceased. From the neuroepithelial layer, gliablasts migrate to the mantle and marginal layers. In the mantle layer, they differentiate into **protoplasmic** and **fibrillar astrocytes** (Fig. 20.11).

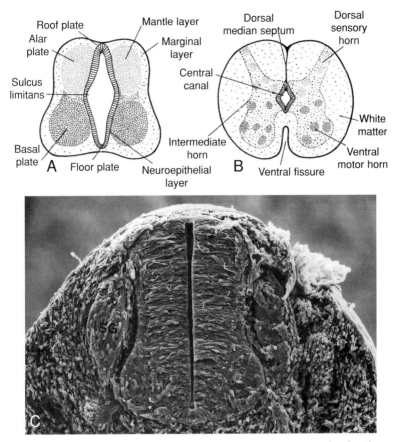

Figure 20.8. **A** and **B.** Diagrams to show two successive stages in the development of the spinal cord. Note formation of ventral motor and dorsal sensory horns and the intermediate column. **C.** Scanning electron micrograph of a section through the spinal cord of a mouse embryo, showing a stage similar to that in **A.** *SG,* spinal ganglion.

Another type of supporting cell possibly derived from gliablasts is the **oligodendroglial cell.** This cell, which is found primarily in the marginal layer, forms myelin sheaths around the ascending and descending axons in the marginal layer.

In the second half of development, a third type of supporting cell, the **microglial cell,** appears in the CNS. This cell type is highly phagocytic and is derived from mesenchyme (Fig. 20.11).

When neuroepithelial cells cease to produce neuroblasts and gliablasts, they finally differentiate into ependymal cells lining the central canal of the spinal cord.

Neural Crest Cells

During folding of the neural plate, a group of cells appears along each edge of the neural groove (Fig. 20.2). These cells, ectodermal in origin and known

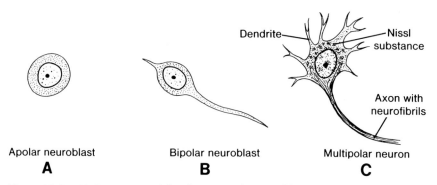

Figure 20.9. Various stages of development of a neuroblast. A neuron is a structural and functional unit consisting of the cell body and all its processes.

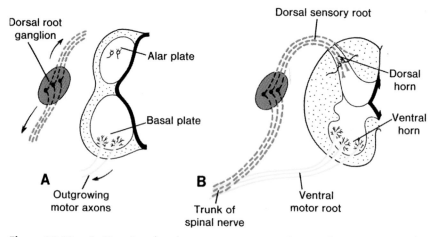

Figure 20.10. A. Drawing showing motor axons growing out from neurons in the basal plate and centrally and peripherally growing fibers of nerve cells in the dorsal root ganglion. B. Nerve fibers of the ventral motor and dorsal sensory roots join to form the trunk of the spinal nerve.

as **neural crest cells,** temporarily form an intermediate zone between the tube and the surface ectoderm (Fig. 20.2, *C* and *E*). This zone extends throughout the length of the neural tube, and crest cells from this region migrate laterally (Fig. 20.2, *D* and *E*). Some of the cells then give rise to **sensory ganglia (dorsal root ganglia)** of the spinal nerves (Fig. 20.2).

During further development, neuroblasts of the sensory ganglia form two processes (Fig. 20.10*A*). The centrally growing processes penetrate the dorsal portion of the neural tube. In the spinal cord they either end in the dorsal horn or ascend through the marginal layer to one of the higher brain centers. These processes are known collectively as the **dorsal sensory root of the spinal nerve** (Fig. 20.10*B*). The peripherally growing processes join fibers of the ventral motor roots and thus participate in formation of the trunk of the spinal

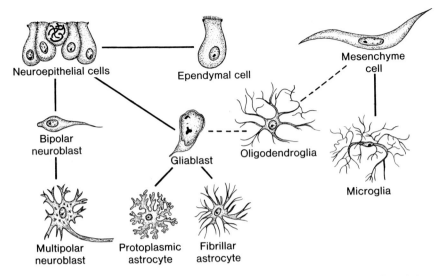

Figure 20.11. Schematic diagram showing the origin of the nerve cell and the various types of glial cells. Neuroblasts, fibrillar and protoplasmic astrocytes, and ependymal cells originate from neuroepithelial cells. Microglia develop from mesenchyme cells. The origin of the oligodendroglia is not clear.

nerve. Eventually, these processes terminate in the sensory receptor organs. Hence, the neuroblasts of the sensory ganglia give rise to the **dorsal root neurons.**

In addition to forming sensory ganglia, cells of the neural crest differentiate into sympathetic neuroblasts, Schwann cells, pigments cells, odontoblasts, meninges, and mesenchyme of the pharyngeal arches.

Spinal Nerves

Motor nerve fibers begin to appear in the 4th week of development, arising from nerve cells located in the basal plates (ventral horns) of the spinal cord. These fibers become collected into bundles known as **ventral nerve roots** (Fig. 20.10). **Dorsal nerve roots** form as collections of fibers originating from cells in **dorsal root ganglia (spinal ganglia).** Central processes from these ganglia form bundles that grow into the spinal cord opposite the dorsal horns. Distal processes join the ventral nerve roots to form a **spinal nerve** (Fig. 20.10). Almost immediately, spinal nerves divide into **dorsal** and **ventral primary rami.** Dorsal primary rami innervate dorsal axial musculature, vertebral joints, and the skin of the back. Ventral primary rami innervate the limbs and ventral body wall and form the major nerve plexuses (cranial, brachial, and lumbosacral).

Myelination

Myelination of peripheral nerves is accomplished by **Schwann cells.** These cells originate from neural crest, migrate peripherally, and wrap themselves around axons, thus forming the **neurilemma sheath** (Fig. 20.12). Beginning at

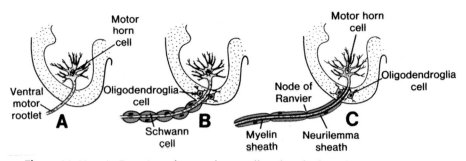

Figure 20.12. **A.** Drawing of motor horn cell with naked rootlet. **B.** In the spinal cord, oligodendroglia cells surround the ventral rootlet; outside the spinal cord, Schwann cells begin to surround the rootlet. **C.** In the spinal cord, the myelin sheath is formed by oligodendroglia cells; outside the spinal cord, the sheath is formed by Schwann cells.

the 4th month of fetal life, many nerve fibers obtain a whitish appearance as a result of deposition of **myelin,** which is formed by repeated coiling of the Schwann cell membrane around the axon (Fig. 20.12*C*).

The myelin sheath surrounding nerve fibers in the spinal cord is of completely different origin, since it is formed by the **oligodendroglial cells** (Fig. 20.12, *B* and *C*). Although myelination of nerve fibers in the spinal cord begins in approximately the 4th month of intrauterine life, some of the motor fibers descending from higher brain centers to the spinal cord do not become myelinated until the 1st year of postnatal life. Tracts in the nervous system become myelinated at about the time they start to function.

POSITIONAL CHANGES OF THE CORD

In the 3rd month of development, the spinal cord extends the entire length of the embryo, and spinal nerves pass through the intervertebral foramina at their level of origin (Fig. 20.13*A*). With increasing age, however, the vertebral column and dura lengthen more rapidly than the neural tube, and the terminal end of the spinal cord gradually shifts to a higher level. At birth, this end is located at the level of the 3rd lumbar vertebra (Fig. 20.13*C*). As a result of this disproportionate growth, spinal nerves run obliquely from their segment of origin in the spinal cord to the corresponding level of the vertebral column. The dura remains attached to the vertebral column at the coccygeal level.

In the adult, the spinal cord terminates at the level of L2-L3. Below this point, a thread-like extension of the pia mater forms the **filum terminale,** which marks the tract of regression of the spinal cord and is attached to the periosteum of the 1st coccygeal vertebra. Nerve fibers below the terminal end of the cord are known collectively as the **cauda equina.** When cerebrospinal fluid is tapped during a **lumbar puncture,** the needle is inserted at the lower lumber level, thus avoiding the lower end of the cord.

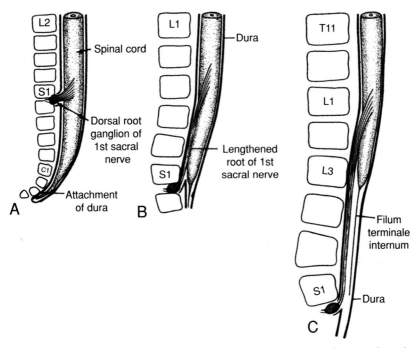

Figure 20.13. Schematic drawing showing the terminal end of the spinal cord in relation to that of the vertebral column at various stages of development. **A.** Approximately the 3rd month. **B.** End of the 5th month. **C.** In the newborn.

CLINICAL CORRELATES

Most defects of the spinal cord result from abnormal closure of the neural folds in the 3rd and 4th weeks of development. The resulting abnormalities are known as **neural tube defects** (NTDs), which also involve the meninges, vertebrae, muscles, and skin.

Spina bifida refers to a splitting of the vertebral arches and may or may not involve underlying neural tissue. The incidence for severe neural tube defects is approximately 1 in 1000 but varies in different populations.

Spina bifida occulta refers to a defect in the vertebral arches that is covered by skin and usually does not involve underlying neural tissue (Fig. 20.14A). It occurs in the lumbosacral region (L4–S1) and is usually marked by a patch of hair overlying the affected region. The defect is due to a lack of fusion of the vertebral arches and is present in about 10% of otherwise-normal people.

Spina bifida cystica is a severe NTD in which neural tissue and/or meninges protrude through a defect in the vertebral arches and skin to form a cyst-like sac (Fig. 20.14). Most are located in the lumbosacral

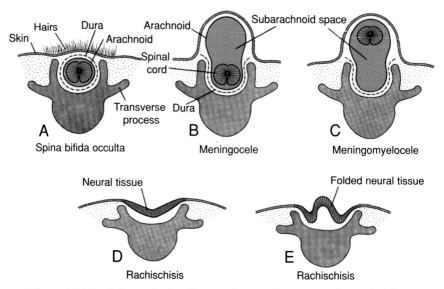

Figure 20.14. Schematic drawings to show various types of spina bifida.

region and result in neurological deficits, but they are usually not associated with mental retardation. In some cases, only fluid-filled meninges protrude through the defect (spina bifida with **meningocele**) (Fig. 20.14*B*), whereas in others, neural tissue is included in the sac (spina bifida with **meningomyelocele**) (Figs. 20.14*C* and 20.15*A*). Occasionally, the neural folds fail to elevate and remain as a flattened mass of neural tissue (spina bifida with **myeloschisis** or **rachischisis**) (Figs. 20.14, *D* and *E,* and 20.15*B*).

Spina bifida cystica can be diagnosed prenatally by ultrasound and by determination of α-fetoprotein (AFP) levels in maternal serum and amniotic fluid. The vertebra can be visualized by 12 weeks of gestation, and defects in closure of the vertebral arches can be detected.

Hyperthermia, valproic acid, and hypervitaminosis A produce NTDs, as do a large number of other teratogens. The origin of most NTDs is multifactorial, and the likelihood of having a child with such a defect increases significantly once one affected offspring is born. Recent evidence indicates that **folic acid (folate)** reduces the incidence of NTDs in certain populations.

Brain

Distinct **basal** and **alar plates,** representing motor and sensory areas, respectively, are found on each side of the midline in the rhombencephalon and

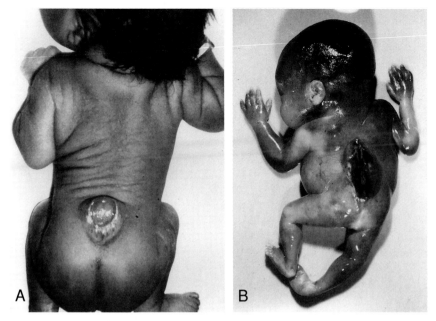

Figure 20.15. Photographs of the lumbosacral region of patients with neural tube defects. **A.** Patient with a large meningomyelocele. **B.** Patient with a severe defect in which the neural folds failed to elevate throughout the lower thoracic and lumbosacral regions, resulting in rachischisis.

mesencephalon (Figs. 20.17 and 20.22). In the prosencephalon, however, the alar plates are accentuated and the basal plates regress.

RHOMBENCEPHALON

The rhombencephalon consists of the **myelencephalon,** the most caudal of the brain vesicles, and the **metencephalon,** which extends from the pontine flexure to the rhombencephalic isthmus (Figs. 20.5 and 20.16).

MYELENCEPHALON

The myelencephalon is a brain vesicle that gives rise to the **medulla oblongata** and differs from the spinal cord in that its lateral walls are everted (Fig. 20.17, *B* and *C*). Alar and basal plates separated by the sulcus limitans can be clearly distinguished. The basal plate, similar to that of the spinal cord, contains motor nuclei. These nuclei are divided into three groups: *(a)* a medial **somatic efferent** group, *(b)* an intermediate **special visceral efferent** group, and *(c)* a lateral **general visceral efferent** group (Fig. 20.17*C*).

The first group contains motor neurons, which form the **cephalic continuation of the anterior horn cells.** Since this somatic efferent group continues rostrally into the mesencephalon, it is referred to as the **somatic efferent motor column.** In the myelencephalon, it includes neurons of the **hypoglossal nerve** that supply the tongue musculature. In the metencephalon and the mesencepha-

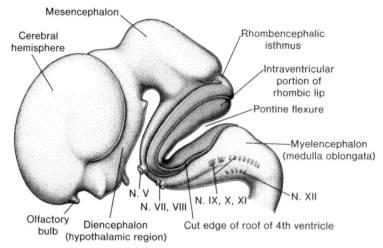

Mesencephalon

Cerebral hemisphere

Rhombencephalic isthmus

Intraventricular portion of rhombic lip

Pontine flexure

Myelencephalon (medulla oblongata)

N. V

N. VII, VIII

N. IX, X, XI

N. XII

Olfactory bulb

Diencephalon (hypothalamic region)

Cut edge of roof of 4th ventricle

Figure 20.16. Lateral view of the brain vesicles in an 8-week embryo (crown-rump length approximately 27 mm). The roof plate of the rhombencephalon has been removed to show the intraventricular portion of the rhombic lip. Note the origin of the cranial nerves.

lon, the column represents neurons of the **abducens** (Fig. 20.18), **trochlear,** and **oculomotor nerves** (Fig. 20.22), respectively. These nerves supply the eye musculature.

The **special visceral efferent** group extends into the metencephalon, thus forming the **special visceral efferent motor column.** Its motor neurons supply **striated muscles** of the pharyngeal arches. In the myelencephalon, the column is represented by neurons of the **accessory, vagus,** and **glossopharyngeal nerves.**

The **general visceral efferent** group contains motor neurons that supply **involuntary musculature** of the respiratory tract, intestinal tract, and heart.

The alar plate contains three groups of **sensory relay nuclei** (Fig. 20.17*C*). The most lateral of these, the **somatic afferent** (sensory) group, receives impulses from the ear and surface of the head by way of the **vestibulocochlear** and **trigeminal nerves.** The intermediate or **special visceral afferent** group receives impulses from taste buds of the tongue and from the palate, oropharynx, and epiglottis. The medial or **general visceral afferent** group receives interoceptive information from the gastrointestinal tract and heart.

The roof plate of the myelencephalon consists of a single layer of ependymal cells covered by vascular mesenchyme, the **pia mater** (Figs. 20.5 and 20.17*B*). The two combined are known as the **tela choroidea.** Because of active proliferation of the vascular mesenchyme, a number of sac-like invaginations project into the underlying ventricular cavity (Figs. 20.17*C* and 20.19*D*). These tuft-like invaginations form the **choroid plexus,** which produces cerebrospinal fluid.

METENCEPHALON

The metencephalon, similar to the myelencephalon, is characterized by basal and alar plates (Fig. 20.18). Two new components, however, are formed: *(a)* the

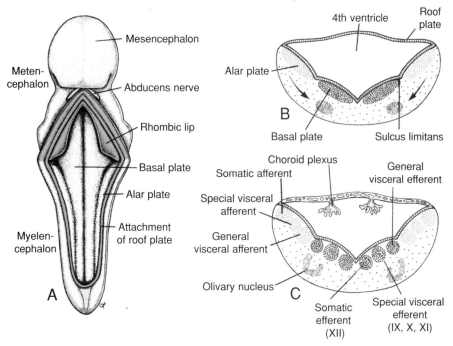

Figure 20.17. **A.** Dorsal view of the floor of the 4th ventricle in a 6-week embryo after removal of the roof plate. Note the alar and basal plates in the myelencephalon. The rhombic lip is visible in the metencephalon. **B** and **C.** Diagrams showing the position and differentiation of the basal and alar plates of the myelencephalon at different stages of development. Note formation of the nuclear groups in the basal and alar plates. *Arrows* indicate the path followed by cells of the alar plate to the olivary nuclear complex. The choroid plexus produces cerebrospinal fluid.

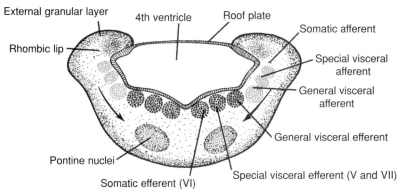

Figure 20.18. Schematic drawing of a transverse section through the caudal part of the metencephalon. Note the differentiation of the various motor and sensory nuclear areas in the basal and alar plates, respectively. Note the position of the rhombic lips, which project partly into the lumen of the 4th ventricle and partly above the attachment of the roof plate.

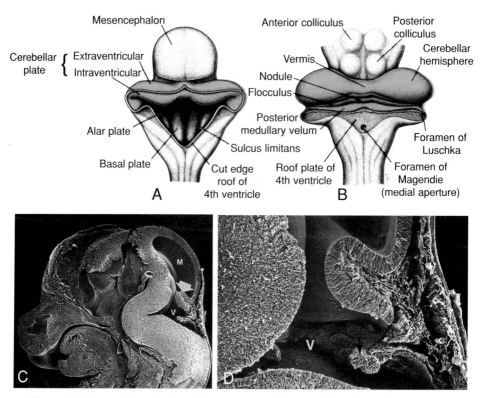

Figure 20.19. A. Dorsal view of the mesencephalon and rhombencephalon in an 8-week embryo. The roof of the 4th ventricle has been removed, allowing a view of the floor of the 4th ventricle. **B.** Similar view in a 4-month embryo. Note the choroidal fissure and the lateral and medial apertures in the roof of the 4th ventricle. **C.** Scanning electron micrograph of a mouse embryo at a slightly younger stage than that in **A,** showing the cerebellar primordium *(arrow)* extending into the 4th ventricle *(V).* M, mesencephalon. **D.** High magnification of the cerebellar region in **C.** The choroid plexus *(arrow)* in the roof of the 4th ventricle *(V)* is also illustrated.

cerebellum, which functions as a coordination center for posture and movement (Fig. 20.19), and *(b)* the **pons,** which serves as the pathway for nerve fibers between the spinal cord and the cerebral and cerebellar cortices.

Each basal plate of the metencephalon (Fig. 20.18) contains three groups of motor neurons: *(a)* the medial **somatic efferent** group, which gives rise to the nucleus of the **abducens nerve;** *(b)* the **special visceral efferent** group, containing nuclei of the **trigeminal** and **facial nerves,** which innervate the musculature of the 1st and 2nd pharyngeal arches; and *(c)* the **general visceral efferent** group, whose axons supply the submandibular and sublingual glands.

The marginal layer of the basal plates of the metencephalon expands as it serves as a bridge for nerve fibers connecting the cerebral cortex and cerebellar cortex with the spinal cord. Hence, this portion of the metencephalon is known as the **pons.** In addition to nerve fibers, the pons contains the **pontine nuclei,** which originate in the alar plates of the metencephalon and myelencephalon (see the *arrow* in Fig. 20.18).

The alar plates of the metencephalon contain three groups of sensory nuclei: *(a)* a lateral **somatic afferent** group, which contains neurons **of the trigeminal nerve** and a small portion of the **vestibulocochlear complex,** *(b)* the **special visceral afferent** group, and *(c)* the **general visceral afferent** group (Fig. 20.18).

CEREBELLUM

The dorsolateral parts of the alar plates bend medially and form the **rhombic lips** (Fig. 20.17). In the caudal portion of the metencephalon the rhombic lips are widely separated, but immediately below the mesencephalon they approach each other in the midline (Fig. 20.19). As a result of a further deepening of the pontine flexure, the rhombic lips become compressed in a cephalo-caudal direction and form the **cerebellar plate** (Fig. 20.19). In a 12-week embryo this plate shows a small midline portion, the **vermis,** and two lateral portions, the **hemispheres.** A transverse fissure soon separates the **nodule** from the vermis and the lateral **flocculus** from the hemispheres (Fig. 20.19*B*). This **flocculonodular** lobe is phylogenetically the most primitive part of the cerebellum.

Initially, the **cerebellar plate** consists of neuroepithelial, mantle, and marginal layers (Fig. 20.20*A*). During further development, a number of cells formed by the neuroepithelium migrate to the surface of the cerebellum to form the **external granular layer.** Cells of this layer retain their ability to divide and form a proliferative zone on the surface of the cerebellum (Fig. 20.20, *B* and *C*).

In the 6th month of development, the external granular layer gives rise to various cell types. These cells migrate toward the differentiating Purkinje cells (Fig. 20.21) and give rise to **granule cells, basket cells,** and **stellate cells.** The cortex of the cerebellum, consisting of Purkinje cells, Golgi II neurons, and neurons produced by the external granular layer, reaches its definitive size after birth (Fig. 20.21*B*). The deep cerebellar nuclei, such as the **dentate nucleus,** reach their final position before birth (Fig. 20.20*D*).

MESENCEPHALON

The mesencephalon is morphologically the most primitive of the brain vesicles (Fig. 20.22). Each basal plate contains two groups of motor nuclei: *(a)* a medial **somatic efferent** group, represented by the **oculomotor** and **trochlear nerves,** which innervate the eye musculature; and *(b)* a small **general visceral efferent** group, represented by the **nucleus of Edinger-Westphal,** which innervates the **sphincter pupillary muscle** (Fig. 20.22*B*). The marginal layer of each basal plate enlarges and forms the **crus cerebri.** These crura serve as pathways for nerve fibers descending from the cerebral cortex to lower centers in the pons and spinal cord. Initially, the alar plates of the mesencephalon appear as two longitudinal elevations separated by a shallow midline depression (Fig. 20.22). With further development, a transverse groove divides each elevation into an **anterior** (superior) and a **posterior** (inferior) **colliculus** (Fig. 20.22*B*). The

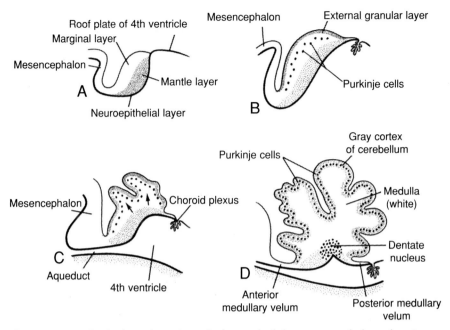

Figure 20.20. Sagittal sections through the roof of the metencephalon, showing development of the cerebellum. **A.** 8 weeks (approximately 30 mm). **B.** 12 weeks (70 mm). **C.** 13 weeks. **D.** 15 weeks. Note formation of the external granular layer on the surface of the cerebellar plate (**B** and **C**). During later stages, cells of the external granular layer migrate inward to mingle with Purkinje cells and thus form the definitive cortex of the cerebellum. The dentate nucleus is one of the deep cerebellar nuclei. Note the anterior and the posterior velum.

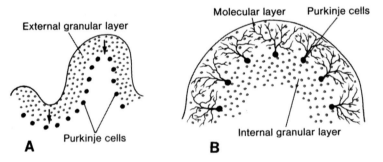

Figure 20.21. Diagrams of stages in development of the cerebellar cortex. **A.** The external granular layer located on the surface of the cerebellum forms a proliferative layer from which granule, basket, and stellate cells arise. They migrate inward from the surface as indicated by the *arrows.* **B.** Postnatal cerebellar cortex showing differentiated Purkinje cells, the molecular layer on the surface, and the internal granular layer beneath the Purkinje cells.

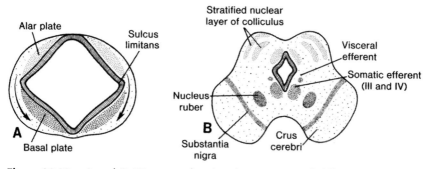

Figure 20.22. A and B. Diagrams showing the position and differentiation of the basal and alar plates in the mesencephalon at various stages of development. *Arrows in A indicate the path followed by cells of the alar plate to form the nucleus ruber and substantia nigra. Note the various motor nuclei in the basal plate.*

posterior colliculi serve as synaptic relay stations for auditory reflexes; the anterior colliculi function as correlation and reflex centers for visual impulses.

The colliculi are formed by waves of neuroblasts migrating into the overlying marginal zone. Here, they become arranged in stratified layers (Fig. 20.22*B*).

DIENCEPHALON

Roof Plate and Epiphysis

The diencephalon develops from the median portion of the prosencephalon (Figs. 20.5 and 20.16) and is thought to consist of a roof plate and two alar plates but to lack floor and basal plates. The roof plate of the diencephalon consists of a single layer of ependymal cells covered by vascular mesenchyme. The two combined give rise to the **choroid plexus** of the 3rd ventricle (Fig. 20.28). The most caudal part of the roof plate develops into the **pineal body** or **epiphysis.** This body initially appears as an epithelial thickening in the midline but by the 7th week begins to evaginate (Figs. 20.23 and 20.24). Eventually, it becomes a solid organ located on the roof of the mesencephalon (Fig. 20.28) and serves as a channel through which light and darkness affect endocrine and behavioral rhythms. In the adult, calcium is frequently deposited in the epiphysis, and it then serves as a landmark on an x-ray of the skull.

Alar Plate, Thalamus, and Hypothalamus

The alar plates form the lateral walls of the diencephalon. A groove, the **hypothalamic sulcus,** divides the plate into a dorsal and a ventral region, the **thalamus** and **hypothalamus,** respectively (Figs. 20.23 and 20.24).

As a result of proliferative activity, the thalamus gradually projects into the lumen of the diencephalon. Frequently, this expansion is so great that thalamic regions from the right and left sides fuse in the midline, thereby forming the **massa intermedia** or **interthalamic connexus.**

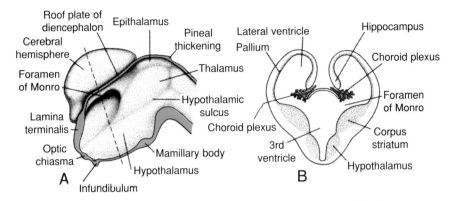

Figure 20.23. A. Diagram of the medial surface of the right half of the prosencephalon in a 7-week embryo. **B.** Transverse section through the prosencephalon at the level of the *broken line* in **A**. The corpus striatum bulges out in the floor of the lateral ventricle and the foramen of Monro.

The hypothalamus, forming the lower portion of the alar plate, differentiates into a number of nuclear areas, which serve as regulation centers of the visceral functions, including sleep, digestion, body temperature, and emotional behavior. One of these groups, the **mamillary body,** forms a distinct protuberance on the ventral surface of the hypothalamus on each side of the midline (Figs. 20.23*A* and 20.24*A*).

Hypophysis or Pituitary Gland

The hypophysis or pituitary gland develops from two completely different parts: *(a)* an ectodermal outpocketing of the stomodeum immediately in front of the buccopharyngeal membrane, known as **Rathke's pouch,** and *(b)* a downward extension of the diencephalon, the **infundibulum** (Fig. 20.25, *A* and *D*).

When the embryo is approximately 3 weeks old, Rathke's pouch appears as an evagination of the oral cavity and, subsequently, grows dorsally toward the infundibulum. By the end of the 2nd month, it loses its connection with the oral cavity and is then in close contact with the infundibulum.

During further development, cells in the anterior wall of Rathke's pouch increase rapidly in number and form the **anterior lobe of the hypophysis** or **adenohypophysis** (Fig. 20.25*B*). A small extension of this lobe, the **pars tuberalis,** grows along the stalk of the infundibulum and eventually surrounds it (Fig. 20.25*C*). The posterior wall of Rathke's pouch develops into the **pars intermedia,** which in humans seems to have little significance.

The infundibulum gives rise to the **stalk** and the **pars nervosa** or **posterior lobe of the hypophysis** (neurohypophysis) (Fig. 20.25*C*). It is composed of neuroglial cells. In addition, it contains a number of nerve fibers that come from the hypothalamic area.

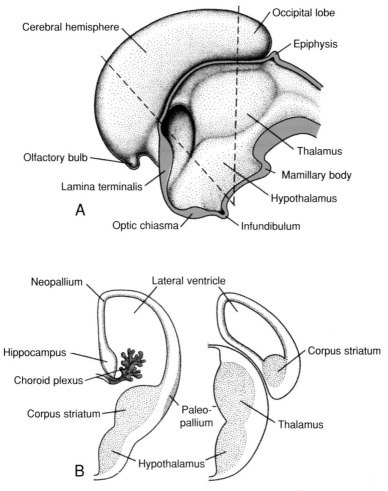

Figure 20.24. **A.** Diagram of the medial surface of the right half of the telencephalon and diencephalon in an 8-week embryo. **B** and **C.** Transverse sections through the right half of the telencephalon and diencephalon at the level of the *broken lines* in **A.**

CLINICAL CORRELATES

Occasionally, a small portion of Rathke's pouch persists in the roof of the pharynx as a **pharyngeal hypophysis.**

Craniopharyngiomas arise from remnants of Rathke's pouch. They may form within the sella turcica or along the stalk of the pituitary but are usually located above the sella. The may cause hydrocephalus and pituitary dysfunction (diabetes insipidus, growth failure, etc.).

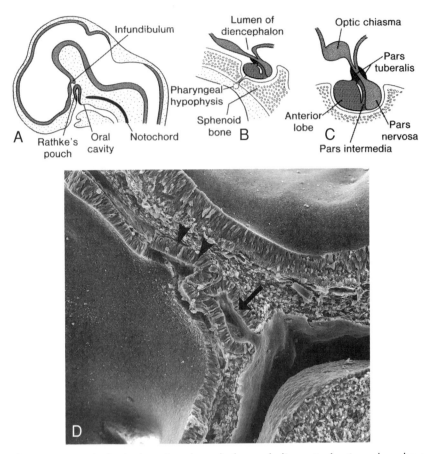

Figure 20.25. **A.** Sagittal section through the cephalic part of a 6-week embryo, showing Rathke's pouch as a dorsal outpocketing of the oral cavity and the infundibulum as a thickening in the floor of the diencephalon. **B** and **C.** Sagittal sections through the developing hypophysis in the 11th and 16th weeks of development, respectively. Note formation of the pars tuberalis encircling the stalk of the pars nervosa. **D.** High-magnification scanning electron micrograph of the region of the developing hypophysis similar to that in **A.** Rathke's pouch *(arrow)* and the infundibulum *(arrowheads)* are visible.

TELENCEPHALON

The telencephalon, the most rostral of the brain vesicles, consists of two lateral outpocketings, the **cerebral hemispheres,** and a median portion, the **lamina terminales** (Figs. 20.4, 20.5, 20.23, and 20.24). The cavities of the hemispheres, the **lateral ventricles,** communicate with the lumen of the diencephalon through the **interventricular foramina of Monro** (Fig. 20.23).

Cerebral Hemispheres

The cerebral hemispheres arise at the beginning of the 5th week of development as bilateral evaginations of the lateral wall of the prosencephalon (Fig.

20.23). By the middle of the 2nd month, the basal part of the hemispheres (i.e., the part that initially formed the forward extension of the thalamus) (Fig. 20.23*A*) begins to increase in size. As a result, this area bulges into the lumen of the lateral ventricle as well as into the floor of the foramen of Monro (Figs. 20.23*B* and 20.24, *A* and *B*). In transverse sections, the rapidly growing region has a striated appearance and is therefore known as the **corpus striatum** (Fig. 20.24*B*).

In the region where the wall of the hemisphere is attached to the roof of the diencephalon, it fails to develop neuroblasts and remains very thin (Fig. 20.23*B*). Here, the hemisphere wall consists of a single layer of ependymal cells covered by vascular mesenchyme, and together they form the **choroid plexus.** The choroid plexus should have formed the roof of the hemisphere, but as a result of the disproportionate growth of the various parts of the hemisphere, it protrudes into the lateral ventricle along a line known as the **choroidal fissure** (Figs. 20.24 and 20.26). Immediately above the choroidal fissure the wall of the hemisphere is thickened, thus forming the **hippocampus** (Figs. 20.23*B* and 20.24*B*). This structure, which mainly has an olfactory function, gradually bulges into the lateral ventricle.

With further expansion, the hemispheres cover the lateral aspect of the diencephalon, mesencephalon, and cephalic portion of the metencephalon (Figs. 20.23–20.28). The corpus striatum (Fig. 20.23*B*), being a part of the wall of the hemisphere, likewise expands posteriorly and is divided into two parts: *(a)* a dorsomedial portion, the **caudate nucleus,** and *(b)* a ventrolateral portion, the **lentiform nucleus** (Fig. 20.26*B*). This division is accomplished by axons passing to and from the cortex of the hemisphere and breaking through the nuclear mass of the corpus striatum. The fiber bundle thus formed is known as the **internal capsule** (Fig. 20.26*B*).

At the same time, the medial wall of the hemisphere and the lateral wall of the diencephalon fuse, and the caudate nucleus and thalamus come into close contact (Fig. 20.26*B*).

Continuous growth of the cerebral hemispheres in anterior, dorsal, and inferior directions results in the formation of frontal, temporal, and occipital lobes, respectively. As growth in the region overlying the corpus striatum slows, however, the area between the frontal and temporal lobes becomes depressed and is known as the **insula** (Fig. 20.27*A*). This region is later overgrown by the adjacent lobes and, at the time of birth, is almost completely covered. During the final part of fetal life, the surface of the cerebral hemispheres grows so rapidly that a great many convolutions (**gyri**) separated by fissures and sulci appear on its surface (Fig. 20.27*B*).

Cortex Development

The cerebral cortex develops from the pallium (Fig. 20.23), which may be divided into two regions: *(a)* the **paleopallium** or **archipallium,** an area located immediately lateral to the corpus striatum (Fig. 20.24*B*), and *(b)* the **neopallium,** between the hippocampus and the paleopallium (Figs. 20.24*B* and 20.26*B*).

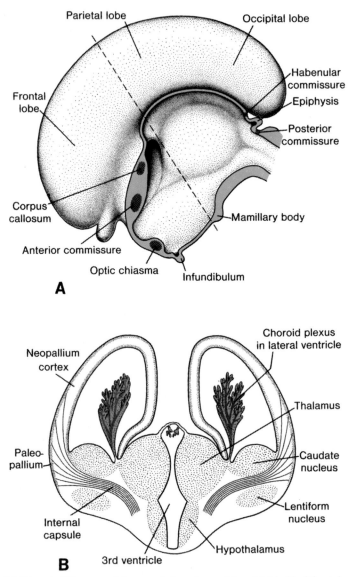

Figure 20.26. **A.** Diagram of the medial surface of the right half of the telencephalon and diencephalon in a 10-week embryo. **B.** Schematic transverse section through the hemisphere and diencephalon at the level of the *broken line* in **A.**

In the neopallium, waves of neuroblasts migrate to a subpial position and then differentiate into fully mature neurons. When the next wave of neuroblasts arrives, they migrate through the earlier formed layers of cells until they reach the subpial position. Hence, the early formed neuroblasts obtain a deep position in the cortex, while those formed at later times obtain a more superficial position.

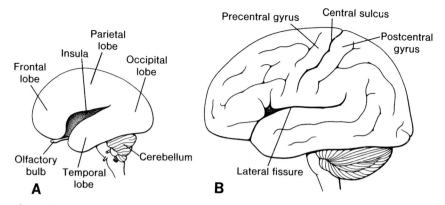

Figure 20.27. Schematic drawings to show development of gyri and sulci on the lateral surface of the cerebral hemisphere. **A.** 7 months. **B.** 9 months.

At birth, the cortex has a stratified appearance due to differentiation of the cells in different layers. The motor cortex contains a large number of **pyramidal cells,** and the sensory areas are characterized by **granular cells.**

Commissures

In the adult, the right and left halves of the hemispheres are connected by a number of fiber bundles, the **commissures,** which cross the midline. The most important fiber bundles make use of the **lamina terminalis** (Figs. 20.23, 20.26, and 20.28). The first of the crossing bundles to appear is the **anterior commissure.** It consists of fibers connecting the olfactory bulb and related brain areas of one hemisphere to those of the opposite side (Figs. 20.26 and 20.28).

The second commissure to appear is the **hippocampal** or **fornix commissure.** Its fibers arise in the hippocampus and converge on the lamina terminalis close to the roof plate of the diencephalon. From here, the fibers continue, forming an arching system immediately outside the choroid fissure, to the mamillary body and the hypothalamus.

The most important commissure is the **corpus callosum.** It appears by the 10th week of development and connects the nonolfactory areas of the right and the left cerebral cortex. Initially, it forms a small bundle in the lamina terminalis. As a result of continuous expansion of the neopallium, however, it extends first anteriorly and then posteriorly, thereby arching over the thin roof of the diencephalon (Fig. 20.28).

In addition to the three commissures developing in the lamina terminalis, three more appear. Two of these, the **posterior** and **habenular commissures,** are located just below and rostral to the stalk of the pineal gland. The third, the **optic chiasma,** appears in the rostral wall of the diencephalon and contains fibers from the medial halves of the retinae (Fig. 20.28).

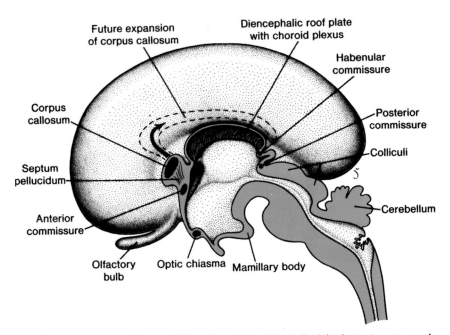

Figure 20.28. View of the medial surface of the right half of the brain in a 4-month embryo, showing the various commissures. *Broken line* indicates the future site of the corpus callosum. The hippocampal commissure is not indicated.

CLINICAL CORRELATES

Meningocele, meningoencephalocele, and **meningohydroencepha-locele** are all caused by an ossification defect in the bones of the skull. The most frequently affected bone is the squamous part of the occipital bone, which may be partially or totally lacking. If the opening of the occipital bone is small, only meninges bulge through it **(meningocele),** but if the defect is large, part of the brain and even part of the ventricle may penetrate through the opening into the meningeal sac (Figs. 20.29 and 20.30). The latter two malformations are known as **meningoen-cephalocele** and **meningohydroencephalocele,** respectively. These defects occur at a rate of 1 in 2000 births.

Exencephaly is characterized by failure of the cephalic part of the neural tube to close. As a result, the vault of the skull does not form, leaving the malformed brain exposed. Later, this tissue degenerates, leaving a mass of necrotic tissue. The defect is referred to as **anen-cephaly,** despite the fact that the brainstem remains intact (Fig. 20.31, *A* and *B*). Since the fetus lacks the mechanism for swallowing, the last 2 months of pregnancy are characterized by **hydramnios.** On an x-ray of the fetus, the abnormality can easily be recognized, since the vault

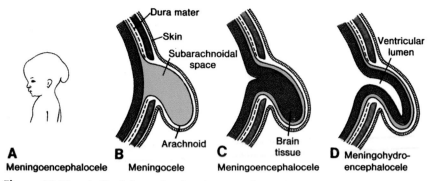

A Meningoencephalocele **B** Meningocele **C** Meningoencephalocele **D** Meningohydro-encephalocele

Dura mater
Skin
Subarachnoidal space
Arachnoid
Ventricular lumen
Brain tissue

Figure 20.29. A–D. Schematic drawings to show the various types of brain herniation due to abnormal ossification of the skull.

of the skull is absent. Anencephalus is a common abnormality (1:1000) and occurs 4 times more frequently in females than in males.

Hydrocephalus is characterized by an abnormal accumulation of cerebrospinal fluid within the ventricular system. In the majority of cases, hydrocephalus in the newborn is due to an obstruction of the **aqueduct of Sylvius (aqueductal stenosis).** This prevents the cerebrospinal fluid of the lateral and 3rd ventricles from passing into the 4th ventricle and from there into the subarachnoid space, where it would be resorbed. As a result, fluid accumulates in the lateral ventricles putting pressure on the brain and bones of the skull. Since the cranial sutures have not yet fused, spaces between them widen as the head expands. In extreme cases, brain tissue and bones become thin, and the head may be very large (Fig. 20.32).

The **Arnold-Chiari malformation** involves caudal displacement and herniation of cerebellar structures through the foramen magnum. The defect occurs in virtually every case of spina bifida cystica and is usually accompanied by hydrocephalus.

Microcephaly refers to a cranial vault that is smaller than normal (Fig. 20.33). Since the size of the cranium is dependent on growth of the brain, the underlying defect is in brain development. Etiology of the abnormality is varied and may be genetic (autosomal recessive) or due to prenatal insults such as infections or exposures to drugs and other teratogens. Impaired mental development occurs in more than half the cases.

The aforementioned abnormalities are, obviously, the most serious ones and may be incompatible with life. A great many other defects of the CNS may occur, however, without much external manifestation. For example, the **corpus callosum** may be partially or completely absent without much functional disturbance. Likewise, partial or

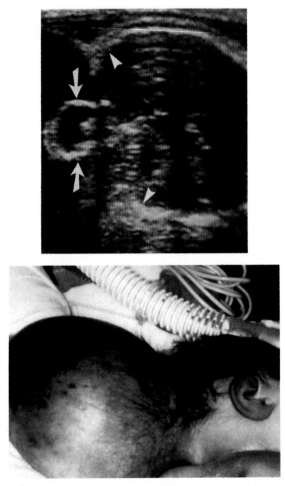

Figure 20.30. Ultrasonogram **(top)** and photograph **(bottom)** of a child with a meningoencephalocele. The defect was detected by ultrasound in the 7th month of gestation and repaired after birth. On ultrasound, brain tissue *(arrows)* can be visualized extending through the bony defect in the skull *(arrowheads)*.

complete absence of the cerebellum may result in only a slight disturbance of coordination. On the other hand, cases of severe **mental retardation** may not be associated with morphologically detectable brain abnormalities. Mental retardation may result from genetic abnormalities (e.g., Down and Klinefelter syndromes) or from exposures to teratogens, including infectious agents (rubella, cytomegalovirus, toxoplasmosis). The leading cause of mental retardation is, however, **maternal alcohol abuse.**

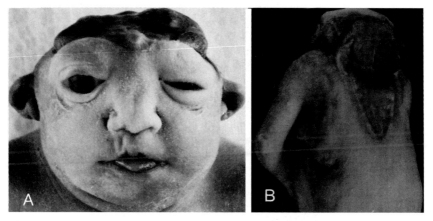

Figure 20.31. **A.** Photograph of an anencephalic child, ventral view. This abnormality occurs frequently (1:1000 births). Usually, the child dies a few days after birth. **B.** Photograph of an anencephalic child with spina bifida in the cervical and thoracic segments, dorsal view.

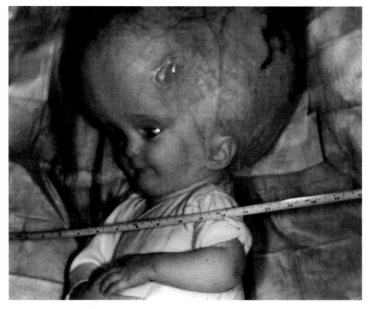

Figure 20.32. Photograph of a child with severe hydrocephalus. Since the cranial sutures had not closed, pressure from the accumulated cerebrospinal fluid enlarged the head, thinning the bones of the skull and cerebral cortex.

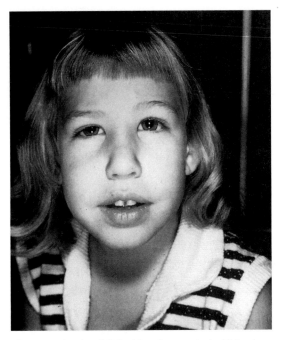

Figure 20.33. Photograph of a child with microcephaly. This abnormality is due to decreased growth of the brain and is frequently associated with mental retardation.

Fetal infection by toxoplasmosis may result in cerebral calcification, mental retardation, hydrocephalus, or microcephaly. Likewise, exposure to radiation during the early stages of development may produce microcephaly. Hyperthermia produced by maternal infections or by sauna baths may cause spina bifida and exencephaly.

CRANIAL NERVES

By the 4th week of development, nuclei for all 12 cranial nerves are present. All except the olfactory (I) and optic (II) nerves arise from the brainstem, and of these only the oculomotor (III) arises outside the region of the hindbrain. In the hindbrain, proliferation centers in the neuroepithelium establish eight distinct segments known as rhombomeres. Pairs of rhombomeres give rise to motor nuclei of cranial nerves IV, V, VI, VII, IX, X, XI, and XII (Figs. 20.16 and 20.34). Establishment of this segmental pattern appears to be directed by mesoderm collected into somitomeres beneath the overlying neuroepithelium.

Motor neurons for cranial nuclei are located within the brainstem, while sensory ganglia are located outside the brain. Thus, the organization of cranial nerves is homologous to spinal nerves, although not all cranial nerves contain both motor and sensory fibers (see Table 20.1).

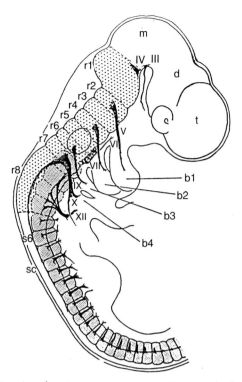

Figure 20.34. Drawing showing segmentation patterns in the brain and mesoderm that appear by the 25th day of development. The hindbrain *(coarse stipple)* is divided into 8 rhombomeres *(r1–r8)*, and pairs of these structures give rise to the motor nerves. Mesoderm segmentation precedes that in the brain. Thus, somitomeres form along the brain, and somites *(fine stipple)* form along the spinal cord *(sc)*. *b1–b4*, pharyngeal arches; *d*, diencephalon; *m*, mesencephalon; *s6*, somite 6; and *t*, telencephalon.

The origin of cranial nerve sensory ganglia is from **ectodermal placodes** and **neural crest cells.** Ectodermal placodes include the nasal, otic, and four **epibranchial placodes** represented by ectodermal thickenings dorsal to the pharyngeal (branchial) arches (see Fig. 16.2 and Table 20.2). Epibranchial placodes contribute to ganglia for nerves of the pharyngeal arches (V, VII, IX, and X). Parasympathetic (visceral efferent) ganglia are derived from neural crest cells, and their fibers are carried by cranial nerves III, VII, IX, and X (see Table 20.1).

Autonomic Nervous System

Functionally, the autonomic nervous system can be divided into two parts: a **sympathetic** portion, which is localized in the thoracolumbar region, and a **parasympathetic** portion, found in the cephalic and sacral regions.

Table 20.1.
Origins of Cranial Nerves and Their Composition

Brain Region	Cranial Nerve	Composition
Telencephalon	Olfactory (I)	Sensory
Diencephalon	Optic (II)	Sensory
Mesencephalon	Oculomotor (III)	Motor and parasympathetic
Metencephalon	Trochlear (IV) (finally located in the mesencephalon)	Motor
	Trigeminal (V) (sensory ganglia arise in the metencephalon and myelencephalon, but a portion later becomes located in the mesencephalon)	Sensory and motor
	Abducens (VI)	Motor
	Facial (VII)	Sensory, motor, and parasympathetic
	Vestibulocochlear (VIII)	Sensory
Myelencephalon	Glossopharyngeal (IX)	Sensory, motor, and parasympathetic
	Vagus (X)	Sensory, motor, and parasympathetic
	Accessory (XI)	Motor
	Hypoglossal (XII)	Motor

SYMPATHETIC NERVOUS SYSTEM

In the 5th week of development, cells originating in the **neural crest** of the thoracic region migrate on each side of the spinal cord toward the region immediately behind the dorsal aorta (Fig. 20.35). Here, they form a bilateral chain of segmentally arranged sympathetic ganglia interconnected by longitudinal nerve fibers. Together, they form the sympathic chains located on each side of the vertebral column. From their position in the thorax, neuroblasts migrate toward the cervical and lumbosacral regions, thus extending the sympathetic chains to their full length. Although, initially, the ganglia are arranged segmentally, this arrangement is later obscured, particularly in the cervical region, by fusion of the ganglia.

Some sympathetic neuroblasts migrate in front of the aorta to form **preaortic ganglia,** such as the **celiac** and **mesenteric** ganglia. Other sympathetic cells migrate to the heart, lungs, and gastrointestinal tract, where they give rise to **sympathetic organ plexuses** (Fig. 20.35).

Once the sympathetic chains have been established, nerve fibers originating in the **visceroefferent column (intermediate horn)** of the thoracolumbar segments of the spinal cord penetrate the ganglia of the chain (Fig. 20.36). Some of these nerve fibers synapse at the same levels in the sympathetic chains or pass through the chains to **preaortic** or **collateral ganglia** (Fig. 20.36). They are known as **preganglionic fibers,** have a myelin sheath, and stimulate the sympathetic ganglion cells. Passing from spinal nerves to the sympathetic ganglia, they form

Table 20.2.
Contributions of Neural Crest Cells and Placodes to Ganglia of the Cranial Nerves

Nerve	Ganglion	Origin
Oculomotor (III)	Ciliary (visceral efferent)	Neural crest at the forebrain-midbrain junction
Trigeminal (V)	Trigeminal (general afferent)	Neural crest at the forebrain-midbrain junction and the trigeminal placode
Facial (VII)	Superior (general and special afferent)	Hindbrain neural crest and 1st epibranchial placode
	Inferior (geniculate) (general and special afferent)	1st epibranchial placode
	Sphenopalatine (visceral efferent)	Hindbrain neural crest
	Submandibular (visceral efferent)	Hindbrain neural crest
Vestibulocochlear (VIII)	Acoustic (cochlear) (special afferent)	Otic placode
	Vestibular (special afferent)	Otic placode and hindbrain neural crest
Glossopharyngeal (IX)	Superior (general and special afferent)	Hindbrain neural crest
	Inferior (petrosal) (general and special afferent)	2nd epibranchial placode
	Otic (visceral efferent)	Hindbrain neural crest
Vagus (X)	Superior (general afferent)	Hindbrain neural crest
	Inferior (nodose) (general and special afferent)	Hindbrain neural crest and 3rd and 4th epibranchial placodes
	Vagal parasympathetic (visceral efferent)	Hindbrain neural crest

the so-called **white communicating rami.** Since the visceroefferent column extends only from the 1st thoracic to the 2nd or 3rd lumbar segment of the spinal cord, white rami are found only at these levels.

Axons of the sympathetic ganglion cells are called **postganglionic fibers** and have no myelin sheath. They pass either to other levels of the sympathetic chain or extend to the heart, lungs, and intestinal tract (*broken lines* in Fig. 20.36). Other fibers known as **gray communicating rami** pass from the sympathetic chain to spinal nerves and from there to peripheral blood vessels, hair, and sweat glands. Gray communicating rami are found at all levels of the spinal cord.

Suprarenal Gland

The suprarenal gland develops from two components: (*a*) a mesodermal portion, which forms the **cortex,** and (*b*) an ectodermal portion, which forms the **medulla.**

During the 5th week of development, mesothelial cells located between the root of the mesentery and the developing gonad begin to proliferate and penetrate

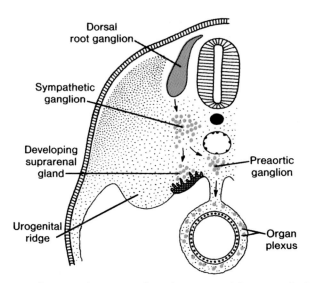

Figure 20.35. Schematic drawing to show formation of the sympathetic ganglia. A portion of the sympathetic neuroblasts migrates toward the proliferating mesothelium to form the medulla of the suprarenal gland.

the underlying mesenchyme (Fig. 20.35). Here, they differentiate into large acidophilic organs, which form the **fetal** or **primitive cortex** of the suprarenal gland (Fig. 20.37A). Shortly afterward, a second wave of cells from the mesothelium penetrates the mesenchyme and surrounds the original acidophilic cell mass. These cells, smaller than those of the first wave, later form the **definitive cortex** of the gland (Fig. 20.37, A and B). After birth, the fetal cortex regresses rapidly except for its outermost layer, which differentiates into the reticular zone. The adult structure of the cortex is not achieved until puberty.

While the fetal cortex is being formed, cells originating in the sympathetic system **(neural crest cells)** invade its medial aspect, where they become arranged in cords and clusters. These cells give rise to the medulla of the suprarenal gland. They stain yellow-brown with chrome salts and, hence, are called **chromaffin cells** (Fig. 20.37). During embryonic life, chromaffin cells are scattered widely throughout the embryo, but in the adult the only persisting group is located in the medulla of the adrenal glands.

PARASYMPATHETIC NERVOUS SYSTEM

Neurons located in the brainstem and the sacral region of the spinal cord give rise to **preganglionic parasympathetic fibers.** Fibers from nuclei in the brainstem travel via the **oculomotor (III), facial (VII), glossopharyngeal (IX),** and **vagus (X) nerves.** Postganglionic fibers arise from neurons (ganglia) derived from **neural crest cells** and pass to the structures they innervate (pupil of the eye, salivary glands, viscera, etc.).

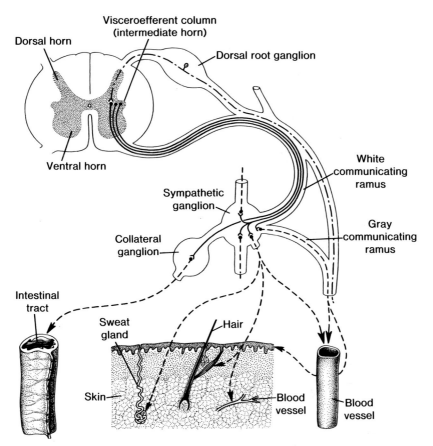

Figure 20.36. Schematic drawing to show the relationship of the preganglionic and postganglionic nerve fibers of the sympathetic nervous system to the spinal nerves. Note the origin of preganglionic fibers in the visceroefferent column of the spinal cord.

CLINICAL CORRELATES

Congenital megacolon (Hirschsprung's disease) results from a failure of neural crest cells to migrate into the wall of part or all of the colon and rectum. Consequently, no parasympathetic ganglia form in affected areas. The rectum is involved in nearly all cases, and the rectum and sigmoid are involved in 80% of affected infants. The transverse and ascending portions of the colon are involved in only 10–20%. The colon is dilated above the affected region, which has a small diameter due to tonic contraction of noninnervated vasculature.

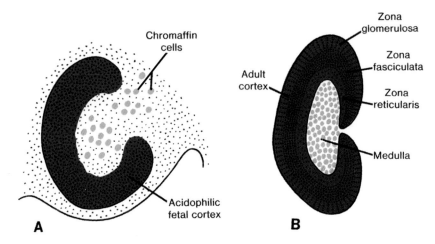

Figure 20.37. **A.** Drawing showing chromaffin (sympathetic) cells penetrating the fetal cortex of the suprarenal gland. **B.** At a later stage of development, the definitive cortex surrounds the medulla almost completely.

SUMMARY

The CNS is of ectodermal origin and appears as the **neural plate** at the middle of the 3rd week (Fig. 20.1). After the edges of the plate become folded, the **neural folds** approach each other in the midline to fuse into the **neural tube** (Figs. 20.2 and 20.3). The cranial end closes approximately at day 25, and the caudal end closes at day 27. The CNS then forms a tubular structure with a broad cephalic portion, the **brain,** and a long caudal portion, the **spinal cord.** Failure of the neural tube to close results in defects such as **spina bifida** (Figs. 20.14 and 20.15) and **anencephaly** (Figs. 20.29–20.31).

The **spinal cord** forms the caudal end of the CNS and is characterized by the **basal plate** containing the **motor neurons,** the **alar plate** for the **sensory neurons,** and a **floor** and a **roof** plate as connecting plates between the two sides (Fig. 20.8). These same basic features can also be recognized throughout most of the brain vesicles. The **brain** forms the cranial part of the CNS and consists originally of three vesicles: the rhombencephalon (hindbrain), mesencephalon (midbrain), and prosencephalon (forebrain).

The **rhombencephalon** is divided into *(a)* the myelencephalon, which forms the **medulla oblongata** [this region has a basal plate for somatic and visceral efferent neurons and an alar plate for somatic and visceral afferent neurons (Fig. 20.17)], and *(b)* the **metencephalon** with its typical basal (efferent) and alar (afferent) plates (Fig. 20.18). This brain vesicle is, in addition, characterized by formation of the **cerebellum** (Fig. 20.19), a coordination center for posture and movement, and the **pons,** the pathway for nerve fibers between the spinal cord and the cerebral and the cerebellar cortices (Fig. 20.18).

The **mesencephalon** or **midbrain** is the most primitive brain vesicle and most resembles the spinal cord with its basal efferent and alar afferent plates. Its alar plates form the inferior and posterior colliculi as relay stations for auditory and visual reflex centers (Fig. 20.22).

The **diencephalon,** the posterior portion of the forebrain, consists of a thin roof plate and a thick alar plate in which the **thalamus** and **hypothalamus** develop (Figs. 20.23 and 20.24). It participates in formation of the pituitary gland, which also develops from Rathke's pouch (Fig. 20.25). Whereas Rathke's pouch forms the **adenohypophysis,** the **intermediate lobe,** and **pars tuberalis,** the diencephalon forms the **posterior lobe,** the **neurohypophysis,** which contains neuroglia and receives nerve fibers from the hypothalamus.

The **telencephalon,** the most rostral of the brain vesicles, consists of two lateral outpocketings, the **cerebral hemispheres,** and a median portion, the **lamina terminalis** (Fig. 20.26). The lamina terminalis is used by the commissures as a connection pathway for fiber bundles between the right and left hemispheres (Fig. 20.28). The cerebral hemispheres, originally two small outpocketings (Figs. 20.23 and 20.24), expand and cover the lateral aspect of the diencephalon, mesencephalon, and metencephalon (Figs. 20.25–20.27). Eventually, nuclear regions of the telencephalon come in close contact with those of the diencephalon (Fig. 20.26).

The ventricular system, containing cerebrospinal fluid, extends from the lumen in the spinal cord to the 4th ventricle in the rhombencephalon, through the narrow duct in the mesencephalon, and subsequently to the 3rd ventricle in the diencephalon. By way of the foramina of Monro, the ventricular system extends from the 3rd ventricle into the lateral ventricles of the cerebral hemispheres. Cerebrospinal fluid is produced in the choroid plexus of the 3rd, 4th, and lateral ventricles. Blockage of cerebrospinal fluid in the ventricular system or subarachnoid space may lead to hydrocephalus.

PROBLEMS TO SOLVE

1. How are cranial nerves and spinal nerves similar? How are they different?

2. At what level is a spinal tap performed? From an embryological standpoint, why is this possible?

3. What is the embryological basis for most neural tube defects? Can they be diagnosed prenatally? Are there any means of prevention?

4. Prenatal ultrasound revealed an infant with an enlarged head with expansion of both lateral ventricles. What is this condition called, and what might have caused it?

SUGGESTED READINGS

Bell JE: The pathology of central nervous system defects in human fetuses of different gestational ages. *Adv Study Birth Defects* 7, 1982.
D'Amico-Martel A: Contributions of placodal and neural crest cells to avian cranial peripheral ganglia. *Am J Anat* 166:445, 1983.

Geelen JAG, Langman J: Closure of the neural tube in the cephalic region of the mouse embryo. *Anat Rec* 189:625, 1977.

Hinrichsen K, Mestres P, Jacob HJ: Morphological aspects of the pharyngeal hypophysis in human embryos. *Acta Morphol Neerl-Scand* 24:235, 1986.

Langman J: Histogenesis of the central nervous system. *In* Bourne GH (ed): *The Structure and Function of Nervous Tissue.* New York, Academic Press, 1968.

Langman J, Geurrant RJ, Freeman BG: Behavior of neuroepithelial cells during closure of the neural tube. *J Comp Neurol* 127:399, 1966.

LeDouarin N, Fontaine-Perus J, Couly G: Cephalic ectodermal placodes and neurogenesis. *Trends Neurosci* 9:175, 1986.

LeDouarin N, Smith J: Development of the peripheral nervous system from the neural crest. *Annu Rev Cell Biol* 4:375, 1988.

Lemire RJ, Loeser JD, Leech RW, Alvord EC: *Normal and Abnormal Development of the Human Nervous System.* New York, Harper & Row, 1975.

Loggie JMH: Growth and development of the autonomic nervous system. *In* Davis JA, Dobbing J (eds): *Scientific Foundations of Pediatrics.* Philadelphia, WB Saunders, 1974.

Lumsden A, Keynes R: Segmental patterns of neuronal development in the chick hindbrain. *Nature (Lond)* 337:424, 1989.

Lumsden A, Sprawson N, Graham A: Segmental origin and migration of neural crest cells in the hindbrain region of the chick embryo. *Development* 113:1281, 1991.

Muller F, O'Rahilly R: Development of anencephaly and its variants. *Am J Anat* 190:193, 1991.

Muller F, O'Rahilly R: The development of the human brain and the closure of the rostral neuropore at stage 11. *Anat Embryol* 175:205, 1986.

Muller F, O'Rahilly R: The development of the human brain from a closed neural tube at stage 13. *Anat Embryol* 177:203, 1986.

Muller F, O'Rahilly R: The first appearance of the future cerebral hemispheres of the human embryo at stage 14. *Anat Embryol* 177:495, 1988.

Noden DM: The control of the avian cephalic neural crest cytodifferentiation. I. Skeletal and connective tissues. *Dev Biol* 67:296, 1978.

O'Rahilly R, Muller F: The first appearance of the human nervous system at stage 8. *Acta Embryol* 163:1, 1981.

O'Rahilly R, Muller F: The meninges in human development. *J Neuropathol Exp Neurol* 45:588, 1986.

Rodier PM, Reynolds SS, Roberts WN: Behavioral consequences of interference with CNS development in the early fetal period. *Teratology* 19:327, 1979.

Sakai Y: Neurulation in the mouse. I. The ontogenesis of neural segments and the determination of topographical regions in a central nervous system. *Anat Rec* 218:450, 1987.

Schoenwolf G: On the morphogenesis of the early rudiments of the developing central nervous system. *Scanning Electron Microsc* 1:289, 1982.

Schoenwolf G, Smith JL: Mechanisms of neurulation: traditional viewpoint and recent advances. *Development* 109:243, 1990.

Waterman RE: Topographical changes along the neural fold associated with neurulation in the hamster and the mouse. *Am J Anat* 146:151, 1976.

PART III

Appendix

Answers to Problems

Chapter 1

1. The most common cause for abnormal chromosome number is nondisjunction during either meiosis or mitosis. For unknown reasons, chromosomes fail to separate during cell division. Nondisjunction during meiosis I or II results in one-half of the gametes with no copy and one-half with two copies of a chromosome. If fertilization occurs between a gamete lacking a chromosome and a normal one, then monosomy results; if it occurs between a gamete with two copies and a normal one, then trisomy results. Trisomy 21 is the most common numerical abnormality resulting in birth defects (mental retardation, abnormal facies, heart malformations), is usually due to nondisjunction in the mother, and occurs more frequently in women over age 35, reflecting the fact that the risk of meiotic nondisjunction increases with increasing maternal age. Other trisomies that result in syndromes of abnormal development involve chromosomes 8, 9, 13, and 18. Monosomies involving autosomal chromosomes are fatal, whereas monosomy of the X chromosome (Turner syndrome) is compatible with life. This condition is usually (80%) a result of nondisjunction during meiosis of paternal chromosomes and is characterized by infertility, short stature, webbing of the neck, and other defects. Karyotyping of embryonic cells obtained by amniocentesis or chorionic villus biopsy (see under "Clinical Correlates" in Chapter 6) can detect chromosome abnormalities prenatally.

2. Chromosome breaks forming pieces of chromosomes that may create partial monosomies or trisomies or may become attached (translocated) to other chromosomes may occur. Translocation of part of chromosome 21 onto chromosome 14, for example, accounts for approximately 4% of cases of Down syndrome. Chromosomes may also be altered by mutations in single genes. The risk of chromosomal abnormalities is increased by advanced maternal and paternal age (over 35).

3. Mosaicism is a condition in which an individual has two or more cell lines that are derived from a single zygote but that have different genetic characteristics. The different cell lines may arise by mutation or by mitotic nondisjunction during cleavage, as in some cases of Down syndrome.

Chapter 2

1. Infertility occurs in approximately 20% of married couples. In women, a major cause of infertility is blockage of the uterine (fallopian) tubes due to scarring from repeated pelvic inflammatory disease; in men, the primary cause is low sperm count. In vitro fertilization (**IVF**) techniques can circumvent these problems, although the success rate (approximately 20%) is low.

2. Pelvic inflammatory diseases, such as gonorrhea, are a major cause of occluded oviducts (uterine tubes). Although the patient may be cured, scarring closes the lumen of the tubes and prevents passage of sperm to the oocyte and of oocytes to the uterine cavity. IVF can overcome the difficulty by fertilizing the woman's oocytes in culture and transferring them to her uterus for implantation. The alternative programs, **gamete intrafallopian transfer (GIFT)** and zygote intrafallopian transfer (ZIFT), would not be possibilities, since both techniques require patent uterine tubes.

Chapter 3

1. It is not clear why the conceptus is not rejected by the maternal system, but it may be that transplantation antigens are absent from the syncytiotrophoblast or that trophoblast cells are resistant to killer cells. In some cases, maternal immunological responses do adversely affect pregnancy, as, for example, in some cases of autoimmune disease. Thus, patients with systemic lupus erythematosus (SLE) have poor reproductive outcomes and histories of multiple spontaneous abortions. It has not been conclusively shown, however, that maternal antibodies can cause birth defects.

2. In some cases, trophoblastic tissue is the only tissue present in the uterus, and embryo-derived cells are either absent or present in small numbers. Such a condition is termed a hydatidiform mole, which, because of its trophoblastic origin, secretes human chorionic gonadotropin (hCG) and mimics the initial stages of pregnancy. Most moles are aborted early in pregnancy, but those containing remnants of an embryo may remain into the 2nd trimester. If pieces of trophoblast are left behind following spontaneous abortion or surgical removal of a mole, then cells may continue to proliferate and form tumors known as invasive moles or as choriocarcinoma. Since early trophoblast development is controlled by paternal genes, it is thought that the origin of moles may be from fertilization of an ovum without a nucleus.

3. The most likely diagnosis is an ectopic pregnancy in the uterine tube, which can be confirmed by ultrasound. Implantation in a uterine tube is due to poor transport of the zygote and may be a result of scarring. As with Down syndrome, the frequency of ectopic pregnancy increases with maternal age over 35.

Chapter 4

1. Unfortunately, consuming large quantities of alcohol at any stage during pregnancy may adversely affect embryonic development. In this case, the woman has exposed the embryo during the 3rd week of gestation (assuming that fertilization occurred at the midpoint of the menstrual cycle) at the time of gastrulation. This stage is particularly vulnerable to insult by alcohol and may result in fetal alcohol syndrome (mental retardation, abnormal facies; see Chapter 8). Although the condition is more common in offspring from alcoholics, no *safe* levels of blood alcohol concentration have been established for embryogenesis. Therefore, since alcohol causes birth defects and is the leading cause of mental retardation, it is recommended that women who are planning a pregnancy or who are already pregnant refrain from use of any alcohol.

2. Such a mass is probably a sacrococcygeal teratoma. These tumors arise as remnants of the primitive streak and usually occur in the sacral region. The term, teratoma, refers to the fact that the tumor contains different types of tissues. Since it is derived from the streak, which contains cells for all three germ layers, it may contain tissues of ectoderm, mesoderm, or endoderm origin. Such tumors are 3 times more common in females than males.

3. The baby has a severe form of caudal dysgenesis called sirenomelia (mermaid-like). Varying degrees of the malformations exist and are probably due to abnormalities in gastrulation in caudal segments. Initially termed caudal regression, it is clear that structures do not regress; they simply do not form. Also, known as caudal agenesis and sacral agenesis, the syndrome is characterized by varying degrees of flexion, inversion, lateral rotation, and occasional fusion of the lower limbs; defects in lumbar and sacral vertebrae; renal agenesis; imperforate anus; and agenesis of internal genital structures except the testes and ovaries. The etiology of the syndrome is unknown. The syndrome occurs sporadically but is most frequently observed among infants of diabetic mothers.

Chapter 5

1. The 3rd to 8th weeks of development are critical because this is the time when cell populations responsible for organ formation are established and when organ primordia are being formed. Early in the 3rd week, gastrulation begins to provide cells that comprise the three germ layers responsible for organogenesis. Late in the 3rd week, differentiation of the central nervous system is initiated, and over the next 5 weeks, all the primordia for the major organ systems will be established. At these times, cells are rapidly proliferating, and critical cell-cell signals are occurring. These phenomena are particularly sensitive to disruption by outside factors such as environmental hazards, pharmaceutical agents, and drugs of abuse. Thus, exposure to such factors may result in abnormalities known as birth defects or congenital malformations.

Chapter 6

1. Neural tube defects, such as spina bifida and anencephaly, produce elevated α-fetoprotein (AFP) levels, as do abdominal defects such as gastroschisis and omphalocele. Maternal serum AFP levels will also be elevated and may be used as a prescreen to be confirmed by amniocentesis. Ultrasonography is utilized to confirm the diagnosis.

2. Since Down syndrome is a chromosomal abnormality resulting most commonly from trisomy 21 (see Chapter 8), cells for chromosomal analysis can be collected by amniocentesis or chorionic villus biopsy (CVS). CVS has the advantage that sufficient cells can be obtained immediately to do the analysis, whereas cells collected by amniocentesis, which is not usually done prior to 14 weeks gestation, must be cultured for approximately 2 weeks to obtain sufficient numbers. The risk of fetal loss following CVS is 1%, which is about twofold higher than that occurring with amniocentesis.

3. Status of the fetus is critical for managing pregnancy, delivery, and postnatal care. Size, age, and position are important for determining the time and mode of delivery. Knowing whether or not birth defects are present is important for planning postnatal care. Tests for determining fetal status are dictated by maternal history and factors that increase risk, such as exposure to teratogens, chromosome abnormalities in either parent, advanced maternal age, or the birth of a previous infant with a birth defect.

Chapter 7

1. An excess of amniotic fluid is called hydramnios or polyhydramnios, and many times (35%) the cause is unknown (idiopathic). A higher incidence (25%), however, is associated with maternal diabetes and with birth defects that interfere with fetal swallowing, such as esophageal atresia and anencephaly.

2. No. She is not correct. The placenta does not act as a complete barrier, and many compounds cross freely, especially lipophilic substances such as toluene and alcohol. Furthermore, during early stages of pregnancy, the placenta has not completed its development, and the embryo is particularly vulnerable. These early weeks are also very sensitive to insult by compounds such as toluene, which causes the toluene embryopathy.

Chapter 8

1. Factors that influence the action of a teratogen are *(a)* genotype of the mother and conceptus, *(b)* dose and duration of exposure to the agent, and *(c)* stage of embryogenesis when exposure occurs. Most major malformations are produced during the embryonic period (teratogenic period) that occurs during the 3rd to 8th weeks of gestation. However, stages prior to this time, including the preimplantation period, and after the 8th week (fetal period) remain susceptible. The brain, for example, remains sensitive to insult throughout the fetal period. Thus, no stage of pregnancy is completely free of risk from teratogenic insult.

2. The woman is correct that drugs may be teratogenic. Severe hyperthermia such as this, however, is known to cause neural tube defects (spina bifida and anencephaly at this stage of gestation). Therefore, one must weigh the risks of the potential teratogenicity of an antipyretic agent with a low teratogenic potential, such as aspirin (in low doses), and the risk of hyperthermia. Interestingly, malformations have been associated with sauna-induced hyperthermia. No information about exercise-induced hyperthermia and birth defects is available, but strenuous physical activity (running marathons) raises body temperature significantly and probably should be avoided during pregnancy.

3. Yes, women over age 35 are at greater risk for having a malformed child. The defects are caused by chromosomal abnormalities such as trisomy 21 (Down syndrome) and can be detected by chromosome analysis from cells collected by chorionic villus biopsy or amniocentesis.

4. The woman's concerns are valid, since infants of insulin-dependent diabetic mothers have an increased incidence of birth defects, including a broad spectrum of minor and major anomalies. Placing the mother under strict metabolic control using multiple insulin injections prior to conception, however, significantly reduces the incidence of abnormalities and affords the greatest opportunity for a normal pregnancy. A similar scenario occurs with women who have phenylketonuria (PKU). In these patients, strict management of their disease prior to conception virtually eliminates the risk of congenital defects occurring in the offspring. Both situations stress the need for planning pregnancies and for avoiding potential teratogenic exposures, especially during the first 8 weeks of gestation, when most defects are produced.

Chapter 9

1. Cranial sutures are fibrous regions between flat bones of the skull. Membranous regions between the flat bones are known as fontanelles, the largest of which is the anterior fontanelle (soft spot). These sutures and fontanelles permit *(a)* molding of the head as it passes through the birth canal and *(b)* growth of the brain. Growth of the skull continues postnatally as the brain enlarges, and is greatest during the first 2 years of life. Premature closure of one or more sutures (craniosynostosis) results in deformities in the shape of the head, depending on which sutures are involved. Craniosynostosis is often associated with other skeletal defects, and evidence suggests that genetic factors are important in the etiology.

2. Defects of the long bones and digits are often associated with other malformations and should serve as a clue to conduct a thorough examination on all systems. Clusters of defects that occur simultaneously with a common etiology are called syndromes, and limb anomalies, especially of the radius and digits, are common components of such clusters. Diagnosis of syndromes is important in determining recurrence risks and, thus, in counseling parents about subsequent pregnancies.

3. Vertebral formation is a complex process involving growth and fusion of the caudal portion of one sclerotome with the cranial portion of an adjacent one. Not surprisingly, mistakes occur resulting in fusions and increases and decreases in the number of vertebrae (Klippel-Feil syndrome). In some cases, only half a vertebra forms (hemivertebra), resulting in asymmetry and lateral curvature of the spine (scoliosis). Scoliosis may also be caused by weakness of muscles of the back.

Chapter 10

1. Partial or complete absence of the pectoralis major muscle is the most likely diagnosis, and the defect is known as Poland anomaly. Absence of the muscle is often associated with shortness of the middle digits (brachydactyly) and digital fusion (syndactyly). Loss of the pectoralis major muscle produces little or no loss of function, since other muscles compensate.

2. Patterning for muscles is dependent on connective tissue that forms from fibroblasts. In the head, with its complicated pattern of muscles of facial expression, patterning is directed by neural crest cells; in cervical and occipital regions, it is directed by connective tissue from somites; and in the body wall and limbs, it is directed by somatic mesoderm.

Chapter 11

1. Failure of the left pleuroperitoneal membrane to close the pericardioperitoneal canal on that side is responsible for the defect. This canal is larger on the left than on the right, closes later, and, therefore, may be more susceptible to abnormalities. The degree of hypoplasia of the lungs, resulting from compression by abdominal viscera, determines the fate of the infant. Treatment requires surgical repair of the defect, and attempts to correct the malformation in utero have been made.

2. The defect is an omphalocele and arises from a failure of loops of bowel, which normally herniate during the 6th week (physiological herniation), to return to the abdominal cavity during the 10th week (see Chapter 14). The defect is associated with other major malformations and chromosomal abnormalities.

Chapter 12

1. In ultrasound scans of the heart, a four-chambered view is sought. The chambers are divided by the atrial septum superiorly, the ventricular septum inferiorly, and the endocardial cushions surrounding the atrioventricular canals laterally. Together, these structures form a cross whose integrity is readily visualized by ultrasound. In this case, however, the fetus probably has a ventricular septal defect (VSD), the most commonly occurring heart malformation, in the membranous portion of the septum. The integrity of the great vessels should also be checked carefully, since the conotruncal septum that divides the aortic and pulmonary channels must contact the region of the membranous portion of the interventricular septum in order for this structure to develop normally.

2. Since neural crest cells contribute to much of the development of the face and to the truncal portion of the conotruncal septum, these cells have probably been disrupted. Crest cells may have failed to migrate to these regions, failed to proliferate, or been killed. Retinoic acid (vitamin A) is a potent teratogen that targets neural crest cells among other cell populations. Since retinoids are effective in treating acne and since acne is common in young women of childbearing age, great care should be employed before prescribing the drug to this cohort.

3. Endocardial cushion tissue is essential for proper development of these structures. In the common atrioventricular canal, the superior, the inferior, and two lateral endocardial cushions divide the opening and contribute to the mitral and tricuspid valves in the left and right atrioventricular canals. In addition, the superior and inferior cushions are essential for complete septation of the atria, by fusion with the septum primum, and of the ventricles, by forming the membranous part of the interventricular septum. Cushion tissue in the conus and truncus forms the conotruncal septum that spirals downward to separate the aorta and pulmonary channels and to fuse with the inferior endocardial cushion to complete the interventricular septum. Therefore, any abnormality of cushion tissue may result in a number of cardiac defects, including atrial and ventricular septal defects, transposition of the great vessels, and other abnormalities of the outflow tract.

4. In the development of the vascular system for the head and neck, a series of arterial arches forms around the pharynx. Most of these arches undergo alterations, including regression, as the original patterns are modified. Two such alterations that produce difficulty swallowing are *(a)* double aortic arch, in which a portion of the right dorsal aorta (that normally regresses) persists between the 7th intersegmental artery and its junction with the left dorsal aorta, creating a vascular ring around the esophagus, and *(b)* right aortic arch, in which the ascending aorta and the arch form on the right. If in such cases the ligamentum arteriosum remains on the left, it passes behind the esophagus and may constrict it.

Chapter 13

1. This infant most likely has some type of tracheoesophageal atresia with or without a tracheoesophageal fistula. The baby cannot swallow, and this results in polyhydramnios. The defect is caused by abnormal partitioning of the trachea and esophagus by the tracheoesophageal septum. These defects are often associated with other malformations, including a constellation of vertebral anomalies, anal atresia, cardiac defects, renal anomalies, and limb defects known as the VACTERL association.

2. Babies born prior to 7 months of gestation do not produce sufficient amounts of surfactant to reduce surface tension in the alveoli to permit normal lung function. Consequently, alveoli collapse, resulting in respiratory distress syndrome (RDS). Recent improvements in artificial surfactants have improved the prognosis for these infants.

Chapter 14

1. The baby most likely has some type of esophageal atresia and/or tracheoesophageal fistula. In 90% of these cases, the proximal part of the esophagus ends in a blind pouch, and there is a fistula present connecting the distal part with the trachea. Polyhydramnios results because the baby cannot swallow amniotic fluid. At birth, aspiration of fluids may result in pneumonia. The defect is caused by an abnormal partitioning of the respiratory diverticulum from the foregut by the esophagotracheal septum.

2. The most likely diagnosis is an omphalocele resulting from a failure of herniated bowel to return to the abdominal cavity at the 10th to 12th weeks of gestation. Since the bowel normally herniates into the umbilical cord, it is covered by amnion. This situation is in contrast to gastroschisis, where loops of bowel herniate through an abdominal wall defect and are not covered by amnion. The prognosis is not good, since 25% of infants with omphalocele die before birth, 40–88% have associated anomalies, and approximately 50% show chromosomal abnormalities. If no other defects are present, however, successful surgical repair is possible, and if this is performed by experienced hands, survival is 100%.

3. This infant has an imperforate anus with a rectovaginal fistula, part of an anorectal atresia complex. She appears to have a high anorectal atresia, since the fistula connects the rectum to the vagina, accounting for meconium (intestinal contents) in this structure. Separation of the cloaca into a urogenital sinus and rectum is accomplished by the urorectal septum, a wedge of mesoderm that grows downward between the urachus and hindgut until it contacts the cloacal membrane to form the perineal body. Ventral displacement of this septum produces an abnormal partitioning of these structures, accounting for the defect.

Chapter 15

1. The three systems to form are the pronephros, mesonephros, and metanephros, and they are derivatives of the intermediate mesoderm. They form in succession in a cranial to caudal sequence. Thus, the pronephros forms in cervical segments at the end of the 3rd week but is rudimentary and rapidly regresses. The mesonephros begins early in the 4th week, extending from thoracic to upper lumbar regions. It is segmented in only its upper portion and contains excretory tubules that connect to the mesonephric (wolffian) duct. This kidney also regresses but may function for a short time. It is more important because the tubules and collecting duct contribute to the genital ducts in the male. Collecting ducts near the testis form the efferent ductules, whereas the mesonephric duct forms the epididymis, ductus deferens, and ejaculatory duct. In the female, these tubules and ducts degenerate, since their maintenance is dependent on testosterone production. The metanephros lies in the pelvic region as a mass of unsegmented mesoderm (metanephric blastema) that forms the definitive kidneys. Ureteric buds grow from the mesonephric ducts and, on contact with the metanephric blastema, induce it to differentiate. The ureteric buds form collecting ducts and ureters, while the metanephric blastema forms nephrons (excretory units), each of which consists of a glomerulus (capillaries) and renal tubules.

2. Both the ovaries and testes develop in the abdominal cavity from intermediate mesoderm along the urogenital ridge. Both also descend by similar mechanisms from their original position, but the uterus prevents migration of the ovary out of the abdominal cavity. In the male, however, a mesenchymal condensation, the gubernaculum (this structure also forms in females but becomes attached to the uterus), attaches the caudal pole of the testis, first to the inguinal region and then to the scrotal swellings. Growth and retraction of the gubernaculum, together with increasing intraabdominal pressure, cause the testis to descend. Failure of these processes causes undescended testes, known as cryptorchism. Approximately 2–3% of term male infants will have an undescended testicle, and in 25% of these the condition will be bilateral. In many cases the undescended testis will descend by age 1. If it does not, testosterone administration (since this hormone is thought to play a role in descent) or surgery may be necessary. Fertility may be affected in cases where the condition is bilateral.

3. Male and female external genitalia pass through an indifferent stage during which it is impossible to differentiate between the two sexes. Under the influence of testosterone, these structures assume a masculine appearance, but the derivatives are homologous between males and females. These homologies include *(a)* the clitoris and penis, derived from the genital tubercle; *(b)* the labia majora and scrotum, derived from the genital swellings that fuse in the male; and *(c)* the labia minora and penile urethra, derived from the urethral folds that fuse in the male. During early stages, the genital tubercle is larger in the female than in the male, and this has led to misidentification of sex by ultrasound.

4. The uterus is formed by fusion of the lower portions of the paramesonephric (müllerian) ducts. Numerous abnormalities have been described, including the most common abnormality consisting of two uterine horns (bicornuate uterus). Complications from this defect include difficulties in becoming pregnant, increased incidence of spontaneous abortion, and abnormal fetal presentations. In some cases, a part of the uterus will end blindly (rudimentary horn), causing problems with menstruation and abdominal pain.

Chapter 16

1. Neural crest cells are important for craniofacial development because they contribute to so many structures in this region. Thus, they form all of the bones of the face and cranial vault except for a small area in the occipital region and the connective tissue that provides patterning of the facial muscles. They also contribute to cranial nerve ganglia, meninges, dermis, odontoblasts, and stroma for glands derived from pharyngeal pouches. In addition, crest cells from the hindbrain region of the neural folds migrate ventrally to participate in septation of the conotruncal region of the heart into aortic and pulmonary vessels.

Unfortunately, crest cells appear to be vulnerable to a number of compounds, including alcohol and retinoids, perhaps because they lack catalase and super-oxide dismutase enzymes that scavenge toxic free radicals. Many craniofacial defects are due to insults on neural crest cells and may be associated with cardiac abnormalities because of the contribution of these cells to heart morphogenesis.

2. The child may have DiGeorge sequence, which is characterized by these types of craniofacial defects and partial or complete absence of thymic tissue. It is the loss of thymic tissue that compromises the immune system, resulting in numerous infections. Damage to neural crest cells is the most likely cause of the sequence, since these cells contribute to development of all these structures, including the stroma of the thymus. Teratogens, such as alcohol, have been shown to cause these defects experimentally.

3. Children with midline clefts of the lip often have mental retardation. Thus, median clefts are associated with loss of other midline structures, including those in the brain. In its extreme form, the entire cranial midline is lost, and the lateral ventricles of the cerebral hemispheres are fused into a single ventricle, a condition called holoprosencephaly. Midline clefts are induced as the cranial neural folds begin to form (approximately days 19–21) and result from the loss of midline tissue in the prechordal plate region.

4. The child most likely has a thyroglossal cyst that results from incomplete regression of the thyroglossal duct. These cysts may form anywhere along the line of descent of the thyroid gland as it migrates from the region of the foramen cecum of the tongue to its position in the neck. A cyst must be differentiated from ectopic glandular tissue that may also remain along this pathway.

Chapter 17

1. Microtia involves defects of the external ear that range from small but well-formed ears, to absence of the ear (anotia). Other defects occur in 20–40% of children with microtia and/or anotia, including the oculoauriculovertebral spectrum (hemifacial microsomia), in which case the craniofacial defects may be asymmetrical. Since the external ear is derived from hillocks on the first two pharyngeal arches, which are largely formed by neural crest cells, this cell population plays a role in most ear malformations.

Chapter 18

1. The lens forms from a thickening of ectoderm (lens placode) adjacent to the optic cup. Lens induction may begin very early, but contact with the optic cup plays a role in this process as well as in maintenance and differentiation of the lens. Therefore, if the optic cup fails to contact the ectoderm or if the molecular and cellular signals essential for lens development are disrupted, then a lens will not form.

---

2. Rubella is known to cause cataracts, micropthalmia, congenital deafness, and cardiac malformations. Exposure during the 4th to 8th weeks would place the offspring at risk for one or more of these birth defects.

3. As the optic cup reaches the surface ectoderm, it invaginates and forms a fissure along its ventral surface that extends along the optic stalk. It is through this fissure that the hyaloid artery reaches the inner chamber of the eye. Normally, the distal portion of the hyaloid artery degenerates, and the choroid fissure closes by fusion of its ridges. If this fusion does not occur, then colobomas occur. These defects (clefts) may occur anywhere along the length of the fissure. If they occur distally, they form colobomas of the iris; if they occur more proximally, they form colobomas of the retina, choroid, and optic nerve, depending on their extent.

Chapter 19

1. Mammary gland formation begins as buds of epidermis into the underlying mesenchyme. These buds normally form in the pectoral region along a thickened ridge of ectoderm, the mammary or milk line. This line or ridge extends from the axilla into the thigh on both sides of the body. Occasionally, accessory sites of epidermal growth occur, such that extra nipples (polythelia) and extra breasts (polymastia) appear. These accessory structures always occur along the milk line and usually in the axillary region. Similar conditions also occur in males.

Chapter 20

1. Cranial and spinal nerves are homologues, but they differ in that cranial nerves are much less consistent in their composition. Motor neurons for both lie in basal plates of the central nervous system, and sensory ganglia derived from the neural crest are located outside the central nervous system. Fibers from sensory neurons synapse on neurons in the alar plates of the spinal cord and brain. Differences occur in that three cranial nerves (I, II, and VIII) are entirely sensory, four are entirely motor (IV, VI, XI, and XII), three have motor, sensory, and parasympathetic fibers (VII, IX, and X), and one has only motor and parasympathetic components (III). In contrast, each spinal nerve has motor and sensory fibers.

2. A spinal tap is performed between vertebra L4 and vertebra L5, since the spinal cord ends at the L2-L3 level. Thus, it is possible to obtain cerebrospinal fluid at this level without damaging the cord. The space is created because after the 3rd month, the cord, which initially extended the entire length of the vertebral column, does not lengthen as rapidly as the dura and vertebral column do, such that in the adult the spinal cord ends at the L2-L3 level.

3. The embryological basis for most neural tube defects is inhibition of closure of the neural folds at the cranial and caudal neuropores. In turn, defects occur in surrounding structures, resulting in anencephaly, some types of encephaloceles, and spina bifida cystica. Severe neurological deficits accompany abnormalities in these regions. Neural tube defects occur in approximately 1 in 1000 births and may be diagnosed prenatally by ultrasound and findings of elevated levels of α-fetoprotein in maternal serum and amniotic fluid. Recent evidence has shown that folate supplements provided prior to conception are effective in preventing some of these defects.

4. This condition is hydrocephalus and results from a blockage in the flow of cerebrospinal fluid from the lateral ventricles through the foramina of Monro and the cerebral aqueduct into the 4th ventricle and out into the subarachnoid space, where it would be resorbed. In most cases, blockage occurs in the cerebral aqueduct in the midbrain and may result from genetic causes (X-linked recessive) or viral infections (toxoplasmosis, cytomegalovirus).

Figure and Table Credits

Printed insert: Susceptibility to Teratogenesis for Selected Organ Systems. Modified from Shenefelt RE: Morphogenesis of malformations in hamsters caused by retinoic acid: relation to dose and stage at treatment. *Teratology* 5:103–188, 1972.

Figure 1.5. Courtesy of Dr. Kathleen Rao, Department of Pediatrics, University of North Carolina

Figure 1.6. From Gelehrter TD, Collins FS: *Principles of Medical Genetics.* Baltimore, Williams & Wilkins, 1990:168.

Figure 1.9. Modified after Ohno et al: Female germ cells in man. *Exp Cell Res* 24:106, 1961

Figure 1.14. From Fawcett DW: *Bloom and Fawcett: A Textbook of Histology.* Philadelphia, WB Saunders, 1986

Figure 1.16. Derived from Clermont and Leblond

Figure 1.17. From Fawcett DW: *Bloom and Fawcett: A Textbook of Histology.* Philadelphia, WB Saunders, 1986

Figure 2.3. From Van Blerkom J, Motta P: *The Cellular Basis of Mammalian Reproduction.* Baltimore, Urban & Schwarzenberg, 1979

Figure 2.5A. Courtesy of Dr. P. Motta

Figure 2.7A. Courtesy of Drs. L. Dickmann and R. Noyes, Vanderbilt University

Figure 2.7B. From Hertig AT, Rock J: Two human ova of the previllous stage, having a developmental age of about seven and nine days, respectively. *Contrib Embryol* 31:65, 1945. Courtesy of Carnegie Institution of Washington, Washington, DC

Figure 2.9. From Gilbert SF: *Developmental Biology.* 4th ed. Sunderland, MA, Sinauer Associates, 1994

Figure 2.10A. From Hertig AT, Rock J, Adams EC: A description of 34 human ova within the first 17 days of development. *Am J Anat* 98:435, 1956. Courtesy of Carnegie Institution of Washington, Washington, DC

Figure 2.10B. Modified after Hertig AT, Rock J: Two human ova of the previllous stage, having a developmental age of about seven and nine days, respectively. *Contrib Embryol* 31:65, 1945. Courtesy of Carnegie

Institution of Washington, Washington, DC

Figure 3.2. From Hertig AT, Rock J: Two human ova of the previllous stage, having a developmental age of about seven and nine days, respectively. *Contrib Embryol* 31:65, 1945. Courtesy of Carnegie Institution of Washington, Washington, DC

Figure 3.5. From Hertig AT, Rock J: Two human ova of the previllous stage, having a developmental age of 11 and 12 days, respectively. *Contrib Embryol* 29:127, 1941. Courtesy of Carnegie Institution of Washington, Washington, DC

Figure 3.7. From Hertig AT, Rock J, Adams EC: A description of 34 human ova within the first 17 days of development. *Am J Anat* 98:435, 1956. Courtesy of Carnegie Institution of Washington, Washington, DC

Figure 3.8. Modified after Hamilton WJ, Mossman HW: *Human Embryology.* Baltimore, Williams & Wilkins, 1972

Figure 4.2C. Courtesy of Dr. K. K. Sulik, Department of Cell Biology and Anatomy, University of North Carolina

Figure 4.3B, D, and F. Courtesy of Dr. K. K. Sulik, Department of Cell Biology and Anatomy, University of North Carolina

Figure 4.4. Courtesy of Dr. K. K. Sulik, Department of Cell Biology and Anatomy, University of North Carolina

Figure 4.5. From Heuser CH: A presomite embryo with a definite chorda canal. *Contrib Embryol* 23:253, 1932. Courtesy of Carnegie Institution of Washington, Washington, DC

Figure 4.11. From King BF, Mias JJ: Developmental changes in rhesus monkey placental villi and cell columns. *Anat Embryol* 165:361–376, 1982

Figure 5.1. From Heuser CH: A presomite embryo with a definite chorda canal. *Contrib Embryol* 23:253, 1932. Courtesy of Carnegie Institution of Washington, Washington, DC

Figure 5.2A. Modified after Davis

Figure 5.2B. Modified after Ingalls

Figure 5.2C. Courtesy of Dr. K. K. Sulik, Department of Cell Biology and Anatomy, University of North Carolina

Figure 5.3E and F. Courtesy of Dr. K. K. Sulik, Department of Cell Biology and Anatomy, University of North Carolina

Figure 5.4. Courtesy of Dr. K. K. Sulik, Department of Cell Biology and Anatomy, University of North Carolina

Figure 5.5A. Modified after Payne

Figure 5.5B. Modified after Corner

Figure 5.6. Courtesy of Dr. K. K. Sulik, Department of Cell Biology and Anatomy, University of North Carolina

Figure 5.7. From Blechschmidt E: *The Stages of Human Development Before Birth.* Philadelphia, WB Saunders, 1961. Courtesy of E. Blechschmidt, Professor of Anatomy, University of Göttingen

Figure 5.8. Modified after Streeter GL: Developmental horizons in human embryos: age group XI, 13–20 somites, and age group XII, 21–29 somites. *Contrib Embryol* 30:211, 1942

Figure 5.10. Courtesy of Dr. K. K. Sulik, Department of Cell Biology and Anatomy, University of North Carolina

Figure 5.18. From Streeter GL: Developmental horizons in human embryos: age groups XV, XVI, XVII, and XVIII [the third issue of a survey of the Carnegie Collection]. *Contrib Embryol* 32:133, 1948. Courtesy of Carnegie Institution of Washington, Washington, DC

Figure 5.19. From Blechschmidt E: *The Stages of Human Development Before Birth.* Philadelphia, WB Saunders, 1961. Courtesy of E. Blechschmidt, Professor of Anatomy, University of Göttingen

Figure 5.20. From Blechschmidt E: *The Stages of Human Development Before Birth.* Philadelphia, WB Saunders, 1961. Courtesy of E. Blechschmidt, Professor of Anatomy, University of Göttingen

Figure 5.21. From Hamilton WJ, Mossman HW: *Human Embryology.* Baltimore, Williams & Wilkins, 1972

Figure 5.22. From Starck D: *Embryologie.* Stuttgart, Georg Thieme, 1965. Courtesy of Dietrich Starck, Professor of Anatomy, University of Frankfurt am Main

Figure 6.4. Courtesy of E. Blechschmidt, Professor of Anatomy, University of Göttingen

Figure 6.7. Courtesy of Dr. Nancy Chescheir, Department of Obstetrics and Gynecology, University of North Carolina

Figure 7.1. Modified after von Ortmann

Figure 7.7. Modified after Ramsey EM: The placenta and fetal membranes. *In* Greenhill JP (ed): *Obstetrics.* Philadelphia, WB Saunders, 1965; and Hamilton WJ, Boyd JD: Trophoblastin human uteroplacental arteries. *Nature* 212:906, 1966

Figure 8.1. From National Center for Health Statistics, Center for Disease Control, Atlanta, GA

Figure 8.2. From National Center for Health Statistics, Center for Disease Control, Atlanta, GA

Figure 8.3. Courtesy of Dr. M. Edgerton, Department of Plastic Surgery, University of Virginia

Figure 8.4. Courtesy of Dr. David Smith, Department of Pediatrics, University of Washington

Figure 8.5. Courtesy of Dr. J. Miller, Department of Neurology, University of Virginia

Figure 8.6. Courtesy of Dr. J. Miller, Department of Neurology, University of Virginia

Figure 8.7. Courtesy of Dr. J. Miller, Department of Neurology, University of Virginia

Figure 8.8. Courtesy of Dr. J. Miller, Department of Neurology, University of Virginia

Figure 8.9. Courtesy of Dr. R. J. Gorlin, Department of Oral Pathology and Genetics, University of Minnesota

Figure 8.10. Courtesy of Dr. R. J. Gorlin, Department of Oral Pathology and Genetics, University of Minnesota

Figure 9.6. Modified from Noden DM: Interactions and fates of avian craniofacial mesenchyme. *Development* 103:121–140, 1988, Company of Cell Biologists, Ltd.

Figure 9.7. Courtesy of Dr. J. Warkany. From Warkany J: *Congenital Malformations.* Chicago, Year Book Medical Publishers, 1971

Figure 9.8. Courtesy of Dr. J. Jane, Department of Neurosurgery, University of Virginia

Figure 9.11. Courtesy of Dr. K. K. Sulik, Department of Cell Biology and Anatomy, University of North Carolina

Figure 9.12. Courtesy of Dr. M. Edgerton, Department of Plastic Surgery, University of Virginia

Figure 9.13A. From Stevenson RE, Hall JG, Goodman RM (eds): *Human Malformations and Related Anomalies.* New York, Oxford University Press, 1993

Figure 9.13B and C. Courtesy of Dr. M. Edgerton, Department of Plastic Surgery, University of Virginia

Figure 9.14. Courtesy of Dr. A. Aylsworth, Department of Pediatrics, University of North Carolina

Figure 9.16. Courtesy of Dr. N. Chescheir, Department of Obstetrics and Gynecology, University of North Carolina

Table 10.1. Adapted from Noden DM: Craniofacial development: new views on old problems. *Anat Rec* 208:1, 1984.

Figure 10.4A and B. From Langman J, Woerdeman MW: *Atlas of Medical Anatomy.* Philadelphia, WB Saunders, 1978

Figure 10.5. Courtesy of Dr. K. K. Sulik, Department of Cell Biology and Anatomy, University of North Carolina

Figure 10.6. Courtesy of Dr. D. Nakayama, Department of Surgery, University of North Carolina

Figure 11.3A and D. Courtesy of Dr. S. Lacey, Department of Surgery, University of North Carolina

Figure 11.3C. Courtesy of Dr. S. Shaw, Department of Surgery, University of Virginia

Figure 12.1. Courtesy of Dr. K. K. Sulik, Department of Cell Biology and Anatomy, University of North Carolina

Figure 12.4. Courtesy of Dr. K. K. Sulik, Department of Cell Biology and Anatomy, University of North Carolina

Figure 12.6A–C. Modified from Kramer TC: The partitioning of the truncus and conus and the formation of the membranous portion of the interventricular septum in the human heart. *Am J Anat* 71:343, 1942

Figure 12.6D and E. Courtesy of Dr. K. K. Sulik, Department of Cell Biology and Anatomy, University of North Carolina

Figure 12.7A and B. Modified after Kramer TC: The partitioning of the truncus and conus and the formation of the membranous portion of the interventricular septum in the human heart. *Am J Anat* 71:343, 1942

Figure 12.7C. Courtesy of Dr. K. K. Sulik, Department of Cell Biology and Anatomy, University of North Carolina

Figure 12.11B and D. Courtesy of Dr. K. K. Sulik, Department of Cell Biology and Anatomy, University of North Carolina

Figure 12.15B and C. Courtesy of Dr. K. K. Sulik, Department of Cell Biology and Anatomy, University of North Carolina

Figure 12.16B. Courtesy of Dr. K. K. Sulik, Department of Cell Biology and Anatomy, University of North Carolina

Figure 12.21. Courtesy of Dr. K. K. Sulik, Department of Cell Biology and Anatomy, University of North Carolina

Figure 12.25. After Kramer TC: The partitioning of the truncus and conus and the formation of the interventricular septum in the human heart. *Am J Anat* 71:343, 1942

Figure 12.28. Courtesy of Dr. Nancy Chescheir, Department of Obstetrics and Gynecology, University of North Carolina

Figure 14.27. From Agur AMR: *Grant's Atlas of Anatomy*. 9th ed. Baltimore, Williams & Wilkins, 1991:123

Figure 14.29B. Courtesy of Dr. S. Shaw, Department of Surgery, University of Virginia

Figure 14.29C. Courtesy of Dr. D. Nakayama, Department of Surgery, University of North Carolina

Figure 14.33. Courtesy of Dr. D. Nakayama, Department of Surgery, University of North Carolina

Figure 15.1. Modified after Heuser

Figure 15.3C. Courtesy of Dr. K. K. Sulik, Department of Cell Biology and Anatomy, University of North Carolina

Figure 15.7. From Stevenson RE, Hall JG, Goodman RM (eds): *Human Malformations and Related Anomalies*. New York, Oxford University Press, 1993

Figure 15.8D and E. From Stevenson RE, Hall JG, Goodman RM (eds): *Human Malformations and Related Anomalies*. New York, Oxford University Press, 1993

Figure 15.9B. Courtesy of Dr. K. K. Sulik, Department of Cell Biology and Anatomy, University of North Carolina

Figure 15.10C. From Stevenson RE, Hall JG, Goodman RM (eds): *Human Malformations and Related Anomalies*. New York, Oxford University Press, 1993

Figure 15.15. From Stevenson RE, Hall JG, Goodman RM (eds): *Human Malformations and Related Anomalies*. New York, Oxford University Press, 1993

Figure 15.16C and D. Courtesy of Dr. K. K. Sulik, Department of Cell Biology and Anatomy, University of North Carolina

Figure 15.17A. After Witchi

Figure 15.22. From George FW, Wilson JD: Sex determination and differentiation. *In* Knobil E, et al (eds): *The Physiology of Reproduction*. New York, Raven Press, 1988:3–26

Figure 15.29C. Courtesy of Dr. K. K. Sulik, Department of Cell Biology and Anatomy, University of North Carolina

Figure 15.31. Courtesy of Dr. K. K. Sulik, Department of Cell Biology and Anatomy, University of North Carolina

Figure 15.32B. Courtesy of Dr. R. J. Gorlin, Department of Oral Pathology and Genetics, University of Minnesota

Figure 15.35. Courtesy of Dr. J. Kitchin, Department of Obstetrics and Gynecology, University of Virginia

Figure 15.36. Courtesy of Dr. J. Kitchin, Department of Obstetrics and Gynecology, University of Virginia

Figure 15.37E. Courtesy of Dr. K. K. Sulik, Department of Cell Biology and Anatomy, University of North Carolina

Figure 16.1. Modified from Noden DM: Interactions and fates of avian craniofacial mesenchyme. *Development* 103:121–140, 1988, Company of Biologists, Ltd.

Figure 16.2A. Courtesy of Dr. K. K. Sulik, Department of Cell Biology and Anatomy, University of North Carolina

Figure 16.2B. Adapted from Noden DM: Interactions and fates of avian craniofacial mesenchyme. *Development* 103:121–140, 1988, Company of Biologists, Ltd.

Figure 16.5C. Courtesy of Dr. K. K. Sulik, Department of Cell Biology and Anatomy, University of North Carolina

Figure 16.6A and B. Courtesy of Dr. K. K. Sulik, Department of Cell Biology and Anatomy, University of North Carolina

Figure 16.13. Courtesy of Dr. A. Shaw, Department of Surgery, University of Virginia

Figure 16.14A. Courtesy of J. Warkany. From Warkany J: *Congenital Malformations*. Chicago, Year Book Medical Publishers, 1971

Figure 16.14B–D. Courtesy of Dr. R. J. Gorlin, Department of Oral Pathology and Genetics, University of Minnesota

Figure 16.15C and D. Courtesy of Dr. K. K. Sulik, Department of Cell Biology and Anatomy, University of North Carolina

Figure 16.18. Courtesy of Dr. A. Shaw, Department of Surgery, University of Virginia

Figure 16.19C. Courtesy of Dr. K. K. Sulik, Department of Cell Biology and Anatomy, University of North Carolina

Figure 16.20C. Courtesy of Dr. K. K. Sulik, Department of Cell Biology and Anatomy, University of North Carolina

Figure 16.21C. Courtesy of Dr. K. K. Sulik, Department of Cell Biology and Anatomy, University of North Carolina

Figure 16.23C and D. Courtesy of Dr. K. K. Sulik, Department of Cell Biology and Anatomy, University of North Carolina

Figure 16.24C and D. Courtesy of Dr. K. K. Sulik, Department of Cell Biology and Anatomy, University of North Carolina

Figure 16.25C. Courtesy of Dr. K. K. Sulik, Department of Cell Biology and Anatomy, University of North Carolina

Figure 16.27A–C. Courtesy of Dr. M. Edgerton, Department of Plastic Surgery, University of Virginia

Figure 16.27D–F. Courtesy of Dr. R. J. Gorlin, Department of Oral Pathology and Genetics, University of Minnesota

Figure 16.31. From Langman J, Woerdeman MW: *Atlas of Medical Anatomy*. Philadelphia, WB Saunders, 1978

Figure 17.1A. Courtesy of Dr. K. K. Sulik, Department of Cell Biology and Anatomy, University of North Carolina

Figure 17.2D and E. Courtesy of Dr. K. K. Sulik, Department of Cell Biology and Anatomy, University of North Carolina

Figure 17.3F and G. Courtesy of Dr. K. K. Sulik, Department of Cell Biology and Anatomy, University of North Carolina

Figure 17.9E–G. Courtesy of Dr. K. K. Sulik, Department of Cell Biology and Anatomy, University of North Carolina

Figure 17.10. Courtesy of Dr. R. J. Gorlin, Department of Oral Pathology and Genetics, University of Minnesota

Figure 18.1D. Courtesy of Dr. K. K. Sulik, Department of Cell Biology and Anatomy, University of North Carolina

Figure 18.2. After Mann IC: *The Development of the Human Eye*. 3rd ed, British Medical Association. New York, Grune & Stratton, 1974

Figure 18.3. Modified after Mann IC: *The Development of the Human Eye*. 3rd ed, British Medical Association. New York, Grune & Stratton, 1974

Figure 18.4. Courtesy of Dr. K. K. Sulik, Department of Cell Biology and Anatomy, University of North Carolina

Figure 18.5. Modified after Mann IC: *The Development of the Human Eye*. 3rd ed, British Medical Association. New York, Grune & Stratton, 1974

Figure 18.10. From Stevenson RE, Hall JG, Goodman RM (eds): *Human Malformations and Related Anomalies*. New York, Oxford University Press, 1993, vols I and II

Figure 20.1A and B. Modified after Ingalls

Figure 20.1C. Courtesy of Dr. K. K. Sulik, Department of Cell Biology and Anatomy, University of North Carolina

Figure 20.2E. Courtesy of Dr. K. K. Sulik, Department of Cell Biology and Anatomy, University of North Carolina

Figure 20.3C. Courtesy of Dr. K. K. Sulik, Department of Cell Biology and Anatomy, University of North Carolina

Figure 20.4. Courtesy of Dr. K. K. Sulik, Department of Cell Biology and Anatomy, University of North Carolina

Figure 20.5. Courtesy of Dr. K. K. Sulik, Department of Cell Biology and Anatomy, University of North Carolina

Figure 20.6B. Courtesy of Dr. K. K. Sulik, Department of Cell Biology and Anatomy, University of North Carolina

Figure 20.8C. Courtesy Dr. K. K. Sulik, Department of Cell Biology and Anatomy, University of North Carolina

Figure 20.15A. Courtesy of Dr. K. K. Sulik, Department of Cell Biology and Anatomy, University of North Carolina

Figure 20.15B. Courtesy of Dr. M. J. Sellers, Division of Medical and Molecular Genetics, Guys Hospital, London

Figure 20.19C and D. Courtesy of Dr. K. K. Sulik, Department of Cell Biology and Anatomy, University of North Carolina

Figure 20.25D. Courtesy of Dr. K. K. Sulik, Department of Cell Biology and Anatomy,

University of North Carolina

Figure 20.30. Courtesy of Dr. Nancy Chescheir, Department of Obstetrics and Gynecology, University of North Carolina

Figure 20.31A. Courtesy of Dr. J. Warkany. From Warkany J: *Congenital Malformations.* Chicago, Year Book Medical Publishers, 1971.

Figure 20.32. Courtesy of Dr. R. J. Gorlin, Department of Oral Pathology and Genet-

ics, University of Minnesota

Figure 20.33. Courtesy of Dr. R. J. Gorlin, Department of Oral Pathology and Genetics, University of Minnesota

Figure 20.34. From Lumsden R: The cellular basis for segmentation in the developing hindbrain. *Trends Neurosci* 13:329, 1990. Elsevier Trends Journals, Cambridge, United Kingdom

Index

Page numbers followed by "f" denote figures; those followed by "t" denote tables.

Angioblasts, 183
  formation of, 78
Angiogenic cells
  clusters of, 78, 184f
  coalescence of, 184f
Angiotensin-converting enzyme inhibitors, 129
Aniridia, 365
Ankyloglossia, 329
Annulus fibrosus, 161
Anomalies
  minor, 122
  structural, 122
Anophthalmia, 365
Anorectal atresia complex, 422
Anorectal canal, 268, 283
Anotia, 424
Anterior chamber, 364f, 366
  development of, 362
Anterior commissure, 399
Anterior horn cells, cephalic continuation of,
  387–388
Antianxiety agents, 129
Antibody, maternal, 109
Anticoagulants, 129
Anticonvulsants
  cleft palate with, 340
  teratogenic, 128–129
Antigen-antibody interaction, 109
Antihypertensive agents, 129
Antimullerian hormone (AMH), 292
Antineoplastic agents, 128
Antipsychotic agents, 129
Antrum, 14, 15f
Anus
  imperforate, 269
  striated muscles of, 168
Aorta
  coarctation of, 229
    preductal and postductal, 216–217
  development of, 421
  dorsal, 183, 214f
    obliteration of, 215
  ventral, 213
Aortic arches
  abnormal right, 229
  changes in, 215–216
  development of, 212–215, 229
  double, 218
  fifth, 215
  first, 213
  fourth, 214
    obliteration of, 219f
  interrupted, 218
  right, 218
  second, 213
  sixth, 215
  system of, 213f
  third, 213
Aortic channel, 203
  formation of, 193

Aortic sac, 212
Aortic valve
  atresia of, 209, 211f
  stenosis of, 208, 211f
Aorticopulmonary septum, 202–203, 213f
  formation of, 229
Aphakia, congenital, 365
Apical ectodermal ridge (AER), 154, 156f
  cell death in, 155
Appendix, 262
  primitive, 261
Appendix epididymis, 293
Appendix testis, 293
Apple peel atresia, 267
Aqueductal stenosis, 401
Archipallium, 397
Arnold-Chiari malformation, 401
Arrector pili muscle, 370
Arterial system
  components of, 219f
  development of, 212–219, 229–230
Arytenoid cartilage, 234, 317
Arytenoid swellings, 327
Association neurons, 380
Associations, 124
Astrocytes, protoplasmic and fibrillar, 380
Atomic bomb explosions, 127
Atresia. See specific forms
Atrial appendage, 197
Atrial septum
  defects of, 194–195, 200
  formation of, 193, 195–197, 228–229
  normal formation of, 201f
Atrichia, 371
Atrioventricular canal, 204f
  abnormalities of, 200–201
  cross section of, 193f
  endocardial cushion fusion in, 201
  endocardial cushions in, 421
  formation of, 186–187, 193
  persistent, 200, 202f
  septum formation in, 197–201, 229
Atrioventricular cushions, 228
Atrioventricular junction, 186–187
  development of, 193
Atrioventricular node, 212
Atrioventricular valves, 197–200
Atrium
  differentiation of, 196–197
  in fetal circulation, 224–226
  formation of, 188–181
  smooth-walled, 197
Auditory meatus, external, 319, 323, 344, 354,
  357–357
Auditory tube, 344, 357. See also Eustachian
  tube
  formation of epithelial lining of, 87
Auditory vesicles, 347
Auricle, 354, 357
  congenital defects of, 357

C cells, 322–323
    formation of, 330
Calcitonin
    secretion of, 323
    source of, 330
Calyx
    major, 274
    minor, 274–276
Cantrell pentalogy, 173
Capacitation, 29
    process of, 39
Capillary system, trophoblastic, 101
Carbohydrate metabolism disturbances, 131–132
Cardiac defects, 124–125
Cardiac loop
    formation of, 186–188, 189f
    formation to left, 210
Cardiac muscle, 166
    development of, 172
Cardiac septum, 191–195
Cardinal vein, 219, 230
    anastomosis between, 221
    anterior, 221
    common, 188–190, 221
    development of, 221–222
    obliteration of, 222
    posterior, 221
Cardiogenic area, 183
    position of, 184f
Cardiovascular system, 183–230. *See also* Heart; Vascular system; specific vessels
Carotid artery
    common, 213, 214
    elongation of, 215
    external, 213
    internal, 213
Carotid duct, 215
Cartilage
    formation of, 79
    hypophyseal, 151
    parachordal, 150–151
Cataracts
    congenital, 365
    with rubella virus, 425
Cauda equina, 384
Caudal dysgenesis, 131–132
Caudal dysplasia, 417
Caudal genital ligament, 306
Caudal regression, 60, 61f
Caudate nucleus, 397
Caval system, 230
Cecal bud, 261
Cecum, mobile, 263
Celiac artery, 216, 229, 253
Celiac ganglia, 406
Cementoblasts, 342, 344
Cementum, 342, 344
Central artery, retinal, 363–364

Central nervous system. *See also* Brain
    defects from rubella, 125
    development of, 87, 374–411
    formation of, 71–74
Centromere, 4
Cephalic flexure, 374
Cephalic folding, 215
Cephalic limb, elongation of, 259–260
Cephalocaudal folding, 79–80, 87, 183–185
    in digestive system formation, 242
    results of, 80–81
    stages of, 80f
Cerebellar plate, 391
Cerebellum, 374, 410
    absence of, 402
    development of, 390, 391
    developmental stages of cortex, 392f
Cerebral hemispheres, 391, 411
    development of, 396–397
    primitive, 374
Cerebrospinal fluid, 411
    accumulation of, 403f
    blockage of, 426
    tapping of, 384
Cerebrum
    calcification of, 404
    cortical development of, 397–399
Cervical cyst, lateral, 324, 325f
Cervical flexure, 374
Cervical sinus, 323
Cervix
    atresia of, 298
    development of, 294
CHARGE association, 124
Cheeks, 332
Chemical agents, 127–130, 141t
Chiasma, 5
Chickenpox, 126
Chlordiazepoxide, 129
Choanae
    definitive, 341
    primitive, 340
Chondrocranium, 148, 150–151, 164
    chordal, 150
    prechordal, 150
Chordae tendineae, 197
    formation of, 200f
Choriocarcinoma, 50
Chorion frondosum, 101–102, 119
Chorion laeve, 101
Chorionic cavity, 44–45, 46, 52
    enlargement of, 63
    formation of, 47
    at 6 weeks, 104f
    yolk sac in, 110
Chorionic gonadotropin, 29
Chorionic plate, 47, 63, 65f, 85f, 101, 103
Chorionic sac, 85f
Chorionic vessels, 105

Gonadal vein, left, 222
Gonadotropin-releasing hormone, 23
Gonadotropin(s), 23
  during ovulation, 26
  syncytiotrophoblast production of, 110
Gonad(s). *See also* specific organs
  development of, 286–291
  indifferent, 287–288, 289t, 309
  streak, 303–304
Graafian follicle, 14, 15f
  before rupture, 24f
Granular cells, 399
Granular layer, 368
Granule cells, 391
Granulosa cells, 14
  fluid-filled spaces between, 14
  following ovulation, 26–28
  surrounding oocyte, 25f
Gray communicating rami, 407
Great veins, 192f
Great vessel transposition, 194–195, 208, 210f, 229
Greater omentum, 243
Growth retardation, 140
Gubernaculum, 306, 307f, 423
Gut
  blood supply to, 259f
  primitive, 242
Gut tube, closure of, 177f
Gyrus, 397
  development of, 399f

Habenular commissure, 399
Hair
  abnormalities of, 371
  development of, 87, 370–371, 373
  formation of, 74
  lanugo, 92, 370, 373
Hair cells, 348
Hair papillae, 370
Hair shaft, 370
Handplates, 155
Hand(s)
  abnormalities of, 159–160
  development of, 157f
Haploid chromosomes, 20, 134
Harlequin fetus, 369, 370f
hCG. *See* Human chorionic gonadotropin
Head
  development of, 312–329, 331–345
  musculature of, 168
  size at developmental stages, 92f
  skeletal structures of, 313f
  vascular system of, 421
Head fold, 80, 81, 87
Heart
  conducting system of, 211–212
  congenital defects of, 173
  development of, 183–212, 228–229
  malformations of, 208–211, 421

muscle of, 172
outflow tract septation of, 325
septum formation of, 191–195, 228
ultrasound scan of, 420
Heart tube, 78
  atrial portion of, 186
  cardiac loop in, 186–188
  conotruncal portion of, 188
  formation and position of, 183–186
  layers of, 185–186
  sinus venosus of, 188–191
Hematopoietic cells, 255, 270
Hematopoietic function, 255
Hemiazygos vein, 222
Hemifacial microsomia, 326, 425
  craniofacial defects in, 327f
Hemivertebra, 419
Hemochorial placenta, 108, 119–120
Hemolytic disease of newborn (HDN), 109
Henle, loop of, 277
Hepatic artery, 253f
Hepatic cells, 254–255
Hepatic diverticulum, 254–255
Hepatic ducts, accessory, 255–256
Hepatic flexure, 261
Hepatic sinusoids, 220
Hepatitis, 126
Hepatoduodenal ligament, 251
Hermaphrodites, 304
Hernia
  congenital diaphragmatic, 180, 181f, 182
  congenital hiatal, 247
  esophageal, 180
  inguinal, 308
  parasternal, 180
  retrocolic, 263
Herniation, physiological, 259–260
Herpes simplex virus, 126
Hiatal hernia, congenital, 247
High-resolution chromosome banding
        techniques, 138
Hindbrain, 374
Hindgut
  cloaca and, 276f
  congenital abnormalities of, 269–270, 271
  development of, 268–268, 271
  formation of, 80, 242
Hindlimb buds, 85
Hip dislocation, congenital, 160
Hippocampal commissure, 399, 400f
Hippocampus, 397
Hirschsprung's disease, 270, 409
His bundle, 212
Holoprosencephaly, 60, 337, 425
Homeobox genes
  activation of, 67
  in digit development, 155
Homologous chromosomes pairs, 20
Hormones
  congenital malformations from, 131, 141t

Measles
congenital malformations with, 124–126
German, 124–125
Meatal plug, 354
Meckel's cartilage, 151, 313–314
Meckel's diverticulum, 258, 265
Meconium aspiration, 97
Medial umbilical ligaments, 216
Median nerve, 169
Medulla, 407
Medulla oblongata, 387, 410
Medullary cords, 288, 291
Megacolon, congenital, 270, 409
Meiosis
nondisjunction during, 415
purpose of, 3
Meiotic division, 20, 21
chromosome abnormalities during, 7–9
chromosomes during, 5–10
first, 5, 6f, 8f
second, 5–7, 30, 38–39
Melanin pigment, 368
Melanocytes, 368, 372
Meninges, 383
formation of, 74
Meningocele, 400
cranial, 152–153
spina bifida with, 386
Meningoencephalocele, 400, 402f
Meningohydroencephalocele, 400
Meningomyelocele, spina bifida with, 386
Menstrual cycle, 38
endometrial changes during, 37, 38f
middle pain during, 26
problems of, 423
Mental retardation, 140
with brain abnormalities, 402
with cleft lip, 337
with lip cleft, 424
with microcephaly, 404f
Meprobamate, 129
Mercury, organic, 132–133
Meromelia, 158
with thalidomide use by mother, 127
Mesencephalon, 378f. See also Midbrain
development of, 387, 391–393, 411
Mesenchymal cells, 161
Mesenchyme, 71
bone-forming capacity of, 147
condensation of, 168
formation of, 76
limb development from, 154
pharyngeal arches from, 313
teeth from, 341
Mesenteric artery
inferior, 216, 229, 268
superior, 216, 229, 253, 258, 259f, 260
origin of, 261–262
Mesenteric ganglia, 406
Mesenteric vein, superior, 220

Mesentery
development of, 242–244
dorsal, 176, 182, 243, 244f
derivatives of, 250f
function of, 242
of intestinal loops, 261–263
proper, 261
ventral, 176, 182, 243, 244f
Mesocardium, dorsal, 185
Mesocolon
dorsal, 243
persistence of, 263
transverse, 251f, 262
Mesoderm
derivatives of, 74–79, 87
displacement of, 71–74
extraembryonic, 51–52
extraembryonic somatopleuric, 44–45, 52
extraembryonic splanchnopleuric, 45, 52
formation of, 53, 64–65
intermediate, 75, 77–78, 87, 272, 422
lateral plate, 312
metanephric, 273–274, 276f
muscular system from, 166, 172
paraxial, 75, 87, 166, 168, 312
parietal and visceral layers of, 78
skeletal system from, 147
somatic, 173, 176, 180
splanchnic, 166, 172, 173, 180
Mesoduodenum, 243
Mesogastrium
dorsal, 243, 248–250
ventral, 248–250, 255
Mesonephric duct, 287f, 291
ureters and, 284f
Mesonephros, 272, 273, 287f, 309, 422–423
Mesothelial membrane, 78
Metabolic exchange, 108–109
Metanephric blastema, 422
Metanephric excretory system, 277
Metanephric tissue
cap, 277
division of, 279
Metanephros, 272, 273–274, 309, 422–423. See
also Kidney
arterial supply of, 279
collecting system of, 274–276
excretory system of, 277
Metaphase plate, 16
Metencephalon, 374, 378f, 410
caudal, 398f
development of, 388–391
dorsal, 399f
roof of, 392f
Microcephaly, 154, 401, 404f
with cytomegalovirus infection, 125
Microdeletions, 138, 139f
Microglial cells, 381
Micromelia, 158
Micropenis, 302

Somite(s), 75–76, 82f, 87, 147
  in cardiac loop formation, 189f
  at day 22, 72f
  development of, 148f
  development stages of, 77f
  differentiation of, 76
  head formation from, 312
  in muscle development, 166, 172
  number of correlated with age, 76t
  occipital, 328–329
  rapidly growing, 79–80, 81
  ribs and vertebral column from, 164
Somitomere(s), 87, 147
  appearance of, 75
  head formation from, 312
  musculature from, 166
Special visceral afferent neurons, 391
Special visceral efferent motor column, 388
Special visceral efferent neurons, 387, 388
  motor, 388, 390
Speech, defective, 335
Sperm
  binding to zona pellucida, 27f
  in determining sex, 31
  fusion with oocyte, 30–31
Spermatic cord hydrocele, 308
Spermatic fascia, 308
Spermatid, 21
  formation of, 18
Spermatocyte, 18
Spermatogenesis, 16–18, 21
Spermatogonia, 16
  type A, 16, 17f
  type B, 16
Spermatozoon, 3, 16
  abnormal, 20
  during fertilization, 29
Spermicide, 32
Spermiogenesis, 19–20, 21
Sphenoid, 151
Sphenomandibular ligament, 151
Sphincter mechanism, 224
Sphincter muscle, 360–361
  pupillary, 391
Spina bifida, 162, 163f, 385, 410, 417
  cystica, 162, 385–386
  occulta, 162, 385
Spinal cord
  defects of, 385–386
  formation of, 70, 410
  histological differentiation of, 377–384
  lumen of, 374–375
    junctional complexes at, 379f
  neuroepithelial, mantle, and marginal layers
    of, 375–376
  plates of, 376–377
  positional changes of, 384
  vertebral column and, 384, 385f
  white matter of, 376
Spinal ganglia, 383

Spinal nerve(s), 162, 406–407, 426
  development of, 383
  dorsal sensory root of, 382–383
  in limb buds, 171f
  in limb musculature development, 169
  ventral motor root of, 379–380
Spinal tap, 425
Spine abnormalities, 162–163. *See also*
    Vertebral column
Spinous layer, 368
Spiral artery, 105–106
Spiral ligament, 347
Spiral limbus, 348
Splanchnic mesoderm, 75, 166, 172, 173
  in body cavity formation, 180
  in digestive tract development, 242, 244f
  of serous membrane, 180
Spleen
  connection to body wall, 249–250
  position at 5th week, 249f
  primordium, 248
Stapedial artery, 213
Stapedius muscle, 351
Stapes, 152, 316, 351, 357
Statoacoustic ganglion, 349
Stellate cell, 391
Stellate reticulum, 341
Stem cell, 16
Sternalis muscle, 168
Sternebrae, 164
Sternocleidomastoid muscle, 324
Sternum
  cleft, 173
  development of, 163–164
  failure to fuse, 175f
Stomach, 182
  congenital abnormalities of, 251
  development of, 247–251, 270
  duplication of, 251
  greater and lesser curvatures of, 248
  position of, 251f
  pyloric and cardiac portions of, 248
  retroperitoneal position of, 250
  rotation of, 247–248
Striated muscle, 388
Stylohyoid ligament, 316
Stylopharyngeus muscle, 316
Subcardinal vein(s), 221
  anastomosis between, 221–222
Subclavian artery(ies), 214
  abnormal origin of right, 217–218
  abnormal right, 229
Subcorium, 369
Subcutaneous fat deposition, 92
Sublingual gland, 390
Submandibular gland, 390
Sulcus
  development of, 399f
  limitans, 376–377
Supracardinal vein, 221

Suprarenal gland, 407–408
Surfactant, 421
  deficiency of, 239
  production of, 237, 240
  in respiration, 238–239
Suspensory ligament
  eye, 361
  ovarian, 309
Sustentacular cell, 16
Suture, newborn skull, 149
Sweat gland, 372, 373
Sylvius, aqueduct of, 375
  obstruction of, 401
Sympathetic ganglia, 408f
Sympathetic nervous system, 405
  development of, 406–408
Sympathetic neuroblasts, 383
Sympathetic organ plexuses, 406
Syncytial knot, 101
Syncytiotrophoblast, 41, 42f, 43f, 45–46, 51
  gonadotropin production by, 110
  human chorionic gonadotropin production by,
    47
  resistant to killer cells, 47–48
Syndactyly, 159, 420
Syndrome, 164
  definition of, 124
Synophthalmia, 365–366
Syphilis, 127
Systemic lupus erythematosus, 416

Tail fold, 80, 87
  formation of, 81
Taste, 329
Tectorial membrane, 348
Teeth
  congenital abnormalities of, 343, 344–345
  deciduous, 344
  deciduous (milk), 343
  development of, 341–343, 344
  formation of enamel of, 74
  incisor, 334
  natal, 343
  permanent, 343, 345
Tela choroidea, 388
Telencephalon, 374, 378f
  congenital abnormalities of, 400–404
  development of, 396–399, 411
  right half of, 395f, 398f
Telophase, 5
Temporal bone, 314
  development of, 151
  styloid process of, 316
Temporal lobe, 397
Temporal muscle, 314
Tensor palatini muscle, 316
Tensor tympani muscle, 316, 351
Teratogenic period, 140
Teratogen(s), 127–130
  associated with malformations, 141t

cardiovascular, 211
in craniofacial defects, 152–154, 424
exposure during 3rd week of development,
  60–61
factors influencing action of, 418–419
identification of, 124
intrauterine growth retardation and, 97
limb abnormalities with, 158
Teratology, 122
  principles of, 133
Teratoma, sacrococcygeal, 61, 62f
Terminal sulcus, 328
Tertiary villi, 61–63
Testicular feminization syndrome, 304–305, 306f
Testis
  abnormal position of, 309
  congenital abnormalities of, 308–309
  descent of, 305–308
  development of, 288–290, 309, 423
  efferent ductules of, 293
  hydrocele of, 308
  undescended, 423
Testis-determining factor (TDF) gene, 286
Testosterone, 310
  in external genitalia, 423
  production of, 290, 292
  receptors for, 293f
  in testicular development, 423
Tetracycline, 343
Thalamus, 411
  development of, 393
Thalidomide, 124
  cardiac malformations with, 211
  congenital malformations from, 127–128
  limb abnormalities with, 158
Theca externa, 14
Theca folliculi, 14
Theca interna, 14
Thoracic cavity
  abnormalities of, 180
  development of, 176–179
  division of, 182
  formation of, 180–182
Thoracic lymph duct, 228, 230
Thoracic muscle, transverse, 168
Thoracopagus twins, 118
Thymic tissue, accessory, 324
Thymus, 321, 344
  migration of, 323f
  stroma of, 424
Thyroglossal cyst, 330, 331f, 425
Thyroglossal duct, 329
Thyroglossal fistula, 330
Thyroid cartilage, 234, 317
Thyroid gland, 344
  abnormalities of, 330, 331f
  development of, 329–330
Thyroid tissue, aberrant, 330
Thyroxine, 330
Toe abnormality, 159